Monitoring the Health of Populations

Monitoring the Health of Populations
Statistical Principles and Methods for Public Health Surveillance

Edited by
RON BROOKMEYER
DONNA F. STROUP

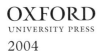
OXFORD
UNIVERSITY PRESS
2004

OXFORD

UNIVERSITY PRESS

Oxford   New York
Auckland   Bangkok   Buenos Aires   Cape Town   Chennai
Dar es Salaam   Delhi   Hong Kong   Istanbul   Karachi   Kolkata
Kuala Lumpur   Madrid   Melbourne   Mexico City   Mumbai
Nairobi   São Paulo   Shanghai   Taipei   Tokyo   Toronto

Copyright © 2004 by Oxford University Press, Inc.

Published by Oxford University Press, Inc.
198 Madison Avenue, New York, New York, 10016
http://www.oup-usa.org

Oxford is a registered trademark of Oxford University Press

Library of Congress Cataloging-in-Publication Data
Monitoring the health of populations : statistical principles and methods
for public health surveillance /
edited by Ron Brookmeyer, Donna F. Stroup.
p. cm.   Includes bibliographical references and index
Includes bibliographical references and index.
ISBN 0-19-514649-2 (cloth)
1. Public health surveillance.   2. Public health surveillance—Statistical methods.
3. Epidemiology.
I. Brookmeyer, Ron. II. Stroup, Donna F., 1951–
RA652.2.P82M66 2004   362.1′07′27—dc21   2003048679

9 8 7 6 5 4 3 2 1

Printed in the United States of America
on acid-free paper

Foreword

Surveillance is the cornerstone of public health practice. Public health surveillance has been defined as the routine, ongoing collection, analysis, and dissemination of data to those in public health who need to know. This connection to practice is essential to the use of these data to prevent and control disease and injury. Appropriate use of statistical methods is essential to surveillance practice. Epidemiologists and statisticians have a rich history of collaboration, and this includes the field of public health surveillance. As public health needs change, surveillance practices change; the statistical methods used must evolve to meet these new challenges. The editors of this volume have successfully conceptualized and completed an excellent text that addresses many of today's critical analytic concerns.

New technologies (e.g., the Internet and Global Information Systems [GIS]) present unprecedented opportunities to conduct surveillance more effectively and efficiently than ever before. The rapidly enlarging global population is in such close contact that new diseases can affect all parts of the globe in hours or days. Motor vehicle and pedestrian injuries are enormous public health concerns in the developing world, not just in traditional industrialized societies. All countries must face the increasing burden of chronic disease and monitor such risk factors as smoking and diet that contribute to that burden. Widening global terrorism brings forth still another challenge to the public health community. All these concerns must also be addressed by surveillance systems.

Data collection for emerging infectious diseases can be made more timely than ever before. Already, electronic laboratory surveillance has enabled epidemiologists to detect epidemics of salmonellosis and *Escherichia coli* O157:H7, and to pave the way to intervention much more rapidly and precisely than in the past. The response to terrorism has created a demand in the United States for real-time data transmission from the physician's office to the response arm of public health. Surveillance systems for injury and chronic diseases are still in early stages of development, but as these conditions are increasingly recognized for their public health importance, the public health system must be able to respond.

The presence of new kinds of data in unprecedented volume produces a demand for better analysis. How can we isolate the most relevant information in the volume of data that will flow from physicians' offices, hospitals, and emergency departments in an effective and timely manner? How can we obtain and use information from new sources of surveillance data (e.g., law enforcement, medical examiners, managed care organizations, and environmental sources) and link it to public health programs? What, in fact, are the analytic questions that must be addressed before useful information will flow from these data and be translated into optimal public health practice? Finally, how can we use new technologies to display and disseminate data that will communicate information most effectively?

Many of these concerns are addressed in this volume. Surveys are used for different surveillance needs, from identifying risk factors for chronic disease to collecting information during epidemics or after a disaster. Will such new technologies as the Internet enhance the effective use of surveys, or will cell phones make survey methods so complicated as to become obsolete? Underreporting and consistency of survey use present critical analytic challenges. The problems that confront epidemiologists in performing analytic studies (e.g., cohort effects and adjustments for incubation period) are also challenging. Defining an epidemic from surveillance, a traditional challenge to the epidemiologist, requires separating true clusters of health events in time and space from apparent epidemics. Aberration detection models and computer software that use these models should enable us to employ such data more effectively. Geographic information systems models will bring new information that can identify risk and help us understand disease patterns embedded in surveillance data. We are only beginning to understand how to use these data more effectively. Identifying the different tools available to the statistician and understanding their appropriate use is essential if we are to respond to today's challenges in public health surveillance.

As useful as this volume should be to public health practice, it should also serve as a stepping stone to further research into future challenges in surveillance. New diseases and risk factors will be identified and will need to be put under surveillance. How will these health events be monitored, and what statistical tools will need to be developed or adapted? How can economic tools be used to assess the cost-effectiveness of surveillance practice, and how can economic burden be monitored within surveillance systems? A critical problem is compatibility among surveillance systems and efficient use of data from multiple sources. As systems are linked, what analytic problems will arise, and how can they be addressed? Can we effectively link risk factor data with outcome data to better understand disease and injury processes and develop better ways to prevent disease or to evaluate intervention activities? Can the patterns of infectious diseases that geographers have studied be adapted to other disease or injury patterns to further our understanding of the relevant public health concerns? These are only some of the challenges confronting statisticians, epidemiologists, and other public health scientists in the coming years. This book illustrates the fruits of such collaborations and should stimulate further joint activity.

Atlanta, Georgia   Stephen B. Thacker
Atlanta, Georgia   Jeffrey P. Koplan

Preface

At the beginning of a new millennium, we face critical public health challenges, ranging from outbreaks of new and old pathogens to the safety of the air we breathe and the water we drink. In the past two decades, infectious disease has re-emerged as a significant threat to global health. This is exemplified by the HIV/AIDS pandemic, the outbreak of Bovine spongiform encephalopathy (mad cow disease), bioterrorism with anthrax, severe acute respiratory syndrome and the emergence and spread of West Nile virus in North America. We have made substantial progress in understanding risk factors for the leading chronic diseases, including heart disease and cancer, and in preventing primary diabetes and stroke, but chronic diseases still pose enormous problems. The twin epidemics of diabetes and obesity continue to grow in the United States, and inexplicable clusters of cancer cases are noted by the media with increasing frequency, causing concern and sometimes needless alarm among the public.

The word *surveillance* is derived from the French word *surveiller*, meaning "to watch over." The origin of the term may suggest that public health surveillance is a passive activity, involving the routine reporting of cases of disease to a public health department. On the contrary, effective public health surveillance must incorporate a range of active and passive approaches to ensure that cases are reported completely, accurately, and without exception. Monitoring may include surveys, active and passive systems for reporting of disease morbidity and mortality, data systems and disease registries with active follow-up, and systems for monitoring risk factors and preventive interventions. Our use of the term *public health surveillance* throughout this monograph includes the entire range of surveillance methods used to monitor the health of populations.

In the past several decades, the information sciences, including the statistical and computer sciences, have advanced in many ways, along with the growth of electronic data storage and sharing. Using these scientific and technological breakthroughs to monitor the health of populations more effectively has been challenging.

Ongoing and systematic monitoring of the health of populations is a central activity of effective public health systems. Modern tools of public health surveillance and sound statistical practices are essential for rapid warning about real public health threats, as well as reducing the resources spent on false alarms. Thus, this volume reviews quantitative and statistical ideas and techniques that underlie modern public health surveillance. We have designed it to be accessible to a wide range of professionals, including public health practitioners, epidemiologists, and statisticians. Many of the chapters feature case studies, worked examples, and descriptions of computing software. The book will be a useful companion to several related monographs, including *Principles and Practice of Public Health Surveillance*, 2nd Edition, edited by Steven M. Teutsch and R. Elliott Churchill (Oxford University Press, 2000); *Prevention Effectiveness A Guide to Decision Analysis and Economic Evaluation*, 2nd Edition, edited by Anne C. Haddix, Steven M. Teutsch, and Phaedra S. Corso (Oxford University Press, 2003); *Field Epidemiology*, 2nd Edition, edited by Michael B. Gregg (Oxford University Press, 2002), and *Statistics in Public Health: Quantitative Approaches to Public Health Problems*, edited by Donna Stroup and Steven Teutsch (Oxford University Press, 1998).

The 13 chapters in the volume provide a broad overview of statistical principles and methods for public health surveillance. In Chapter 1, Donna Stroup, Ron Brookmeyer, and William Kalsbeek give examples of public health surveillance in action and introduce a new framework for public health surveillance activities. They apply this framework to cardiovascular disease surveillance, and they list several publicly available data sources for monitoring health. In Chapter 2, William Kalsbeek reviews the use of surveys and survey research methods in monitoring the health of populations and in identifying groups at high risk for adverse health events.

In Chapter 3, Owen Devine describes statistical approaches for exploratory analysis of public health surveillance data to identify spatial and temporal patterns.

Chapters 4, 5, and 6 concern temporal trends in disease incidence and prevalence. In Chapter 4, Theodore Holford reviews statistical approaches to understanding and disentangling age, period, and cohort effects, and he applies them to lung cancer rates in Connecticut. Ron Brookmeyer considers the effect of the incubation period of disease on temporal patterns in disease surveillance in Chapter 5, and he illustrates his points with a discussion of three diseases that have widely differing incubation periods: HIV/AIDS, Bovine spongiform encephalopathy, and anthrax. In Chapter

6, Ruth Etzioni, Larry Kessler, and Dante di Tommaso show that trends in morbidity and mortality can provide information about the efficacy of control measures. They describe a case study of the effect of screening tests for prostate-specific antigen on trends in prostate cancer incidence and mortality, using data from the Surveillance, Epidemiology and End Results (SEER) program of the National Cancer Institute.

Chapters 7, 8, and 9 focus on detecting disease outbreaks and clusters using surveillance data. In Chapter 7, Lance Waller comprehensively reviews the statistical approaches to detecting disease clusters in time, in space, or in both. In Chapter 8, Paddy Farrington and Nick Andrews consider statistical methods for rapidly detecting outbreaks prospectively. In Chapter 9, Peter Diggle, Leo Knorr-Held, Barry Rowlingson, Ting-li Su, Peter Hawtin, and Trevor Bryant discuss methodological approaches for using a web-based reporting system to identify anomalies in the space-time distribution of incident cases of gastrointestinal infections in the United Kingdom.

In Chapter 10, Scott Zeger, Francesca Dominici, Aidan McDermott, and Jonathan Samet analyze the effects of particulate air pollution on mortality in urban centers using Bayesian hierarchical models. They use data from the 88 largest cities in the United States to develop models for multisite time series studies. Additional models for spatial temporal analysis of surveillance data are considered by Andrew Lawson in Chapter 11. Sander Greenland discusses ecologic inference problems inherent in the analysis of public health surveillance data in Chapter 12. A critical issue for some surveillance data systems is the completeness of reporting, and Ernest Hook and Ronald Regal address this issue by reviewing in Chapter 13 the role of capture–recapture methods in public health surveillance.

We hope that this book will be of value to public health practitioners who use quantitative methods for monitoring health. We also hope that it will stimulate statisticians, epidemiologists, and public health scientists to conduct new methodologic research that addresses our global public health challenges.

We acknowledge the many contributions of Tom Lang and Laurie Yelle, who provided superb editorial work on complex material, Dr. Rick Hull and Evelyn Cater of the Centers for Disease Control and Prevention who managed a complex array of draft chapters, and Patty Hubbard and Becky Newcomer, of the Johns Hopkins Bloomberg School of Public Health, for administrative assistance.

Baltimore, Maryland   R.B.
Atlanta, Georgia   D.S.

Contents

Contributors

NICK ANDREWS
Communicable Disease Surveillance
  Center
London, United Kingdom

RON BROOKMEYER
Department of Biostatistics
Johns Hopkins University
Baltimore, Maryland

TREVOR N. BRYANT
School of Medicine Information and
  Computing
University of Southampton
Southampton, United Kingdom

OWEN DEVINE
National Center for Birth Defects &
  Developmental Disabilities
Centers for Disease Control and
  Prevention
Atlanta, Georgia

DANTE DI TOMMASO
Fred Hutchinson Cancer Research
  Center
Seattle, Washington

PETER DIGGLE
Medical Statistics Unit
Lancaster University
Lancaster, United Kingdom

FRANCESCA DOMINICI
Department of Biostatistics
Johns Hopkins University
Baltimore, Maryland

RUTH ETZIONI
Cancer Prevention, Translational
  Outcomes Research
Fred Hutchinson Cancer Research
  Center
Seattle, Washington

PADDY FARRINGTON
Department of Statistics
The Open University
Milton Keynes, United Kingdom

SANDER GREENLAND
Department of Epidemiology
University of California, Los Angeles
Los Angeles, California

PETER HAWTIN
Southampton Public Health
  Laboratory Service
Southampton, United Kingdom

THEODORE R. HOLFORD
Division of Biostatistics
Yale University
New Haven, Connecticut

ERNEST B. HOOK
School of Public Health
University of California, Berkeley
Berkeley, California

WILLIAM D. KALSBEEK
Survey Research Unit
Department of Biostatistics
University of North Carolina
Chapel Hill, North Carolina

LARRY KESSLER
Visiting Scientist
Fred Hutchinson Cancer Research
   Center
Seattle, Washington

LEO KNORR-HELD
Ludwig-Maximilians University
Munich, Germany

JEFFREY P. KOPLAN
Vice President for Academic Health
   Affairs
Emory University
Atlanta, Georgia

ANDREW B. LAWSON
Department of Epidemiology and
   Biostatistics
Arnold School of Public Health
University of South Carolina
Columbia, South Carolina

AIDAN MCDERMOTT
Department of Biostatistics
Johns Hopkins University
Baltimore, Maryland

RONALD R. REGAL
Department of Mathematics and
   Statistics
University of Minnesota
Duluth, Minnesota

BARRY ROWLINGSON
Medical Statistics Unit
Lancaster University
Lancaster, United Kingdom

JONATHAN M. SAMET
Department of Epidemiology
Johns Hopkins University
Baltimore, Maryland

DONNA F. STROUP
National Center for Chronic Disease
   Prevention & Health Promotion
Centers for Disease Control
Atlanta, Georgia

TING-LI SU
Medical Statistics Unit
Lancaster University
Lancaster, United Kingdom

STEPHEN B. THACKER
Epidemiology Program Office
Centers for Disease Control and
   Prevention
Atlanta, Georgia

LANCE A. WALLER
Department of Biostatistics
Rollins School of Public Health
Emory University
Atlanta, Georgia

SCOTT L. ZEGER
Department of Biostatistics
Johns Hopkins University
Baltimore, Maryland

Monitoring the Health
of Populations

1

Public Health Surveillance in Action: A Framework

DONNA F. STROUP, RON BROOKMEYER,
WILLIAM D. KALSBEEK

Public health surveillance is the ongoing systematic collection, analysis, interpretation, and dissemination of health data for the purpose of preventing and controlling disease, injury, and other health problems (Thacker, 2000). In recent years, the science of public health surveillance has changed in response to new public health concerns, such as bioterrorist events (Khan et al., 2000; CDC, 2001). Relatively new diseases and epidemics, such as acquired immunodeficiency syndrome (AIDS), the new variant Creutzfeldt Jakob disease (vCJD), and severe acute respiratory syndrome (SARS), have also brought new demands to the practice of surveillance. Furthermore, recent technological innovations have advanced the science of public health surveillance. These innovations include real-time on-line monitoring (Koo et al., 2001), large data sets in readily accessible formats, advances in geographic information systems (Boulos et al., 2001), sophisticated statistical methods, and the computational tools to apply those methods (Boulos et al., 2001).

Public health policy frequently is based on public health surveillance data. Accordingly, quantitative and statistical methods that allow the most information to be gleaned from surveillance data are critical tools for evaluating public health policy issues. This book describes several such statistical and quantitative methods.

THE BEGINNINGS OF PUBLIC HEALTH SURVEILLANCE

Public health surveillance has a long history (Thacker, 2000). In the mid-1800s, William Farr worked in the Registrar General's office of England and Wales. He collected and analyzed vital statistics data and plotted the rise and fall of smallpox, cholera, and other epidemics of infectious diseases of his time. Farr was the first to systematically collect data about smallpox deaths, and he became one of the founding fathers of public health surveillance (Eyler, 1970).

In the 1940s, Alexander Langmuir became the first chief epidemiologist of the Communicable Disease Center (now the Centers for Disease Control and Prevention [CDC]) in the United States and is credited with conceptualizing modern disease surveillance (Langmuir, 1963). The National Notifiable Disease Reporting System and the current *Morbidity and Mortality Weekly Reports* grew from his deep commitment to furthering the science and practice of public health surveillance. Langmuir broadened the concept of surveillance beyond simply watching individuals at risk for a disease at quarantine stations. He emphasized rapid collection and analysis of data with quick dissemination of the findings to those who needed to know (Langmuir, 1963).

USES OF PUBLIC HEALTH SURVEILLANCE

Public health surveillance systems can serve many purposes. First, they can be used to detect new outbreaks or epidemics. The quicker outbreaks can be detected, the more effectively disease prevention and control programs can prevent further morbidity or mortality. In the fall of 2001, an outbreak of inhalational anthrax occurred in the United States (CDC, 2001a). An astute clinician identified the first clinical case and promptly reported it to public health officials, enabling prophylactic antibiotics to be distributed to exposed individuals soon thereafter.

Second, public health surveillance data can provide information about the natural history of disease. For example, transfusion-associated AIDS cases reported in the 1980s provided the earliest hint of the long incubation period of HIV infection (Brookmeyer and Gail, 1994). Third, public health surveillance data can be used to project the size and scope of an epidemic, as has been done with the vCJD, AIDS, and SARS epidemics (Mertens, 1996; CDC, 2003).

Finally, public health surveillance can be used to evaluate the impact of health interventions, especially those guided by evidence-based practice standards for clinical care (Cochrane Collaboration, 2003; Harris et al.,

2001). Comprehensive surveillance systems and appropriate analytic tools are critical for effectively monitoring the impact of these standards on the health of the public (Anderson and Knickman, 2001).

Surveillance data must be disseminated quickly to public health practitioners, including those who originally gathered the data, as well as to decision makers throughout the public health organization and, depending on the character of the information, to other public service agencies and the community. The dissemination of surveillance data frequently stimulates the search for additional data that may come from other sources.

This chapter gives some examples of the importance of statistical and quantitative reasoning in public health surveillance, provides a framework for understanding the sort of data that can be compiled from an effective public health surveillance system, and identifies some useful sources of worldwide public health surveillance data.

STATISTICAL REASONING: PUBLIC HEALTH SURVEILLANCE IN ACTION

Blood Lead Levels in Children

Elevated blood lead levels in children are related to problems in mental and behavioral development (Moreira et al., 2001). In the mid-1980s the petroleum and related industries in the United States used approximately 1.3 million metric tons of lead annually and about half of this amount was released into the environment. Almost all of the lead entering the atmosphere came from the combustion of leaded gasoline.

The second National Health and Nutrition Examination Survey (NHANES II) conducted from 1975 to 1981 by the National Center for Health Statistics (NCHS) of the CDC provided the data needed to analyze the blood lead levels of the U.S. population (Annest et al., 1983). A detailed statistical analysis revealed that blood lead levels fell in the 1970s (Fig. 1–1), and an explanation was sought for the decrease. One hypothesis was that the decrease was related to the declining use of lead in gasoline. Data from the Environmental Protection Agency (EPA) on lead in gasoline were used to investigate this hypothesis by evaluating the correlations between blood lead levels and the lead content in gasoline. Detailed statistical analyses were performed on the data sets, including techniques to control for the introduction of unleaded paint.

Although the analyses could not prove cause and effect, they did support the hypothesis that the reduction in lead additives in gasoline was a plausible explanation for the concomitant reduction in blood lead in the

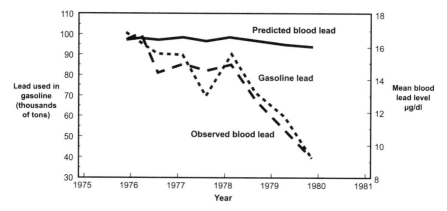

Figure 1–1 The relationship between declines in the lead content of gasoline and lead levels from children's blood, 1975 to 1981—National Health and Nutrition Examination Survey. *Source:* Reprinted with permission from: Pirkle, J.L., Brody, D.J., Gunter, E.W., Kramer, R.A., Paschal, D.C., Flegal, K.M., and Matte, T.D. (1994). The decline in blood levels in the United States. The National Health and Nutrition Examination Surveys (NHANES). *Journal of the American Medical Association* **272,** 284–291.

population. This study was presented in hearings called by the EPA to address a proposal to *increase* the lead content in gasoline. As a result, the final policy required the complete *removal* of lead from gasoline in the United States (Pirkle et al., 1994).

The Increasing Problem of Diabetes

In the 1990s dramatic increases in diabetes and obesity occurred in the United States, and at the same time Americans as a whole did little to improve their eating habits or increase their physical activity (Mokdad et al., 2001; Wang et al., 2002). Diabetes complications can be reduced with treatments such as blood pressure and lipid control and with screening for eye, kidney, and foot disease (U.K. Prospective Diabetes Study Group, 1998). Surveillance data from health plan surveys, medical records, administrative sources, and patient surveys was used to design the Translating Research Into Action for Diabetes (TRIAD) study (The TRIAD Study Group, 2002). The hypothesis of this study was that structural and organizational characteristics of health systems can influence the quality and cost of health care. By combining data from health plans, provider groups, and diverse populations, the study offers opportunities to understand barriers and enabling factors for diabetes care.

The AIDS Epidemic

The first AIDS cases were described in the early 1980s (CDC, 1982). Early in the epidemic, surveillance data were among the most reliable tools for monitoring and tracking its course (Brookmeyer and Gail, 1994). The surveillance definition for these cases allowed sophisticated registries to be created for tracking and counting these cases in many countries (CDC, 1991).

Simple graphical displays of the increase in AIDS cases over time were an invaluable tool for monitoring the epidemic. Statistical methods were developed to correct for reporting delays and were used to show graphically the growth of the epidemic to public health officials, the media, and the general public.

Subsequently, more sophisticated statistical techniques, such as back calculation methods (Brookmeyer and Gail, 1994), were developed to increase understanding of the epidemic. The method of back-calculation used AIDS surveillance data (cases reported over time) with the incubation period distribution to reconstruct the distribution of the rate of infections. From these analyses, not only could the number of HIV-infected individuals in a population be estimated, but the short-term incidence of AIDS could also be projected. Early forecasts of the scope of the epidemic using these statistical methods called worldwide attention to it and helped to garner the resources necessary to develop HIV treatment and prevention programs.

A FRAMEWORK FOR UNDERSTANDING PUBLIC HEALTH SURVEILLANCE DATA

In this book, public health surveillance data is defined broadly to include all types of data collected from populations that could be useful in guiding public health activities. These data may include counts of disease-specific cases of morbidity and mortality as reported to a registry, the spatial and temporal distribution of these cases, representative surveys of populations with regard to health-related behaviors or health status, and other surveys of exposure or hazards in a population or environment.

In this regard, a framework for understanding public health surveillance data is proposed (Fig. 1–2) that portrays the relationships between the population and types of data collection in terms of opportunities for prevention, levels of intervention, and important health outcomes. Types of data are organized by time from earliest prevention opportunity: hazard surveillance, surveillance of health care interventions and public health activ-

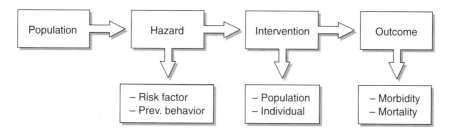

Figure 1–2 A framework for understanding public health surveillance data.

ities, and surveillance of health outcomes. The category of hazard surveillance, includes surveillance of both risk factors and preventive behaviors. Surveillance of health-care interventions and public-health activities consists of obtaining data on interventions directed to populations or individuals. Finally, surveillance of health outcomes includes collecting morbidity and mortality data.

Illustration of the Scope of Public Health Surveillance Data: Cardiovascular Disease

The framework in Figure 1–2 is used to illustrate the scope of public health surveillance data for cardiovascular disease in the United States (Table 1–1). Cardiovascular disease (CVD) is the major cause of death in the United States, accounting for approximately 40% (950,000) of all deaths each year (Fig. 1–3). This condition is increasingly burdensome as the expected life span lengthens and the number of people surviving to age 85

Table 1–1 Public health surveillance framework for cardiovascular disease

Population	Hazard	Intervention	Outcome
U.S. Census	CDC's Behavioral Risk Factor Surveillance System (BRFSS)	POPULATION-BASED Community Programs	American Heart Association
	CDC's National Center for Health Statistics (NCHS)	INDIVIDUAL-BASED National Health and Nutrition Examination Survey (NHANES)	National Hospital Discharge Survey (NHDS) Morbidity and Mortality Weekly Report (MMWR)
	World Health Organization (WHO) Global Youth Tobacco Survey (GYTS)	BRFSS	

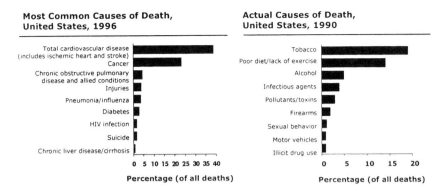

Figure 1–3 Nine leading causes of death and actual causes of death in the United States during the 1990s. *Source:* Reprinted with permission from McGinnis, J.M. and Foege, W.H. (1993). Actual causes of death in the United States. *Journal of the American Medical Association* **270,** 2207–2212.

increases (Kesteloot et al., 2002). When asked about important health problems in the United States in 2001, respondents included heart disease among the top three health concerns (Blendon et al., 2001), illustrating populationwide concern. Cardiovascular disease death rates and preventive services differ substantially by race, age, sex, place of residence, and other demographic factors (Fig. 1–4) (Weber, 1991; Marmot et al., 1978).

Hazard surveillance

Modifiable risk factors for cardiovascular disease include individual health behaviors (tobacco use, physical inactivity, and improper nutrition), health status (hypertension, hyperlipidemia, obesity, diabetes), and policies (smoking policies in restaurants and work sites). In cardiovascular disease prevention, hazard surveillance can include any of these factors. The CDC's Behavioral Risk Factor Surveillance System (BRFSS) provides state-specific prevalence data for major behavioral risks associated with premature morbidity and mortality in adults (Nelson et al., 1998). These data have been used to support tobacco control legislation in most states. In California, the data were influential in supporting the passage of Proposition 99, Tobacco Tax legislation, which generated millions of dollars in state funds to support health education and chronic disease prevention programs. The BRFSS data have also been used to evaluate intervention activities in states participating in the Rocky Mountain Tobacco-Free Challenge. In addition, BRFSS data have illustrated the growing epidemic of overweight among young people (Dietz and Chen, 2002; Mokdad et al., 2001) (Fig. 1–5) and the declining level of physical activity in adults (Wang et al., 2002).

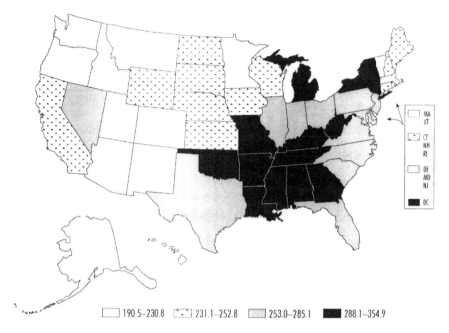

	MA
	VT
⋰	CT
	NH
	RI
	DE
	MD
	NJ
■	DC

☐ 190.5–230.8   ⋰ 231.1–252.8   ▨ 253.0–285.1   ■ 288.1–354.9

Figure 1–4 Death rates of heart disease in the United States, 1999. (Number of deaths per 100,000 people, age-adjusted to 2000 total U. S. Population, for ICD-10 codes 100 through 109, 111, 113, and 120 through 151.) *Source:* National Vital Statistics System.

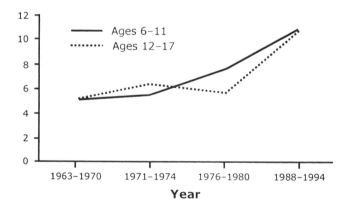

Figure 1–5 Percentage of overweight adolescents in the United States, 1963 through 1994. (Overweight is defined as the top 5% of age- and sex-specific body mass index. [1963–1970 data, age-adjusted].) *Source:* National Center for Health Statistics, unpublished data.

National estimates of the health-related behaviors of U.S. adults are also available from surveys conducted by the CDC's National Center for Health Statistics (NCHS). The National Health Interview Survey (NHIS) conducts face-to-face interviews in a nationally representative sample of households. Each week people selected in a probability sample of the non-institutionalized, civilian population are interviewed by the U.S. Bureau of the Census. Although the NHIS data have the advantage (over the BRFSS) of face-to-face data collection, they cannot be used to provide state-specific estimates (Botman et al., 2000) so both surveys are necessary for surveillance activities. Additionally, period surveys (see Chapter 2) have been used to track these data at a community level (Sturm, 2002).

Internationally, the World Health Organization (WHO) and the CDC have developed the Global Youth Tobacco Survey (GYTS) to track tobacco use by young people in different countries with a common methodology and core questionnaire. The GYTS surveillance system is intended to enhance the capacity of countries to design, implement, and evaluate tobacco control and prevention programs (CDC, 1999).

Intervention surveillance

Cardiovascular disease can be prevented effectively by population-based efforts and individual interventions. At the population level, surveillance of interventions to increase physical activity is illustrated by the Prevention Center at the University of South Carolina, which assesses community indicators promoting physical activity. Geographic Information System (GIS) techniques were applied to validate perceptions of survey participants about the location of environmental features that support physical activity in their communities (Croner and Decola, 2001). Spatial and network analysis and the GIS database were used to validate survey about the perceived accessibility of environmental features, as well as landscape features and established physical activity sites (Hopkins and Fielding et al., 2001). Community programs to reduce tobacco use, school health programs to prevent tobacco use and addiction, and counter-marketing attempts to promote cessation and to decrease the likelihood of initiation are other examples of population-level interventions that can benefit from surveillance (CDC, 1999).

Surveillance data for individual-level interventions for cardiovascular disease includes the prevalence of screening programs for conditions such as hypertension, hyperlipidemia, obesity, and diabetes that are available from the NHIS, the National Health and Nutrition Examination Survey (NHANES), and the BRFSS (Graves, 2000).

Health outcome surveillance

Surveillance for health outcomes should include morbidity and mortality for cardiovascular disease. In 2000, an estimated 12.9 million Americans were living with coronary heart disease, and approximately 250,000 fatal events will occur out of the hospital (U.S. Department of HHS, 2003); in 1998, heart disease was reported as the underlying cause of more than 40% of all deaths (CDC, 2001b). Data from the CDC's National Hospital Discharge Survey (NHDS) (Gillum et al., 2000) and National Health Interview Survey (NHIS) (CDC, 2001) can also be used to assess the burden of cardiovascular disease. These data sources show that major CVD conditions are particularly burdensome for women with diabetes.

Limitations of data sources

The framework shown in Figure 1–2 allows limitations of the model or the data sources to be examined. Because cardiovascular disease is not a single disease, but rather numerous conditions with different causes, risks, and interventions, trends or patterns can be interpreted only by examining specific types of cardiovascular disease (e.g., congenital heart disease). Many types of cardiovascular disease have long latency periods, so several years may pass before changes in behavior or clinical practice affect mortality. In addition, some types of cardiovascular disease (e.g., congenital heart disease) are not amenable to primary prevention or screening. Finally, cause of death listed on the death certificate may be inaccurate (Will et al., 2001).

Sources of Public Health Surveillance Data

The Internet has made many data sets readily available for public health surveillance. In Table 1–2, we present selected sources for public health surveillance categorized by data collection methodology: registries of specific health outcomes, ongoing data collection not using probability sampling, and surveys using some form of probability sampling. These sources are used in subsequent chapters. Features listed for the sources in Table 1–2 include the primary mode of data collection, the scope (national or other), the target population represented, the frequency of data collection, a Web link URL (current as of the date of this printing) if available, and references for additional information.

A key feature of any surveillance system is how it identifies subjects to be monitored, which may vary by type of system. In registries, case ascertainment is determined by the medical definition of a case (e.g., born with a birth defect) and the infrastructure by which cases are ascertained (e.g., a network of reporting hospitals). In surveys, subject identification in some instances employs probability sampling methods, in which those targeted may be chosen with of a formal random selection process. Most of the surveillance surveys in Table 1–2 (22 of 30) were found to use some form of probability sampling. The other eight surveys select subjects by applying a set of eligibility criteria to a selection infrastructure, such as registries. For instance, the Childhood Blood Lead Surveillance (CBLS) System searches for elevated lead levels in blood samples taken from children under 16 years of age through an organized system of reporting laboratories in each of the 28 participating states.

Probability sampling is widely used in public health research because it provides an explicit statistical basis for learning about a population from a sample (Kalsbeek and Heiss, 2000). Random sampling gives each member of the population a known probability of selection. In contrast, in nonprobability methods, the decision to include a population member is left to the judgment of the investigator (e.g., convenience sampling) or the respondent (e.g., self-selected samples in clip-out newspaper surveys).

The *mode* of data collection for a surveillance system, defined by the nature of the information exchange between the investigator and respondent, also varies somewhat by type of system. Surveys using probability sampling typically rely on interviews (telephone or in person) to gather their data, whereas most other surveillance systems use reporting networks of health professionals. Of the 22 surveys using probability sampling in Table 1–2, 15 rely mainly on interviews (11 in person and 4 by telephone); the other 7 are a mixture of self-administered questionnaires (4) and record abstraction (3). Depending on the mode of data collection, planning for surveillance systems may include developing questionnaires or other data-gathering instruments, collecting data (including recruiting, training, and monitoring data gatherers), and preparing data for analysis. These nonsampling activities in surveillance may involve a broad spectrum of workers, from subject-matter experts to survey methods specialists to statisticians.

The scope of a surveillance system may be local, state, national, international, or any combination. Most of the surveillance systems in Table 1–2 are national in scope, although some like the BRFSS, the Youth Risk Behavior Survey (YRBS), and the Youth Tobacco Survey (YTS) monitor at both state and national levels.

The target population of a surveillance system may vary by type of system. Registries tend to target more narrowly defined segments of the population (e.g., those logged through the vital registration system, or those having blood samples analyzed by laboratories), whereas surveys more typically focus on the general residential population. The frequency of data gathering also varies by system. In Table 1–2, the 55 registries and 10 surveys without probability sampling are more likely to be conducted quarterly, monthly, weekly, or continuously, whereas the 30 surveys using probability samples are more likely to be conducted annually or less often.

It has been said that surveillance is the ground cover for public health practice (James S. Marks, personal communication); it is the essential activity that allow other public health actions to have effect. The methods

Table 1-2 Selected data sources for public health surveillance

Surveillance system	Primary mode	Scope	Target population	Frequency	Web link URL*	Reference
1. REGISTRIES OF SPECIFIC HEALTH OUTCOMES						
121 Cities Mortality Reporting System (121 CMRS)	Reporting Network	United States (Urban areas)	Decedents	Weekly	http://www.cdc.gov/epo/dphsi/121hist.htm	Centers for Disease Control and Prevention (1996) *121 Cities Mortality Reporting System Manual of Procedures.* Atlanta: U.S. Department of Health and Human Services, Public Health Service, CDC, October 1996.
Active Bacterial Core Surveillance (ABCS)	Reporting Network	United States (Emerging Infections Program sites)	Patients (Laboratory identified)	At least monthly	http://www.cdc.gov/ncidod/dbmd/abcs	Schuchat, A., Hilger, T., Zell, E., Farley, M.M., Reingold, A., Harrison, L., Lefkowitz, L., Danila, R., Stefonek, K., Barrett, N., Morse, D., and Pinner, R. (2001). Active Bacterial Core Surveillance Team of the Emerging Infections Program Network. Active bacterial core surveillance of the emerging infections program network. *Emerging Infectious Diseases* 7, 92–99.
Adoption and Foster Care Analysis and Reporting System (AFCARS)	Reporting Network	State	Children (in foster care or adopted under the auspices of the State Child welfare agency)	Semiannually	http://www.hhs.gov	Maza, P.L. (2002). Using administration data to reward agency performance: the case of the federal adoption incentive program. *Child Welfare* **79**, 444–456. Barach, C.A., Feigelman, W., Chandra, A., Wilson, J. (1995). Using Archival datasets to study adoption-related questions. *Adoption Research Newsletter*, 1.

System	Method	Geographic Coverage	Population	Frequency	URL	Reference
Alaska Occupational Injury Surveillance System (AOISS)	Reporting Network	State	Decedents (work-related traumatic injuries)	Continuously	http://www.cdc.gov/niosh	Garrett, L.C., Conway, G.A., Manwaring, J.C. (1998). Epidemiology of work-related aviation fatalities in Alaska, 1990–94. *Aviation Space and Environmental Medicine* **69,** 1131–1136.
Adult Spectrum of Disease (ASD)	Record abstraction	United States (10 project areas)	Patients (with HIV infection)	6 months	http://www.cdc.gov/nchs/data	Smith, D. (1998). The HIV Epidemiology Research Study; HIV Out-Patient Study, and the Spectrum of Disease Studies. *Journal of Acquired Immune Deficiency Syndromes,* **17,** *Suppl 1* S17–S19.
AIDS Public Use	Reporting Network	State/Local	Patients	Monthly	http://wonder.cdc.gov	Statistics and Data Management Branch, Division of HIV/AIDS Prevention, Mailstop E-48, Centers for Disease Control and Prevention, Atlanta, GA 30333, telephone (404) 639-2020. Copies are also available from the CDC National AIDS Clearinghouse, telephone (800) 458-5231. If you are calling the Clearinghouse, please ask for inventory number D206. You can also download the software from the internet by linking to http://www.cdc.gov/nchstp/hiv_aids/software/apids/apidsof.htm
Birth Defects Monitoring Program (BDMP)	Reporting Network	United States	Infants (Still- and live-born)	Continuously	http://www.cdc.gov/mmwr	Edmonds, L.D. and James, L.M. (1990). Temporal trends in the prevalence of congenital malformations at birth based on the Birth Defects Monitoring Program, United States, 1979–1987. *MMWR Surveillance Summaries* **39(SS-4),** 19–23.

(continued)

Table 1-2 Selected data sources for public health surveillance (Continued)

Surveillance system	Primary mode	Scope	Target population	Frequency	Web link URL*	Reference
Bureau of the Census	Registration	U.S. Civilian	U.S. Civilian population	Decennially	http://www.census.gov	*Census Catalog and Guide*
California Birth Defects Monitoring Program (CBDMP)	Reporting Network	California	Infants (Still- and live-born)	Continuously	http://www.cbdmp.org	Croen, L.A., Shaw, G.M., and Wasserman, C.R., Tolarova, M.M. (1998). Racial and ethnic variations in the prevalence of orofacial clefts in California, 1983–1992. *American Journal of Medical Genetics* **79**, 42–47, 1998
Congenital Syphilis (CS) Cases Investigation and Report (Form CDC-73.126) (CSCIR)	Record Abstraction	United States	Patients (live-born/ stillborn infants with CS)	Continuously	http://www.cdc.gov/nchstp	CDC. (2001). Congenital syphilis—United States, 2000. *MMWR. Morbidity and Mortality Weekly Report* **50**, 573–577.
Drug and Alcohol Services Information System (DASIS)	Record Abstraction and Telephone Interview	United States	Patients (Substance abuse)	Continuously for client admission, annually for facility census	http://www.drugabuse statistics.samhsa.gov	Hopfer, C.J., Mikulich, S.K., and Crowley, T.J. (2000). Heroin use among adolescents in treatment for substance use disorders. *Journal of the American Academy of Child and Adolescent Psychiatry*, **39**, 1316–1323.
Early Childhood Longitudinal Study	Birth Record Abstraction, interviews with mothers, child assessment	U.S. subset	15,000 Infants born during 2001	Irregularly	http://www.cdc.gov/nchs; http://www.doe.gov	Blackwell, D.L., Hayward, M., and Crimmins, E. (2001). Does childhood health affect chronic morbidity in later life? *Social Science and Medicine* **52**, 1269–1284.
End Stage Renal Disease (ESRD) Program Management and Medical Information System (PMMIS)	Record Abstraction	United States	ESRD patients (Medicare-beneficiaries)	Continuously	http://www.niddk.nih.gov	Calvert, G.M., Steenland, K., and Palu, S. (1997). End-stage renal disease among silica-exposed gold miners. A new method for assessing incidence among epidemiologic cohorts. *Journal of the American Medical Association* **277**, 1219–1223.

System	Type	Location	Population	Frequency	URL	Reference
Fatality Assessment and Control Evaluation Project (FACE)	Reporting Network	State	Workers	Continuously	http://www.cdc.gov/niosh/face/	CDC (2000). Baler and compactor-related deaths in the workplace—United States, 1992–2000. *MMWR—Morbidity and Mortality Weekly Report.* **50,** 309–313.
Fatal Analysis Reporting System (FARS)	Reporting Network	United States	Fatal traffic crashes	Continuously	http://www.nhtsa.dot.gov	Cayten, C.G., Quervalu, I., and Agarwal, N. (1999). Fatality Analysis Reporting System demonstrates association between trauma system initiatives and decreasing death rates. *Journal of Trauma, Injury, Infection, and Critical Care* **46,** 751–755; discussion 755–756.
Foodborne-Disease Outbreak Surveillance System (FBDOSS)	Reporting Network	United States	Patients (Laboratory identified)	Continuously	http://www.cdc.gov/mmwr/preview/mmwrhtml/ss4901a1.htm	Olsen, S.J., MacKinnon, L.C., Goulding, J.S., Bean, N.H., and Slutsker L. (2000). Surveillance for foodborne-disease outbreaks—United States, 1993–1997. *Morbidity and Mortality Weekly Report. CDC Surveillance Summaries.* **49,** 1–62.
Hazardous Substance Release/Health Effects	Reporting Network	Selected states	Facilities	Irregularly	http://www.cdc.gov/HS/atsdr	Hazardous Substances Emergency Events Surveillance (HSEES), Annual Report, 1998.
Gonococcal Isolate Surveillance Project (GISP)	Reporting Network	United States (24 sentinel sites)	Patients (men with gonorrhea)	Monthly (Quarterly for laboratories)	http://www.cdc.gov/ncid	Gorwitz, R.J., Nakashima, A.K., Moran, J.S., and Knapp, J.S. (1993). Sentinel surveillance for antimicrobial resistance in Neisseria gonorrhoeae—United States, 1988–1991. The Gonococcal Isolate Surveillance Project Study Group. *Morbidity and Mortality Weekly Report. CDC Surveillance Summaries* **42,** 29–39.

(continued)

Table 1–2 Selected data sources for public health surveillance (Continued)

Surveillance system	Primary mode	Scope	Target population	Frequency	Web link URL*	Reference
HIV/AIDS Reporting System (HARS)	Reporting Network	United States	Patients	Continuously	http://www.cdc.gov/scientific.htm	Olsen, S.J., MacKinnon, L.C., Goulding, J.S., Bean, N.H., and Slutsker, L. (2000). Surveillance for foodborne-disease outbreaks—United States, 1993–1997. *Morbidity and Mortality Weekly Report. CDC Surveillance Summaries* **49**, 1–62.
International Vital Statistics	Reporting Network & Record Abstraction	International	Decedents Live Births	Annually	http://www.who.int	Anderson, R.N. (2001). Deaths: leading causes for 1999. *National Vital Statistics Reports* **49**, 1–87.
Linked Birth/Infant Death Program	Reporting Network & Record Abstraction	United States	Live Births and Infant Deaths	Annually	http://www.cdc.gov/nchs	Herrchen, B., Gould, J.B., and Nesbitt, T.S. (1997). Vital Statistics linked birth/infant death and hospital discharge record linkage for epidemiologic studies. *Computers and Biomedical Research* **30**, 290–305.
Metropolitan Atlanta Congenital Defects Program (MACDP)	Reporting Network	Georgia	Infants (Still- and live-born)	Continuously	http://www.cdc.gov/ncbddd	Anonymous. (1993). Metropolitan Atlanta Congenital Defects Program surveillance data, 1988–1991. *Teratology* **48**, 695–709.
Medicare Provider Analysis and Review File (MEDPAR)	Record Abstraction	United States	Patients In inpatient hospital and Skilled Nursing Facility)	Quarterly	http://www.os.dhhs.gov/progorg/aspe/minority/minhcf11.htm	Studnicki, J., Schapira, D.V., Straumfjord, J.V., Clark, R.A., Marshburn. J., and Werner, D.C. (1994). A national profile of the use of intensive care by Medicare patients with cancer. *Cancer* **74**, 2366–2373.
National Antimicrobial Resistance Monitoring System (NARMS)	Reporting Network	State	Patients (Laboratory identified)	Continuously	http://www.cms.hhs.gov	Marano, N.N., Rossiter, S., Stamey, K., Joyce, K., Barrett, T.J., Tollefson, L.K., and Angulo, F.J. (2000). The National Antimicrobial Resistance Monitoring System (NARMS) for enteric bacteria, 1996–1999: surveillance for action. *Journal of the American Veterinary Medical Association* **217**, 1829–1830.

Name	Type	Location	Unit	Frequency	URL	Reference
National Automotive Sampling System	Reporting Network				http://www.nrd.nhsta.dot.gov/departments/nrd-30/ncsa/NASS.html	
National Claims History (NCH) 100% Nearline File and Standard Analytical Files (SAFs)	Reporting Network	United States	Patients (Physician/supplier claims)	Daily/weekly	http://www.cms.hhs.gov	Parente, S.T., Weiner, J.P., Garnick, D.W., Richards, T.M., Fowles, J., Lawthers, A.G., Chandler, P., and Palmer, R.H. (1995). Developing a quality improvement database using health insurance data: a guided tour with application to Medicare's National Claims History file. *American Journal of Medical Quality* **10**, 162–176.
National Congenital Rubella Syndrome Registry (NCRSR)	Reporting Network	United States	Congenital rubella syndrome patients	Weekly	http://www.cdc.gov/nip	CDC (1997). Rubella and congenital rubella syndrome—United States, 1994–1997. *MMWR. Morbidity and Mortality Weekly Report* **46**, 350–354.
National Death Index	Reporting Network	United States	All Deaths	Annually	http://www.cdc.gov/nchs	Doody, M.M., Hayes, H.M., and Bilgrad, R. (2001). Comparability of national death index and standard procedures for determining causes of death in epidemiologic studies. *Annals of Epidemiology* **11**, 46–50.
National Drug and Therapeutic Index	Reporting Network	United States	Prescriptions	Annually	http://www.imshealth.com	Zell, E.R., McCaig, L.F., Kupronis, B., Besser, R.E., and Schuchat, A. (2001). Comparison of the National Drug and Therapeutic Index and the National Ambulatory Medical Care Survey to evaluate antibiotic usage. 2000 Proceedings of the Section on Survey Methods Research. Alexandria, VA: *American Statistical Association.* 840–845.

(continued)

Table 1–2 Selected data sources for public health surveillance (Continued)

Surveillance system	Primary mode	Scope	Target population	Frequency	Web link URL*	Reference
National Exposure Registry (NER)	Reporting Network & interview (telephone)	United States	Persons exposed to a hazardous environmental substance	Biennially	http://www.cdc.gov/atsdr	Burg, J.R. and Gist, G.L. (1995). The National Exposure Registry: procedures for establishing a registry of persons environmentally exposed to hazardous substances. *Toxicology and Industrial Health* **11**, 231–248.
National Fire Incident Reporting System					http://www.fema.gov	The many uses of the National Fire Incident Reporting System. FEMA/USDA Publication number FA 171, 1977. Available at http://www.usfa.fema.gov/dhtml/insideOusfa/nfirs3.cfm (Accessed 9/26/02).
National Giardiasis Surveillance System (NGSS)	Reporting Network	State	Patients	Continuously	http://www.cdc.gov/epo/mmwr/preview/mmwrhtml/ss4907a1.htm	Furness, B.W., Beach, M.J., and Roberts, J.M. (2000). Giardiasis surveillance—United States, 1992–1997. *Morbidity and Mortality Weekly Report. CDC Surveillance Summaries* **49**, 1–13.
National Institute on Drug Abuse (NIDA)					http://www.nih.nida.gov	
National Malaria Surveillance System (NMSS)	Reporting Network	United States	Patients	Continuously	http://www.cdc.gov/mmwr/preview/mmwrhtml/ss5001a2.htm	Williams, H.A., Roberts, J., Kachur, S.P., Barber, A.M., Barat, L.M., Bloland, P.B., Ruebush, T.K., and Wolfe, E.B. (1999). Malaria surveillance—United States, 1995. *Morbidity and Mortality Weekly Report. CDC Surveillance Summaries.* **48**, 1–23.
National Notifiable Disease Surveillance System (NNDSS) & National Electronic Telecommunication Surveillance System (NETSS)	Reporting Network	United States	Patients	Weekly	http://www.cdc.gov/epo/dphsi	CDC. (1997). Demographic differences in notifiable infectious disease morbidity—United States, 1992–1994. *MMWR. Morbidity and Mortality Weekly Report* **46**, 637–641.

System	Method	Coverage	Population	Frequency	Website	Reference
National Occupational Mortality Surveillance System (NOMS)	Reporting Network and Record Abstraction	State	Decedents	Continuously	http://www.cdc.gov/niosh	Wagener, D.K., Walstedt, J., Jenkins, L., et al. (1997). Women: work and health. *Vital and Health Statistics* **3**.
National Program of Cancer Registries—Cancer Surveillance System (NPCR–CSS)	Reporting Network	United States	Patients	Annually	http://www.cdc.gov/cancer	Izquierdo, J.N. and Schoenbach, V.J. (2000). The potential and limitations of data from population-based state cancer registries. *American Journal of Public Health* **90**, 695–697.
National Respiratory and Enteric Virus Surveillance System (NREVSS)	Reporting Network	United States (Laboratories)	Patients (Laboratory identified)	Weekly	http://www.cdc.gov/ncid	CDC. (2001). From the Centers for Disease Control and Prevention. Respiratory syncytial virus activity—United States, 1999–2000 season. *Journal of the American Medical Association* **285**, 287–288.
National Salmonella Surveillance System (NSSS)	Reporting Network	United States	Patients (Laboratory identified)	Continuously	http://www.cdc.gov/ncid	Mermin, J., Hoar, B., and Angulo, F.J. (1997). Iguanas and Salmonella marina infection in children: a reflection of the increasing incidence of reptile-associated salmonellosis in the United States. *Pediatrics* **99**, 399–402.
National Surveillance System for Pneumoconiosis Mortality (NSSPM)	Record Abstraction	United States	Decedents (pneumoconiosis)	Annually	http://www.cdc.gov/ncid	Bang, K.M., Althouse, R.B., Kim, J.H., and Games, S.R. (1999). Recent trends of age-specific pneumoconiosis mortality rates in the United States, 1985–1996: coal workers' pneumoconiosis, asbestosis, and silicosis. *International Journal of Occupational and Environmental Health* **5**, 251–255.

(continued)

Table 1–2 Selected data sources for public health surveillance (Continued)

Surveillance system	Primary mode	Scope	Target population	Frequency	Web link URL*	Reference
National Traumatic Occupational Fatality Surveillance System (NTOFSS)	Reporting Network and Record Abstraction	United States	Decedents (>=16 years old)	Annually	http://www.cdc.gov/niosh	CDC. (2001). Fatal occupational injuries—United States, 1980–1987. *MMWR. Morbidity and Mortality Weekly Report* **50**, 317–320.
National Vital Statistics System (NVSS)	Reporting Network and Record Abstraction	United States & State	Decedents Live Births	Annually	http://www.cdc.gov/nchs	Hoyert, D.L. and Martin, J.A. (2002). Vital statistics as a data source. *Seminars in Perinatology* **26**, 12–16.
Pregnancy Mortality Surveillance System (PMSS)	Reporting Network and Record Abstraction	United States	Decedents (Females at reproductive age)	Not applicable	http://www.cdc.gov/nccdphp/drh	Koonin, L.M., MacKay, A.P., Berg, C.J., Atrash, H.K., and Smith, J.C. (1997). Pregnancy-related mortality surveillance—United States, 1987–1990. *Morbidity and Mortality Weekly Report CDC Surveillance Summaries* **46**, 17–36.
Runaway and Homeless Youth Management Information System (RHYMIS)	Reporting Network	United States	Youth (Run-away or homeless, under the age of 27)	Quarterly	http://aspe.hhs.gov/datacncl/datadir/acf.htm	U.S. Department of Health and Human Services, Administration for Children and Families, Administration on Children, Youth and Families (1995). *Report to the Congress on the Youth Programs of the Family and Youth Services Bureau for Fiscal Year 1995.* Prepared by Johnson, Bassin, and Shaw, Inc. Contract No. 105-92-1709.
Surveillance, Epidemiology, and End Results Program (SEER)	Reporting Network	United States	Cancer patients	Not applicable	http://seer.cancer.gov	Brooks, J.M., Chrischilles, E., Scott, S., Ritho, J., and Chen-Hardee, S. (2000). Information gained from linking SEER Cancer Registry Data to state-level hospital discharge abstracts. *Surveillance, Epidemiology, and End Results. Medical Care* **38**, 1131–1140.

System	Type	Level	Population	Frequency	URL	Reference
Sentinel Event Notification Systems for Occupational Risks—Silicosis (SENSOR Silicosis)	Reporting Network	State	Patients (occupational silicosis)	Annually	http://www.cdc.gov/mmwr/preview/mmwrthm1/00046046.htm	Maxfield, R., Alo, C., Reilly, M.J., Rosenman, K., Kalinowski, D., Stanbury, M., Valiante, D.J., Jones, B., Randolph, S., Socie, E., Gromen, K., Migliozzi, A., Willis, T.M., Schnitzer, P., Perrotta, D.M., Gruetzmacher, G., Anderson, H., Jajosky, R.A., Castellan, R.M., and Game, S. (1997). Surveillance for silicosis, 1993—Illinois, Michigan, New Jersey, North Carolina, Ohio, Texas, and Wisconsin, *Morbidity and Mortality Weekly Report. CDC Surveillance Summaries* **46**, 13–28.
Sentinel Event Notification Systems for Occupational Risks—Work-Related Asthma (SENSOR WRA)	Reporting Network	State	Patients (work-related asthma)	Annually	http://www.cdc.gov/niosh	Jajosky, R.A., Harrison, R., Reinisch, F., Flattery, J., Chan, J., Tumpowsky, C., Davis, L., Reilly, M.J., Rosenman, K.D., Kalinowski, D., Stanbury, M., Schill, D.P., and Wood, J. (1999). Surveillance of work-related asthma in selected U.S. states using surveillance guidelines for state health departments—California, Massachusetts, Michigan, and New Jersey. 1993–1995. *Morbidity and Mortality Weekly Report. CDC Surveillance Summaries* **48**, 1–20.
Sexually Transmitted Disease Surveillance (STDS)	Reporting Network	United States	Patients	Monthly, quarterly, and annually	http://www.cdc.gov/nchstp/Rpt.	Centers for Disease Control and Prevention. *Sexually transmitted disease surveillance 1999.* Division of STD Prevention, Department of Health and Human Services, CDC. Atlanta, Georgia. September 2000.

(continued)

Table 1-2 Selected data sources for public health surveillance (Continued)

Surveillance system	Primary mode	Scope	Target population	Frequency	Web link URL*	Reference
Tuberculosis National Surveillance System (SURVS-TB)	Reporting Network	United States	Patients	Monthly	http://www.cdc.gov/nchstp	CDC. (1998). Tuberculosis morbidity—United States, 1997. *MMWR. Morbidity & Mortality Weekly Report* **47**, 253–257.
Traumatic Brain Injury in the United States (TBISS)	Record Abstraction	State	Patients (hospitalized or fatal traumatic brain injuries)	Annually	http://www.cdc.gov/ncipc	Centers for Disease Control and Prevention. (1997). Traumatic brain injury, Colorado, Missouri, Oklahoma, and Utah—1990–1993. *Morbidity and Mortality Weekly Report* **46**, 8–11.
Toxic Exposure Surveillance System (TESS)	Reporting Network	State	Poison exposure reports	Not applicable	http://www.aapcc.org	Litovitz, T.L., Klein-Schwartz, W., White, S., Cobaugh, D.J., Youniss, J., Drab, A., and Benson, B.E. (2000). 1999 annual report of the American Association of Poison Control Centers Toxic Exposure Surveillance System. *American Journal of Emergency Medicine* **18**, 517–574.
Vaccine Adverse Event Reporting System (VAERS)	Reporting Network	United States	Patients	Not applicable	http://www.fda.gov	Singleton, J.A., Lloyd, J.C., Moorrey, G.T., Salive, M.E., and Chen, R.T. (1999). An overview of the vaccine adverse event reporting system (VAERS) as a surveillance system. VAERS Working Group. *Vaccine* **17**, 2908–2917.

Name	Type	Coverage	Population	Frequency	URL	Citation
Vaccine Safety Datalink Project (VSD)	Reporting Network	United States (7 HMOs)	Patients	Annually	http://www.cdc.gov/nip	Chen, R.T., Glasser, J.W., Rhodes, P.H., Davis, R.L., Barlow, W.E., Thompson, R.S., Mullooly, J.P., Black, S.B., and Shinefield, H.R., Vadheim, C.M., Marcy, S.M., Ward, J.I., Wise, R.P., Wassilak, S.G., and Hadler, S.C. (1997). Vaccine Safety Datalink project: a new tool for improving vaccine safety monitoring in the United States. The Vaccine Safety Datalink Team. *Pediatrics* **99**, 765–773.
Waterborne-disease Outbreaks Surveillance System (WBDOSS)	Reporting Network	United States	Patients	Not applicable	http://www.cdc.gov/epo/mmwr/preview/mmwrhtml/00055820.htm	Barwick, R.S., Levy, D.A., Craun, G.F., Beach, M.J., and Calderon, R.L. (2000). Surveillance for waterborne-disease outbreaks—United States, 1997–1998. *Morbidity and Mortality Weekly Report* **49**, 1–21.
West Nile Virus Surveillance System (WNVSS)	Reporting Network	State	Patients	Weekly	http://nationalatlas.gov/virusintro.html	CDC. (2001). Human West Nile virus surveillance—Connecticut, New Jersey, and New York, 2000. *Morbidity and Mortality Weekly Report* **50**, 265–268.

2. SURVEYS NOT UTILIZING PROBABILITY SAMPLING

Name	Type	Coverage	Population	Frequency	URL	Citation
Adult Blood Lead Epidemiology and Surveillance Program (ABLES)	Reporting Network	State	Adult residents	Quarterly	http://www.cdc/gov/niosh	CDC. (1998). Adult blood lead epidemiology and surveillance—United States, fourth quarter, 1997. *MMWR. Morbidity and Mortality Weekly Report* **47**, 570–573.
Ambulatory Sentinel Practice Network (ASPN)	Reporting Network	Selected Clinical Practice		Irregularly	http://www.aspen.denver.co.us	Nutting, P.A., Beasley, J.W., and Werner, J.J. (1999). Practice-based research networks answer primary questions *Journal of the care American Medical Association* **281**, 686–688.

(continued)

Table 1-2 Selected data sources for public health surveillance (Continued)

Surveillance system	Primary mode	Scope	Target population	Frequency	Web link URL*	Reference
Childhood Blood Lead Surveillance (CBLS)	Reporting Network	State	Children (<16 years old)	Quarterly	http://www.cdc.gov/nceh	CDC. (2000). Blood lead levels in young children—United States and selected states, 1996–1999. *MMWR. Morbidity and Mortality Weekly Report* **49**, 1133–1137.
Dialysis Surveillance Network (DSN)	Reporting Network	United States (Dialysis centers)	Hemodialysis patients	Monthly	http://www.cdc.gov/ncid	Surveillance for bloodstream and vascular access infections in outpatient hemodialysis centers: Procedure manual. Hospital Infections Program, Centers for Disease Control and Prevention, Public Health Services, Department of Health and Human Services. Atlanta, Georgia
National Aging Programs Information System—State Performance Reports (NAPIS/SPR)	Reporting Network	United States	Residents (>=60 years old)	Annually	http://www.hhs.gov/aging	Wiener, J.M. and Tilly, J. (2002). Population ageing in the United States of America: implications for public programmers. *International Journal of Epidemiology* **31**, 776–781.
National Child Abuse and Neglect Data System (NCANDS)	Reporting Network	State	Children (<18 years old)	Annually	http://www.hhs.gov/children	U.S. Department of Health and Human Services, Administration on Children, Youth and Families. *Child Maltreatment 1999.* Washington, DC: U.S. Government Printing Office, 2001
National Nosocomial Infections Surveillance System (NNIS)	Reporting Network	United States (Hospitals)	Inpatients (at high risk of infection)	Not applicable	http://www.cdc.gov/ncid	Emori, T.G., Culver, D.H., Horan, T.C., Jarvis, W.R., White, J.W., Olson, D.R., Banerjee, S., Edwards, J.R., Martone, W.J., and Gaynes, R.P. (1991). National nosocomial infections surveillance system (NNIS): description of surveillance methods. *American Journal of Infection Control* **19**, 19–35.

Name	Type	Coverage	Population	Frequency	URL	Reference
Pediatric Nutrition Surveillance System (PedNSS)	Reporting Network	United States	Children (Low-income)	Monthly or quarterly	http://www.cdc.gov/nccdphp/dnpa	Centers for Disease Control and Prevention. (1998). *Pediatric Nutrition Surveillance, 1997 full report.* Atlanta: U.S. Department of Health and Human Services, Centers for Disease Control and Prevention. (1996).
Pregnancy Nutrition Surveillance System (PNSS)	Reporting Network	State	Female residents (Low-income pregnant and postpartum)	Quarterly	http://www.cdc.gov/nccdphp/dnpa	Centers for Disease Control and Prevention. (1996). *Pregnancy Nutrition Surveillance, 1996 full report.* Atlanta: U.S. Department of Health and Human Services, Centers for Disease Control and Prevention.
Pulsenet	Reporting Network	State labs	Lab results from pulse-field gel electrophoresis		http://www.cdc.gov/ncid	Centers for Disease Control and Prevention. Surveillance for Food-borne Disease Outbreaks—United States 1993–1997. (2000). *Mortality and Morbidity Weekly Report* **49**, 1–51.

3. SURVEYS UTILIZING SOME FORM OF PROBABILITY SAMPLING

Name	Type	Coverage	Population	Frequency	URL	Reference
Behavioral Risk Factor Surveillance System (BRFSS)	Interview (Telephone)	United States and State	Adult residents (>=18 years old)	Monthly	http://www.cdc.gov/nccdphp/brfss	Center for Disease Control and Prevention. (1998). *Behavioral Risk Factor Surveillance System User's Guide.* Atlanta: U.S. Departmental of Health and Human Services, Centers for Disease Control and Prevention.
Department of the Interior Water Quality	Samples subjected to lab tests	50 major river basins and aquifers in the United States		Cyclical, every 3–4 years	http://www.usgs.gov	Spruill, T.B. and Candela, L. (1990). *Two Approaches to Design of Monitoring Networks.* Ground Water.
Drug Abuse Warning Network (DAWN)	Record Abstraction	United States	Patients and Decedents (Drug-related)	Continuously	http://www.hhs.gov/drugs	Roberts, C.D. (1996). Data quality of the Drug Abuse Warning Network. *American Journal of Drug and Alcohol Abuse* **22**, 389–401.

(continued)

Table 1–2 Selected data sources for public health surveillance (Continued)

Surveillance system	Primary mode	Scope	Target population	Frequency	Web link URL*	Reference
Medicare Current Beneficiary Study (MCBS)	Interview (in-person)	United States	Medicare beneficiaries	3 times a year	http://www.cms.gov	U.S. Dept. of Health and Human Services, Health Care Financing Administration. (1992). Medicare Current Beneficiary Survey, Calendar Year 1991: [UNITED STATES] [Computer file]. Baltimore, MD: U.S. Dept. of Health and Human Services, Health Care Financing Administration.
Medical Expenditure Panel Survey (MEPS)	Interview (In-person & telephone)	United States	All residents	Annually	http://www.cms.gov	Cohen, J.W., Monheit, A.C., Beauregard, K.M., Cohen, S.B., Lefkowitz, D.C., Potter, D.E., Sommers, J.P., Taylor, A.K., and Arnett, R.H. 3rd. (1996–97). The Medical Expenditure Panel Survey: a national health information resource. *Inquiry* **33**, 373–389.
National Ambulatory Medical Care Survey (NAMCS)	Interview (In-person) during office visit	United States	Patients (Ambulatory care)	Annually	http://www.cdc.gov/nchs	Woodwell, D.A. (2000). National Ambulatory Medical Care Survey: 1998 Summary. Advance Data from Vital and Health Statistics of the Centers for Disease Control and Prevention/National Center for Health Statistics No. 315.
National Agricultural Workers Survey (NAWS)	Interview (In-person)	United States	Adult residents (>=18 years old, working in agriculture)	3 cycles a year	http://www.dol.gov	Mehta, K., Gabbard, S.M., Barrat, V., Lewis, M., Carroll, D, and Mines, R. (2000). Findings from the National Agricultural Workers Survey (NAWS): A Demographic and Employment Profile of United States Farmworkers. U.S. Department of Labor, Office of the Assistant Secretary for Policy, Office of Program Economics, Research Report No. 8. March 2000.

Survey	Method	Country	Population	Frequency	Website	Reference
National Electronic Injury Surveillance System (NEISS)	Record Abstraction	United States	All residents	Not applicable	http://www.cpsc.gov	Quinlan, K.P., Thompson, M.P., Annest, J.L., Peddicord, J., Ryan, G., Kessler, E.P., and Mcdonald, A.K. (1999). Expanding the national electronic injury surveillance system to monitor all nonfatal injuries treated in US hospital emergency departments. *Annals of Emergency Medicine* **34**, 637–645.
National Hospital Ambulatory Medical Care Survey (NHAMCS)	Interview (In-person) during hospital visit	United States	Patients (Ambulatory care in 600 hospitals)	Annually	http://www.cdc.gov/nchs	Slusarcick, A.L. and McCaig, L.F. (2000). National Hospital Ambulatory Medical Care Survey: 1998 Outpatient Department Summary. Advanced Data from Vital and Health Statistics of the Centers for Disease Control and Prevention/National Center for Health Statistics No. 317, July 27.
National Health and Nutrition Examination Survey (NHANES)	Interview (In-person)	United States	Residents (2 months of age or older; oversampling for adolescents, blacks, Mexican Americans, pregnant women	Irregularly	http://www.cdc.gov/nchs	Plan and operation of the Third National Health and Nutrition Examination Survey, 1988–1994. (1994). National Center for Health Statistics. *Vital and Health Statistics* 1.
NHANES I Epidemiologic Followup Study (NHEFS)	Interview (In-person & telephone) record abstraction, death certificates	United States	Persons aged 25–74 from 1971 to 1975 NHANES I, oversampling in poverty areas	Special cohort study	http://www.cdc.gov/nchs	Cox, C.S., Mussolino, M.E., Rothwell, T., et al. (1997). Plan and operation of the NHANES I Epidemiologic Followup Study, 1992. *Vital and Health Statistics Series: Programs and Collections Procedures* **35**, 1–231.

(continued)

Table 1–2 Selected data sources for public health surveillance (Continued)

Surveillance system	Primary mode	Scope	Target population	Frequency	Web link URL*	Reference
National Hospital Discharge Survey (NHDS)	Record Abstraction	United States	Hospital inpatients	Annually	http://www.cdc.gov/nchs	Dennison, C. and Pokras, R. (2000). Design and operation of the National Hospital Discharge Survey: 1988 redesign. *Vital and Health Statistics* 1.
National Health Care Survey					http://www.cdc.gov/nchs	Woodwell, D.A. (1999). National Ambulatory Medical Care Survey 1997 Summary. *Advance Data* **305,** 1–28.
National Home and Hospice Care Survey (NHHCS)	Interview (In-person)	United States	Patients (Home and hospice care agencies)	Biennially (last conducted in 2000)	http://www.cdc.gov/nchs	Haupt, B.J. and Jones, A. (1999). National Home and Hospice Care Survey: Annual Summary, 1996. National Center for Health Statistics. *Vital and Health Statistics* 13.
National Health Interview Summary (NHIS)	Interview (In-person)	United States	All residents	Annually	http://www.cdc.gov/nchs	Botman, S.L., Moore, T.F., Moriarity, C.L., and Parsons, V.L. (2000). Design and estimation for the National Health Interview Survey, 1995–2004. National Center for Health Statistics. *Vital and Health Statistics* 2.
National Health Interview Survey on Disability (NHIS-D)	Interview (In-person) and follow-up	United States	All residents	Biannual (1994–1995)	http://www.cdc.gov/nchs	Todorov, A. and Kirchner, C. (2000). Bias in proxies' reports of disability: data from the National Health Interview Survey on disability. *American Journal of Public Health* **90,** 1248–1253.
National Household Survey on Drug Abuse (NHSDA)	Interview (In-person and self-administered)	United States	Residents (>=12 years older)	Annually	http://www.hhs.gov/drugs	Gfroerer, J., Lessler, J., and Parsley, T. (1997). Studies of nonresponse and measurement error in the national household survey on drug abuse. *NIDA Research Monograph* **167,** 273–295.

Survey	Country	Population	Frequency	Method	Website	References
National Immunization Survey (NIS)	United States	Residents (19–35 months of age)	Continuous with Quarterly 12-month moving averages	Interview (Telephone); provider record check	http://www.cdc.gov/nip	Ezzati-Rice, T.M., Zell, E.R., Battaglia, M.P., Ching, P.L., and Wright, R.A. (1995). The design of the National Immunization Survey. *ASA Proceedings of the Section on Survey Research Methods* 668–672.
National Maternal and Infant Health Survey	United States	Live births, fetal deaths, infant deaths, mothers	1998 and Irregularly thereafter	Record abstraction, mail questionnaire	http://www.cdc.gov/nchs	Sanderson, M. and Gonzalez, J.F. (1998). 1998 National Maternal and Infant Health Survey. Methods and response characteristics. *Vital and Health Statistics. Series 2: Data Evaluation and Methods Research* **125**, 1–39.
National Longitudinal Study of Adolescent Health (Add Health)	United States	Adolescents (Grades 7–12)	Irregularly	Interview (In-person and self-administered)	http://www.cpc.unc.edu/projects/addhealth	Resnick, M.D., Bearman, P.S., Blum, R.W., Bauman, K.E., Harris, K.M., Jones, J., Tabor, J., Beuhring, T., Sieving, R.E., Shew, M., Ireland, M., Bearinger, L.H., and Udry, J.R. (1997). Protecting adolescents from harm. Findings from the National Longitudinal Study on Adolescent Health (see comments). *Journal of the American Medical Association* **278**, 823–832.
National Mortality Followback Survey (NMFS)	United States	Decedents (>=15 years old)	Irregularly	Interview (Telephone)	http://www.cdc.gov/nchs	Bild, D. and Stevenson, J. (1992). Frequency of reporting of diabetes on U.S. death certificates: analysis of the 1986 National Mortality Followback Survey. *Journal of Clinical Epidemiology* **45**, 275–281.

(continued)

Table 1-2 Selected data sources for public health surveillance (Continued)

Surveillance system	Primary mode	Scope	Target population	Frequency	Web link URL*	Reference
National Nursing Home Survey (NNHS)	Self-Administered Questionnaire	United States	Patients (Nursing homes)	Irregularly	http://www.cdc.gov/nchs	Gabrel, C. and Jones, A. (2000). The National Nursing Home Survey: 1997 summary. National Center for Health Statistics. *Vital and Health Statistics* 13.
National Survey of Ambulatory Surgery (NSAS)	Record Abstraction	United States	Surgery visits to 750 facilities	Annual through 1996; irregular thereafter	http://www.cdc.gov/nchs	Hau, M.J. and Lawrence, L. (1998). Ambulatory Surveying in the United States 1996. *Advance Data* **300**, 1–16.
National Survey of Family Growth (NSFG)	Interview (In-person)	United States	Female residents (15–44 years old)	Irregularly 3 and 4 years—2002 & 2005	http://www.cdc.gov/nchs	Abma, J, Chandra, A., Mosher, W., Peterson, L., and Piccinino, L. (1997). Fertility, family planning, and women's health: new data from the 1995 National Survey of Family Growth. National Center for Health Statistics. *Vital and Health Statistics* **23**.
National Weather Service—Air Quality	Environmental monitoring	United States	Selected Locations	Monthly	http://www.nws.ncaa.gov	National Weather Service. Office of Meterology. Technical Procedures Series No. 415. Available at: http://www.nws.noaa.gov/om/tpb/415.htm.
Pregnancy Risk Assessment Monitoring System (PRAMS)	Self-Administered Questionnaire	State	Female residents (with a recent live birth)	Annually	http://www.cdc.gov/ncdphp/drh/srv_prams.htm#1	Lipscomb, L.E, Johnson, C.H., Morrow, B., Colley Gilbert, B., Ahluwalia, I.B., Beck, L.F., Gaffield, M.E., Rogers, M., and Whitehead, N. (2000). *PRAMS 1998 Surveillance Report*. Atlanta: Division of Reproductive Health, National Center for Chronic Disease Prevention and Health Promotion, Centers for Disease Control and Prevention.

Survey	Method	Coverage	Population	Frequency	Website	Reference
Second Supplement on Aging (SOAII)	Interview (Telephone) with linkage to administrative files	United States	Persons aged 70 and over at time of NHIS-D (1994–1996)	Baseline, plus 3 wavers, each at 2-year intervals	http://www.hhs.gov/aging	Desai, M.M., Lentzner, H.R., and Weeks, J.D. (2001). Unmet need for personal assistance with activities of daily living among older adults. *Gerontologist* **41**, 82–88.
State and Local Area Integrated Telephone Survey (SLAITS)	Interview (Telephone)	United States	All residents	Not applicable	http://www.cdc.gov/nchs	Ezzati-Rice T.M., Cynamon, M., Blumberg, S.J., and Madans, J.H. (1999). Use of an existing sampling frame to collect broad-based health and health-related data at the State and Local level. From the Proceedings of the 1999 Federal Committee on Statistical Methodology Research Conference.
Youth Risk Behavior Surveillance System (YRBSS)	Self-Administered Questionnaire	United States and State	Students (Grades 9–12)	Biennially	http://www.cdc.gov	Grunbaum, J.A., Kann, L., Kinchen, S.A., Ross, J.G., Gowda, V.R., Collins, J.L., and Kolbe, L.J. (2000). Youth risk behavior surveillance. National Alternative High School Youth Risk Behavior Survey, United States, 1998. *Journal of School Health* **70**, 5–17. Kann, L., Kinchen, S.A., Williams, B.I., Ross, J.G., Lowry, R., Grunbaum, J.A., and Kolbe, L.J. (2000). Youth Risk Behavior Surveillance—United States, 1999. State and local YRBSS Coordinators. *Journal of School Health* **70**, 271–285.

(continued)

Table 1–2 Selected data sources for public health surveillance (Continued)

Surveillance system	Primary mode	Scope	Target population	Frequency	Web link URL*	Reference
Youth Tobacco Surveys (YTS)	Self-Administered Questionnaire	United States and State	Students (Grade 6–12)	National-based: biennially State based: annually or biennially	http://www.cdc.gov/tobacco	CDC. (2000). Youth tobacco surveillance—United States, 1998–1999. *Morbidity and Mortality Weekly Report. CDC Surveillance Summaries* **49**, 1–94.
4. OTHER USEFUL SURVEILLANCE SOURCES						
Healthy People 2010				National Health Objectives designed to identify preventable health problems	http://www.heath.gov/healthypeople	Klein, R.J, Proctor, S.E., Boudreault, M.A, Turczyn, K.M. (2002). Healthy People 2010—Criteria for data suppression. Healthy People 2010. Statistical Notes. From the Centers for Disease Control and Prevention **24**, 1–12.
International Classification of Disease (ICD) codes				Coding system for diseases and injuries	http://www.cdc.gov/nchs/about/major/dvs	Barbon, J.A. and Weiderpass, E. (2000). An introduction to epidemiology research with medical data-bases. *Annals of Epidemiology* **10**, 200–204.
Morbidity and Mortality Weekly Report				CDC's Weekly Publication Highlighting latest health studies	http://www.cdc.gov/mmwr	

*Current as of date of printing.

presented in this volume are based on rigorous science that can be translated into practice. The new challenges brought by emerging health issues and bioterrorist threats make effective public health surveillance even more critical. As the utility of the data for decision making is increased, the role of surveillance will be heightened even further.

REFERENCES

Anderson, G. and Knickman, J.R. (2001). Changing the chronic care system to meet people's needs. *Health Affairs* **20,** 126–160.

Annest, J.L., Pirkle, J.L., Makuc, D., Neese, J.W., Bayse, D.D., Kovar, M.G. (1983). Chronological trend in blood lead levels between 1976 and 1980. *New England Journal of Medicine* **308,** 1374–1377.

Blendon, R.J., Scoles, K., DesRoches, C., Young, J.T., Herrmann, M.J., Schmidt, J.L., and Kim, M. (2001). American's health priorities: curing cancer and controlling costs. *Health Affairs* **20,** 222–223.

Botman, S.L., Moore, T.F., Moriarity, C.L., and Parsons, V.L. (2000). Design and estimation for the National Health Interview Survey, 1995–2004. National Center for Health Statistics. *Vital and Health Statistics* **2,** 130.

Boulos, M.N.K., Roudsari, A.V., and Carson, E.R. (2001). Health geomatics: an enabling suite of technologies in health and healthcare. *Journal of Biomedical Isoformation* **34,** 195–219.

Brookmeyer, R. and Gail, M.H. (1994). *AIDS Epidemiology: A Quantitative Approach.* New York: Oxford University Press.

Centers for Disease Control and Prevention (1982). A Cluster of Kaposi's Sarcoma and Pneumocystis carinii Pneumonia among Homosexual Male Residents of Los Angeles and range Counties, California. *Morbidity and Mortality Weekly Report* **31,** 305.

Centers for Disease Control and Prevention (1991). Review of draft for revision of HIV infection classification system and expansion of AIDS surveillance case definition. *Morbidity and Mortality Weekly Report* **40,** 787.

Centers for Disease Control and Prevention (1999). Best practices for comprehensive tobacco control programs—August 1999. Atlanta GA: U.S. Department of Health and Human Services, Centers for Disease Control and Prevention, National Center for Chronic Disease Prevention and Health Promotion, Office on Smoking and Health, August 1999 (http://www.cdc.gov/tobacco).

Centers for Disease Control and Prevention (2001a). Update: Investigation of Bioterrorism-Related Anthrax and Interim Guidelines for Exposure Management and Antimicrobial Therapy, October 2001. *Morbidity and Mortality Weekly Report* **50,** 909–919. (www.cdc.gov/mmwr accessed 12/31/01).

Centers for Disease Control and Prevention (2001b). Mortality From Coronary Heart Disease and Acute Myocardial Infarction—United States, 1998. *Morbidity and Mortality Weekly Report* **5,** 90–93.

Centers for Disease Control and Prevention (2003). Updated Interim Surveillance Case Definition for Severe Acute Respiratory Syndrome (SARS)—United States, April 29, 2003. *Morbidity and Mortality Weekly Report* **52,** 391.

Cochrane Collaboration (2003). Handbook. Available: http://www.cochranelibrary.com (accessed 06/12/03).

Croner, C.M. and DeCola, I. (2001). *Visualization of disease surveillance data with Geostatstics.* Session on Methodological Issues Involving Integration of Statistics and Geography. Tallinn, Estonia: Statistical Division of the United Nations Economic Commission on Europe, September 25–28.

Dietz, W.H., Chen, C., Eds. (2002) Obesity in Childhood and Adolescence Nestle Nutrition Workshop Series. Vol. 49. Philadelphia: Lippincott, Williams and Wilkins.

Eyler, J.M. (1970). *Victorian Social Medicine: The Ideas and Methods of William Farr.* Baltimore, MD: Johns Hopkins University Press.

Gillum, R.F., Mussolino, M.E., and Madans, J.H. (2000). Diabetes mellitus, coronary heart disease incidence, and death from all causes in African American and European American women—The NHANES I Epidemiologic Follow-up Study. *Journal of Clinical Epidemiology* **53,** 5:511–518.

Graves, J.W. (2000). Management of difficult to control hypertension. *Mayo Clinic Proceedings* **75,** 256–284.

Harris, J.R., Holman, P.B., Carande-Kulis, V.G. (2001). Financial impact of health promotion: we need to know much more, but we know enough to act. *American Journal of Health Promotion* **15,** 378–382.

Hopkins, D.P., Fielding, J.E., and the Task Force on Community Preventive Services. (2001). The Guide to Community Preventive Services: Tobacco Use Prevention and Control—Reviews, Recommendations, and Expert Commentaries. *American Journal of Preventive Medicine* **20,** (2S).

Kalsbeek, W. and Heiss, G. (2000). Building Bridges Between Populations and Samples in Epidemiological Studies. *Annual Review of Public Health* **21,** 1–23.

Kesteloot, H., Sans, S., and Kromhout, D. (2002). Evolution of all-causes and cardiovascular mortality in the age-group 75–84 years in Europe during the period 1970–1996. *European Heart Journal* **23,** 384–398.

Khan, A.S., Levitt, A.M., and Sage, M.J. (2000). Biological and chemical terrorism: strategic plan for preparedness and response. Recommendations of the CDC strategic planning workgroup, *Morbidity and Mortality Weekly Report,* **49,** RR-4.

Koo, D., O'Carroll, P., Laventure, M. (2001). Public Health 101 for Informaticians. *Journal of the American Medical Informatics Association* **8,** 585–597.

Langmuir, A.D. (1963). The surveillance of communicable diseases of national importance. *New England Journal of Medicine* **268,** 182–192.

Marmot, M.G., Rose, G., Shipley, M., and Hamilton, P.J.S. (1978). Employment grade and coronary heart disease in British civil servants. *Journal of Epidemiology and Community Health* **32,** 244–249.

Mertens, T.E., Low-Beer, D. (1996). HIV and AIDS: where is the epidemic going? *Bulletin of the World Health Organization* **74,** 2:121–129.

Mokdad, A.H., Bowman, B.A., Ford, E.S., Vinicor, F., Marks, J.S., and Koplan, J.P. (2001). The continuing epidemics of obesity and diabetes in the United States. *Journal of the American Medical Association* **286,** 1195–1200.

Moreira, E.G., Vassilieff, I., and Vassilieff, V.S. (2001). Developmental lead exposure: behavioral alterations in the short and long term. *Neurotoxicoloy and Teratology* **23,** 489–495.

Nelson, D.E., Holtzman, D., Waller, M., Leutzinger, C.L., and Condon, K. (1998). Objectives and design of the Behavioral Risk Factor Surveillance System. Proceedings of the section on survey methods. American Statistical Association National Meeting, Dallas, Texas, 1998.

Pirkle, J.L., Brody, D.J., Gunter, E.W., Kramer, R.A., Paschal, D.C., Flegal, K.M., and Matte, T.D. (1994). The decline in blood levels in the United States. The National Health and Nutrition Examination Surveys (NHANES). *Journal of the American Medical Association* **272,** 284–291.

Sturm, R. (2002). The effects of obesity, smoking, and drinking on medical problems and costs. *Health Affairs* **21,** 245–253.

Thacker, S.B. (2000). Historical Development. In Teutsch, S.M. and Churchill, R.E., eds. *Principles and Practice of Public Health Surveillance*, second edition. New York: Oxford University Press. pp 1–16.

The TRIAD Study Group. (2002). The Translating Research Into Action for Diabetes (TRIAD) Study. *Diabetes Care* **25,** 386–389.

U.K. Prospective Diabetes Study Group. (1998). Intensive blood-glucose control with sulphonylureas or insulin compared with conventional treatment and risk of complications in patients with type 2 diabetes. *Lancet* **352,** 837–853.

U. S. Department of Health and Human Services. (2003). A Public Health Action Plan to Prevent Heart Disease and Stroke. Atlanta, GA: US Department of Health and Human Services, Centers for Disease Control and Prevention (available at http://www.cdc.gov/cvh; accessed 06/02/03).

Wang, G., Zheng, Z.J., Heath, G., Macera, C., Pratt, M., Buchner, D. (2002). Economic burden of cardiovascular disease associated with excess body weight in U.S. adults. *American Journal of Preventive Medicine* **23**(1), 1–6.

Weber, M.A. (1991). Cardiovascular and metabolic characteristics of hypertension. *American Journal of Medicine* **91,** (Suppl 1A), 4S.

Will, J.C., Vinicor, F., and Stevenson, J. (2001). The recording of diabetes on death certificates: has it improved? *Journal of Clinical Epidemiology* **54,** 239–244.

2

The Use of Surveys in Public Health Surveillance: Monitoring High-Risk Populations

WILLIAM D. KALSBEEK

A primary goal of public health surveillance is to improve disease preven-tion and control by identifying health risks in populations. A method of gaining information about such risks is to identify, study, and monitor those who are at greatest risk within those populations. This chapter reviews the use of surveys and survey research in monitoring the well-being of the pub-lic and its constituencies and in identifying groups at increased risk for ad-verse health outcomes.

The following section describes the use of surveys as tools of the pub-lic health surveillance system for identifying and monitoring people at in-creased risk. The third section discusses the selection of subjects to be mon-itored, as well as the design and implementation of surveys and some of the statistical problems related to the interpretation of survey data. The next section explores several issues that nonresponse and measurement er-rors raise for survey surveillance systems and reviews methods for dealing with these issues. The final section briefly describes event-related surveil-lance of world events that pose serious health risks. To illustrate many points, I use the Youth Tobacco Survey (YTS), a surveillance system from the National Centers for Disease Control and Prevention (CDC), which consists of a national survey—the National Youth Tobacco Survey (NYTS)—and several periodic statewide surveys (CDC, 2000d). The YTS highlights several statistical issues typical of surveillance monitoring that focuses on people at increased risk within a specific population.

The NYTS is designed to monitor the use of tobacco products and to identify predictors among middle school students (grades 6 to 8) and high school students (grades 9 to 12) in public and private schools in the United States. To date well over 40 states have completed a YTS. The NYTS and most statewide surveys use a stratified multistage cluster sample of students. Participants complete an anonymous, self-administered 30- to 40-minute questionnaire about their tobacco use, exposure to secondhand smoke, access to tobacco products, tobacco-related knowledge and attitudes, and familiarity with messages from the media for and against tobacco.

SURVEYS AND SURVEILLANCE

In their descriptions of public health surveillance, Buehler (1998) and Thacker (2000) cite the CDC's definition of *surveillance*:

The *ongoing, systematic* collection, analysis, and interpretation of health data essential to the planning, implementation, and evaluation of public health practice, closely integrated with the *timely dissemination* of these data to those who need to know. The final link of the surveillance chain is the application of these data to *prevention and control*. A surveillance system includes a functional capacity for data collection, analysis, and dissemination *linked to public health programs*

CDC, 1988 (emphasis added).

According to this definition, surveillance must include the ability to study those in the general population who are at risk for experiencing preventable or controllable adverse health outcomes and not just those who actually experience them. Systematic surveillance implies well-designed and orderly data collection, and ongoing surveillance implies the need to study those targeted periodically over time. Clearly, the CDC definition encompasses the survey, which is defined by the American Statistical Association (1998) as "a method of gathering information from a sample of individuals," in which the sample is "usually just a fraction of the population being studied" and the approaches to sample selection and measurement are thoughtfully designed and carefully implemented.

Surveys are useful in public health surveillance because they can measure the nature, extent, treatment, and costs of illness as well as assess health-related attitudes, knowledge, and behavior that affect the stability of health and susceptibility to illness. They can also produce findings quickly enough that action can be taken to improve health. Particularly useful are continuous surveys (those gathering data without interruption) and periodic surveys (those gathering data at intervals over time).

A public health surveillance system and a survey are not synonymous. The survey is a tool of the surveillance process, as are disease registries and related data systems. For example, a one-time, cross-sectional health survey is not a surveillance system because its primary purpose does not extend beyond the time in which it is conducted. On the other hand, a registry, as a network that monitors disease through the routine reporting of cases by hospitals, physician practices, testing laboratories, and public health agencies, is a type of surveillance system but most would not be considered surveys. The targeted population differs for a survey and a registry. Surveys typically focus on the general population, whereas registries tend to be more narrowly focused exclusively on those with specific diagnoses or health-related conditions. The approach to identifying subjects to be monitored may also differ. For registries, case ascertainment is determined by the medical definition of a case (e.g., born with a birth defect) and an associated infrastructure (e.g., a network of reporting hospitals). For some complete-enumeration surveys, subjects may be identified by applying a set of eligibility criteria to define a targeted population, as in registries. For most surveys, identification involves probability sampling, where subjects are chosen by a strategically developed random selection process.

In public health surveillance, *risk* is defined as the likelihood of an adverse health outcome. This definition goes well beyond the classic epidemiologic definition of risk as the incidence of disease (Gordis, 2000). Outcome likelihood is the probability of a certain health outcome projected from known determinants of disease, rather than from the rate of disease itself, particularly in the case of chronic illness (e.g., the likelihood of lung cancer might be projected from tobacco smoking). These risk indicators are typically measures of behavior, knowledge, and attitudes. Thus, by monitoring, and perhaps controlling, risk factors associated with disease, the disease itself might ultimately be controlled. All surveillance systems address disease risk, by monitoring either those with physical manifestations of disease, as in registries, or those exposed to disease risk factors, as in surveys.

Among the measures of risk reported in the YTS system (CDC, 2000d), for example, are rates of behaviors related to tobacco use, such as current tobacco use, exposure to secondhand smoke, and number of attempts to quit smoking. Linking these system findings to the design of cessation programs, community smoking awareness programs, and counter-marketing efforts is thought to reduce tobacco use and lower the associated risk of lung cancer.

Survey-based surveillance systems can identify those at higher risk for adverse health outcomes. One method of identifying those at higher risk is to compare risk ratios or descriptive differences among subgroups defined by candidate indicators. Such descriptive comparison provides a simple, if sometimes crude, indication of the role of a personal characteristic in increasing risk (Gordis, 2000). For instance, the role of school grade, sex, and race/ethnicity in determining the risk of currently using any tobacco product might be explored by analyzing differences in exposure rate among subgroups defined by these characteristics (Table 2–1).

The descriptive approach is limited because it does not account for other important differences among subgroups with potential risk factors and thus only explains marginal effects on risk. Standardizing subgroups on variables that explain marginal differences is one way to overcome this limitation, but a better one is regression analysis (Rothman and Greenland, 1998). Regression analysis follows an appropriate model-fitting strategy for a standard logistic regression model, with dichotomous risk outcome (i.e., with or without outcome) as the dependent variable and potential indicators as independent variables. Such analyses allow significant indicators of risk to be identified while controlling for (in effect, standardizing) the effects of other independent variables on the risk indicator. Risk ratios or odds ratios are typically reported when modeling is used.

Key indicators of health risk can be used to help identify groups at higher risk. These higher-risk groups may then become the object of pro-

Table 2–1 Prevalence rates of any tobacco use from the fall 1999 National Youth Tobacco Survey*

	Rate in Percent (Margin of Error[†])
MIDDLE SCHOOL	
Gender	
Male	14.2 ($\pm$2.2)
Female	11.3 ($\pm$2.2)
Race/ethnicity	
White	11.6 ($\pm$2.3)
Black	14.4 ($\pm$2.7)
Hispanic	15.2 ($\pm$5.2)
Total, middle school	12.8 ($\pm$2.0)
HIGH SCHOOL	
Gender	
Male	38.1 ($\pm$3.2)
Female	31.4 ($\pm$3.1)
Race/ethnicity	
White	39.4 ($\pm$3.2)
Black	24.0 ($\pm$4.2)
Hispanic	30.7 ($\pm$4.4)
Total, high school	34.8 ($\pm$2.6)

Source: http://www.cdc.gov/tobacco/global/GUTS.htm.

*Current use of cigarettes or cigars or smokeless tobacco or pipies or bidis or kreteks on $\geq$1 of the 30 days preceding the survey.

[†]Half-width of a 95% confidence interval.

gram and policy efforts to reduce risk or the focus of more intensive study. For example, the focus on teenagers in tobacco use research was triggered by earlier studies of the general population, which documented elevated risks in this group and highlighted the importance of reaching teenagers for reducing tobacco use among all ages (U.S. Department of Health and Human Services, 1994). The YTS and its affiliated surveys were then established to monitor the risks of teenage tobacco use by tracking known indicators of risk and to search for new indicators (CDC, 2000d).

Survey-based surveillance systems often track progress toward public health goals, such as the Healthy People 2010 Objectives for the Nation (U.S. Department of Health and Human Services, 2000). Tracking helps establish the usefulness of efforts to increase overall quality of life, and it also gauges progress in eliminating health disparities among groups with different demographic, geographic, economic, and lifestyle characteristics. For example, the YTS measures progress towards meeting the dozen or so Healthy People 2010 objectives that are related to adolescent tobacco use, and can also identify the types of teenagers who lag behind and need greater attention. Several Healthy People 2010 objectives are aimed at specific groups defined by age, race/ethnicity, education, family income, sex, and level of urbanization. Monitoring disparities in health risk thus helps to sharpen the focus of surveillance and to achieve a broader reduction in health risk.

Surveillance on higher-risk people means that data are collected either exclusively for the higher-risk (targeted) group, or that a broader sample is chosen and efforts are made to assure adequate sample sizes for those segments of the population where risk is to be compared. Although sampling people at higher risk is a global consideration in surveillance, the means by which it is accomplished vary by the type of surveillance system. No disproportionate sampling of those at higher risk is needed in registries because those with clinical symptoms already disproportionately reflect those at higher risk. Some surveys not using probability sampling target higher-risk populations by using more selective inclusion criteria that disproportionately include those in the general population who are at higher risk. For example, the National Nosocomial Infections Surveillance System (NNIS) monitors nosocomial infections in the higher-risk population of persons who have been hospitalized.

Surveys with random sampling often use strategies to sample higher-risk groups disproportionately. An overview of some of these strategies is presented in the next section. Besides representing small percentages of the general population, many higher-risk groups present unique sampling challenges because of their comparatively high geographic dispersion and mobility.

ISSUES OF SUBJECT SELECTION

Sampling in health surveillance has two countervailing cost implications. Data from a targeted population can be collected at lower cost than data from everyone of interest. However, the reduced monetary cost is countered by the increased cost of statistical uncertainty about the numerical findings projected from the sample (Kalsbeek and Heiss, 2000). Samples after all are only fractions of populations, regardless of how well they are chosen, so information derived from them provides only a representation of what is happening in the sampled population.

The way uncertainty tied to sample-derived findings is conceived depends on whether inference to the sampled population is design-based or model-based. When statistical inference is design-based, uncertainty from sampling error, (the difference between the sample-based estimate of a population characteristic and the characteristic itself), depends on specific features of the sample design and how the estimate is calculated from the sample data. In contrast, uncertainty linked to model-based inference reflects the ability of the model to specify the observed sample data, which likewise partially depends on the sample design. For simplicity, design-based inference is assumed in the remainder in this chapter.

Important Features of Sample Designs

Cluster sampling and stratification are two design features that affect the inferences which can be drawn from surveillance samples. With regard to the first of these two features, area units such as counties, small groups of neighboring counties, and block groups may serve as sampling clusters for so-called "area samples," whereas organizations such as schools, hospitals, and nursing homes may be randomly chosen in identifying the sample for institutional surveys.

Sometimes samples are chosen at more than one level of a social or geographic hierarchy to produce what is called a multistage cluster sample. Because clusters in most human populations may vary considerably in size, samples of clusters in the early stages of multistage designs are often randomly chosen with probabilities proportional to size (pps), where size is some measure of the number of targeted population members in the cluster. Choosing the NYTS sample of middle and high school students by selecting classrooms, within a sample of schools, within a sample of county groups is an example of a three-stage sample design. Moreover, recent middle and high school enrollment figures by race/ethnicity are used to construct weighted measures of size favoring blacks and Hispanics during the first-stage sample of county groups (see the description of the survey at the end of this section).

Stratified sampling is often used to choose clusters or individuals randomly by strategically subdividing the list of sampling units into population subgroups called strata, allocating the desired sample among strata, and then separately applying an appropriate random selection method in each statum. Stratification is used to make overall population samples more representative and to isolate and control sample sizes for important segments of the population (e.g., age or racial/ethnic groups).

Surveillance samples may have other features to improve their utility, such as partial sample overlap to improve measuring changes over time (Kish, 1987a). More on these and other basic sampling strategies can be found in several excellent sampling texts (e.g., see Kish, 1965; Levy and Lemeshow, 1991; Lohr, 1999).

Also affecting uncertainty in probability samples is the nature of the sampling frame: the population list (or lists) used to choose the sample. Particularly relevant in evaluating the utility of frames is the linkage between entries on the frame and members of the target population (Lessler and Kalsbeek, 1992). In an incomplete frame, some population members are unlisted, whereas in a cluster frame, entries are linked to multiple population members.

These features of sampling frames affect the quality of sample estimates. When inference is design-based, the completeness of the frame and the difference between those covered and those not covered determines the extent of estimation bias for estimates from the samples it yields. Estimates obtained from a sample drawn from a cluster frame tend to be less precise than those chosen from a list of individual members, because of a cluster effect called intraclass correlation. This effect reflects the degree to which clusters are dissimilar, and thus members of the same sample cluster tend to be more alike than those in the population as a whole. The magnitude of intraclass correlation for estimating the prevalence of tobacco use from the school-based NYTS, for instance, is directly related to the amount of variation in prevalence rates among schools.

For surveillance of mobile populations, the dynamic linkage between frame entries and population members may have important statistical drawbacks, and also potential benefits (Kalton, 1991). In sampling more elusive higher-risk groups, some population members may be linked to multiple frame entries if sampling and data gathering span a longer period of time. The resulting frame multiplicity can bias estimates from the resulting samples if multiple selection opportunities are not dealt with during selection or estimation. On the positive side, multiplicity creates more opportunities for selection, which may help in sampling higher-risk groups that are both mobile and relatively rare, such as gay and bisexual men sampled through the places where they congregate (Stueve et al., 2001) and migrant farm workers sampled through their places of employment (Kalsbeek, 1988).

The content of the frame also determines whether pps sampling is a viable option and how the sample might be stratified to improve representation or be expanded to sample important subgroups. Because higher-risk groups are often relatively small minorities in the population surveyed, proportionately allocated samples may not produce sufficient sample sizes for monitoring. Some form of disproportionate sampling, or oversampling, is thus needed to increase sample sizes to more adequate levels. The approach to oversampling depends mainly on how much information about those to be oversampled is available on the frame or frames used to choose the sample. It also depends on the cost of oversampling. Most oversampling strategies involve disproportionate sampling and screening, where information to determine membership status in the group to be oversampled is gathered from a sample before data collection.

Individuals with a higher-risk trait are sometimes easily oversampled by applying strategically varying sampling rates to a stratified sample. When sampling stems from a member list that gives the trait information for each member, oversampling is accomplished simply by isolating the higher-risk group in one or more sampling strata and then applying relatively higher sampling rates to these strata.

In many instances, higher-risk groups cannot be completely isolated on the frame or frames. This situation is typical when clusters of population members are sampled or when member lists lack information that identifies persons with the higher-risk trait. It may be more difficult to oversample in cluster sampling designs since higher risk groups are generally defined by person-level traits (e.g., race/ethnicity, disability status, age, or sex) and clusters are mixtures of those at higher and lower risk. If reasonable measures of the concentration of those at higher risk are available for clusters, oversampling can be accomplished by stratifying on concentration level, disproportionately sampling the high concentration strata, and then screening for those at higher risk in the member-selection stage of sampling. For example, oversampling blacks and Hispanics in the NYTS involved disproportionately sampling county groups and schools with higher enrollments of these groups, and then proportionately sampling all students within selected schools.

An optional oversampling approach, is to alter the pps size measure to favor oversampled groups. This approach was used in the NYTS to sample both blacks and Hispanics. Based on simulated sample draws,

$Mos_i = 2Mos_{i,B} + 3Mos_{i,H} + Mos_{i,O}$ was the weighted size measure used to choose the i-th county group for the first stage sample for the NYTS, where the Mos used to calculate the final measure are recent population counts for blacks (B), Hispanics (H), and all other racial/ethnic groups (O). Using Mos_i for cluster sampling thus favors the selection of areas with larger numbers of blacks and Hispanics over areas where those in other groups predominate. A similar approach was used to choose National Youth Risk Behavior Survey sample schools. Probabilities proportional to size sampling is conceptually similar to clusters using weighted measures of size and disproportionately sampling clusters from strata with higher concentrations of those at higher risk. In both cases, selection probabilities are relatively higher for clusters with higher concentrations of those being oversampled.

Screening for those at higher risk may also be part of an oversampling plan. This feature is applied just before data collection by determining whether each member of an initial at-large sample is a member of the oversampled higher-risk group and then randomly retaining some portion of those found not to be at higher risk. The degree of oversampling is inversely related to the retention rate for those screened out of the sample. At the extremes, retaining none of those screened out means that the final sample will include only those at higher risk, whereas retaining all of those screened out makes the sample proportionate at that point.

The groups oversampled in each of the surveys described in Table 2–2 are those known or expected to be at higher risk for the health-related outcomes studied (e.g., blacks and Hispanics for tobacco use in the NYTS). Procedurally, several surveys disproportionately sample from a list of members; e.g., Medicare beneficiaries within a sample of area clusters, students within a sample of schools, death certificates, and birth certificates. Other surveys (e.g., the National Health Interview Survey) oversample their higher-risk groups by choosing a disproportionately stratified sample of area clusters. Several surveys also weight size in sampling clusters with pps.

The quantitative impact of oversampling can be assessed by comparing the percentages of the sample and populations at higher risk. For example, in the Fall 1999 NYTS (CDC, 2000b), the U.S. Department of Education public middle and high school data from the NCES Public Elementary/Secondary School Universe Survey for the 1999–2000 school year showed that 16.0% of these students were black and 15.5% were Hispanic. By comparison, 16.0% of Fall 1999 NYTS respondents were black and 21.2% were Hispanic. Although strict comparability is lost because private schools were excluded from the NCES figures, as were differential response rates by race/ethnicity, the weighted Mos_i had little effect in increasing the sample size for blacks, relative to a proportionately allocated sample. This oversampling procedure was more effective for Hispanics,

Table 2-2 Oversampling in existing United States surveillance systems

Surveillance system	General sampling approach	Oversampled subpopulation	Type of oversampling	Brief description of oversampling process
Drug Abuse Warning Network (DAWN)	Single-stage stratified optimal allocation cluster sampling	Hospitals reporting 80,000 or more annual ED visits, hospitals located in the 21 DAWN metropolitan areas	DSS (List)*	The PSUs of DAWN are non-Federal, short-stay general surgical and medical hospitals in the coterminous United States that have a 24-hour ED, stratified by hospital size, hospital location, and whether the hospital had an organized outpatient department or a chemical/alcohol inpatient unit. Hospitals in the 21 metropolitan areas were oversampled, and hospitals reporting 80,000 or more annual ED visits were sampled with certainty as a separate stratum. The sample sizes for the metropolitan areas and the National Panel were determined to achieve the specified levels of precision in estimates. The number of sample units in non-certainty strata was allocated based on the theory of optimal allocation. All drug abuse episodes identified within the participating facilities were selected.
Medicare Current Beneficiary Study (MCBS)	Two-stage stratified cluster systematic sampling	Disabled (<65 years of age) and oldest-old (>=85 years of age)	DSS (List)*	MCBS draws its sample from the Health Care Financing Administration's Medicare enrollment file. The PSU is a geographic group of counties, 107 in total to represent the Nation. The beneficiaries residing in these areas are selected in the 2nd stage by systematic random sampling within age strata. Sampling rates varied by age (0–44, 45–64, 65–69, 70–74, 75–79,

80–84, and 85 or over) in order to represent the disabled (under 65 years of age) and the oldest-old (85 years of age or over) by a factor of approximately 1.5.

National Health and Nutrition Examination Survey (NHANES)	Four-stage stratified pps cluster sampling	Young children, older persons, black persons, and Mexican-Americans	DSS (Screening)[†]	The NHANES III applied a stratified multistage probability design. The PSU for NHANES is mostly single counties, stratified and selected with pps and without replacement. The area segments, comprising city or suburban blocks, or combinations of blocks etc., are selected in the second stage, stratified by percent of Mexican Americans. Households and group quarters were sampled in the 3rd stage, sampled pps to household size of area segments, with higher subsampling rates for the geographic strata with high minority concentrations. Persons within the sample of households or group quarters were the 4th stage sampling units. All eligible members within a household were listed, and a subsample of individuals was selected based on sex, age, and race or ethnicity, with the large oversampling of the very young, the very old, black persons, and Mexican Americans.

(continued)

Table 2-2 Oversampling in existing United States surveillance systems (Continued)

Surveillance system	General sampling approach	Oversampled subpopulation	Type of oversampling	Brief description of oversampling process
National Household Survey on Drug Abuse (NHSDA)	Three-stage stratified pps cluster sampling	Youth (12–17 years old) and young adults (18–25 years old)	DSS (List)	The NHSDA utilized a deeply stratified, multistage, area probability design for year 1999 through 2003. The 1st stage sampling units were area segments, stratified by states, socioeconomic status indicator, and percentage of non-Hispanic white. The strata in this stage were field interviewer (FI) regions, contiguous geographic areas designed to yield the same number of interviews on average. Area segments, the PSUs of the survey, were combined adjacent Census blocks within the FI region. The PSUs were sampled with probability proportional to population size. Listed dwelling units and potential dwelling units were randomly selected within area segments in the 2nd stage. Lastly, persons were randomly selected based on all persons aged 12 and over residing in the identified dwelling unit. Sampling rates were preset by age group and state. Younger age groups (12–17, 18–25 years) were oversampled at the 3rd stage, but race/ethnicity groups were not purposely oversampled for the 1999 main study, as was done on prior NHSDAs, due to the large sample size.

Survey	Sampling design	Oversampled groups	Type	Description
National Mortality Followback Survey (NMFS)	Single-stage stratified random sampling	Decedents of black, female, under age 35, or over age 99	DSS (List)	The sampling frame for the 1993 NMFS was the 1993 current Mortality Sample (CMS), a 10% systematic random sample of death certificates received by the vital statistics offices. The death certificates were stratified by age, race, gender, and causes of death. Twelve of 50 defined strata were selected with certainty. Black decedents, female decedents, decedents under age 35, and decedents over age 99 were oversampled to obtain reliable estimates.
National Longitudinal Study of Adolescent Health (Add Health)	Three-stage stratified pps cluster sampling	Ethnic-group of Blacks from well-educated families, Chinese, Cuban, and Puerto Rican adolescents, students in 16 schools, disabled adolescents, and siblings	DSS (List)	The sample of students in the Add Health study represents U.S. schools with respect to region of country, urbanicity, school type, ethnicity, and school size. PSUs were high schools with an 11th grade and a minimum enrollment of 30 students, stratified by region, urbanicity, school size, school type, and percent white and black. Schools with a 7th grade "feeding" selected high schools were then selected, with probability proportional to the number of students it contributed to the high school. After the self-administered in-school questionnaire for all students in grades 7–12 on the roster, students in grades 7–12 were randomly selected for a subsequent in-home interview. Four types of students (blacks from well-educated family, Chinese, Cuban, and Puerto Rican adolescents), disabled adolescents, siblings residing in the same household were oversampled in this stage.

(continued)

Table 2-2 Oversampling in existing United States surveillance systems (Continued)

Surveillance system	General sampling approach	Oversampled subpopulation	Type of oversampling	Brief description of oversampling process
National Survey of Family Growth (NSFG)	Four-stage stratified pps systematic sampling	Black and Hispanic women	DSS (List)	The NSFG in 1995 selected women 15–44 years of age from the responded household of the 1993 NHIS. The first 3 sampling stages are the same as the NHIS design (see NHIS). Women at reproductive age (15–44 years old) from the households in which a member had responded to the NHIS were subsampled in the 4th stage. All households with black and Hispanic women in the 1993 NHIS sample were included in the NSFG to obtain a sufficient number of black and Hispanic women.
National Youth Risk Behavior Surveys (NYRBS)	Three-stage stratified pps cluster sampling	Black and Hispanic students	Weighted Mos‡ and DSS (Screening)	The 1999 NYRBS employed a 3-stage cluster sample design to produce a nationally representative sample of students in grades 9–12. The sample design is similar to the NYTS. The PSU consisted of large counties or groups of smaller, adjacent counties, stratified by degree of urbanization and the relative percentage of black and Hispanic students, selected with pps to weighted school enrollment. Schools were selected in the 2nd stage, with pps to weighted school enrollment. Schools with substantial numbers of black and Hispanic students were sampled at higher rates than all other schools to enable separate analysis of data for black and Hispanic students. One or two intact classes of a required subject were then randomly selected across grades 9–12, with all students in the selected classes eligible to participate in the survey.

*DSS (List): Disproportionate sampling from a list of members

†DSS (Screening): Disproportionate stratified sample of clusters

‡Weighted Mos: Weighted size measure for oversampling

PSU, primary sampling unit; pps, probability proportionate to measure of size.

where the realized sample size was about 37% higher than the sample size that would have been realized in a proportionately allocated sample.

Estimation and Precision

Although surveillance samples are often disproportionate for reasons other than oversampling (e.g., optimum allocation of sampling strata or outdated size measures for sampling clusters), oversampling implies varying selection probabilities. These variable probabilities are important in estimation but can adversely affect the statistical quality of estimates derived from the samples. Varying selection probabilities are accommodated through the use of sample weights whose variation can reduce the precision of estimates. Because the amount of disproportionality in the sample from oversampling is often controlled by the system designer, the relative utility of oversampling must also be considered.

The need for sample weights arises from the definition of probability sampling, the utility of weighted estimates to estimate populations totals, and the fact that rates and many other variables in monitored populations are functions of totals. The selection probability for the i-th among n members of a probability sample (π_i) is known and nonzero, so the sample weight used (in the absence of nonresponse or other practical difficulties) is simply, $\omega_i = \pi_i^{-1}$, which can be viewed as the number among all N members of the targeted population that the i-th sample member represents. Horvitz and Thompson (1952) showed that an unbiased estimate of the sum total (y) for some measurement in a population one can be made with the well-known Horvitz-Thompson estimator,

$$\hat{y}_{HT} = \sum_{i=1}^{n} \omega_i y_i \qquad (2\text{--}1)$$

where y_i is the referent measure for the i-th sample member. To estimate the overall prevalence rate for some adverse health outcome in the population, $p = y/N$, one might use the simple weighted estimate, $\hat{p} = \sum_{i=1}^{n}\omega_i y_i / \sum_{i=1}^{n}\omega_i$, where $y_i = 1$, if the i-th sample member experiences this outcome, $y_i = 0$ if not, and the sum of weights in the denominator of $\hat{p}$ estimates N. Unlike $\hat{y}_{HT}$, $\hat{p}$ is not usually unbiased, although for large enough sizes (n) in well-designed samples it is effectively unbiased. The main design concern for surveillance systems using $\hat{p}$ to estimate p is not so much bias in estimated prevalence rates but the increases in the variances (i.e., losses in the statistical precision or quality of $\hat{p}$) due to variable weights and other design features.

For cluster sample designs with variable weights, the multiplicative increase in the variance of $\hat{p}$, relative to the variance for a comparable unclustered sample with equal weights, is called the *design effect* (*deff*) for $\hat{p}$. One conservative model for *deff* ($\hat{p}$), posed by Kish (1987d) and justified by Gabler et al. (1999) through a model-based argument, assumes constant unit variances, i.e., that $Var(y_i) = \sigma^2$, $\forall i$:

$$deff(\hat{p}) = \left\{ n \frac{\sum\limits_{i=1}^{n} \omega_i^2}{\left(\sum\limits_{i=1}^{n} \omega_i\right)^2} \right\} \{1 + \rho(\bar{n} - 1)\} = meff_w meff_{cs} \qquad (2\text{--}2)$$

where ρ is the intraclass correlation for clusters in the population and $\bar{n} = n/m$ is the average sample size among the m selected clusters in the surveillance sample. The first right term in Eq. 2–2 is the multiplicative effect of variable weights ($meff_w$), and the second term is the effect of cluster sampling ($meff_{cs}$). This model, in assuming that $Var(y_i) = \sigma^2$ $\forall i$, provides a basis for measuring the effect of variable sample weights on sample effectiveness.

The variation in sample weights, and the corresponding effect on variance associated with designs with oversampling, depends on how effectively those groups to be oversampled can be isolated among sample strata. For unclustered samples from population lists containing current information on membership in the subgroup being oversampled, strata containing all subgroup members or nonmembers can be formed. If uniformly higher sampling rates are applied to strata with subgroup members and uniformly lower rates are applied to the others, there will be no variation in sample weights among the oversampled group, but there will be variation for the sample overall and for subgroups that cross stratum boundaries. When sampling clusters that are mixtures of members and nonmembers of the oversampled group, the overall sample and all subgroup samples, including the one being oversampled, will have variable weights.

Using a sample design model first suggested by Waksberg (1973) and adapted by Kalsbeek (2003) for oversampling Hispanics, expected relative gains for parts of samples in surveillance designs with oversampling can be determined. Here below we extend this approach to the case where blacks are oversampled. Waksberg's model presumes stratified, simple, random with-replacement sampling from two strata, each of which is a mixture of the higher-risk group to be oversampled (domain 1) and the rest of the target population (domain 2). All members of the sample from stratum 1, strategically formed to have a higher concentration of those to be oversampled, are assigned the same relatively high selection probability (i.e.,

$\pi_i = \pi_o^{(1)}$, $\forall i$ in stratum 1); and all members of the sample from stratum 2 (with a lower concentration of those to be oversampled) are assigned a lower common selection probabilities (i.e., $\pi_i = \pi_o^{(2)}$, $\forall i$ in stratum 2). If $\theta_{\alpha\beta}$ denotes the proportion of the population consisting of members of domain β assigned to stratum α, and $\theta_{\alpha+} = \theta_{\alpha1} + \theta_{\alpha2}$ is the proportion of the population in stratum α, then $u = (\theta_{11}/\theta_{1+})/(\theta_{21}/\theta_{2+})$ can be used to measure the relative stratum concentrations of those to be oversampled, $v = \theta_{2+}/\theta_{1+}$ to indicate the relative sizes of the strata, and $r = \pi_o^{(1)}/\pi_o^{(2)}$ to depict the relative intensity of sampling in the two strata. Fixing domain sample sizes at their expected values for each stratum and holding the nominal overall sample size constant over values of r, the effect of variable weights for prevalences estimates of the total population is

$$meff_{\omega,all}^{(DSS)} = \{(1 + rv)(r + v)\}/\{r(1 + v)^2\} \tag{2–3}$$

and the comparable effect for prevalence estimates of those oversampled (domain 1, or blacks) is

$$meff_{\omega,black}^{(DSS)} = \{(u + rv)(ur + v)\}/\{r(u + v)^2\} \tag{2–4}$$

Eqs. 2–3 and 2–4 show that the ability of the two strata to isolate those to be oversampled (measured by u) influences the effect of variable weights for the sample of those to be oversampled but not for the overall sample.

By generally defining the realized sample size provided by oversampling involving disproportionate stratified sampling (DSS) relative to the sample size with no oversampling under proportionate stratified sampling (PSS) as $ratio_n = n^{(DSS)}/n^{(PSS)}$, and by noting that $meff_{\omega,d} = 1$ for domain (d) in a PSS design, one can directly obtain ratios of the following sample sizes under comparable DSS and PSS allocation schemes:

Black Nominal: $\qquad ratio_{n_{black}}^{(nom)} = \dfrac{(1 + v)(ur + v)}{(u + v)(r + v)}$ $\qquad\qquad$ (2–5)

Black Effective: $\qquad ratio_{n_{black}}^{(eff)} = \dfrac{ratio_{n_{black}}^{(nom)}}{meff_{\omega,black}} = \dfrac{r(u + v)(1 + v)}{(u + rv)(r + v)}$ $\qquad$ (2–6)

Overall Effective: $\qquad ratio_{n_{all}}^{(eff)} = \dfrac{1}{meff_{\omega,all}^{(DSS)}}$ $\qquad\qquad\qquad$ (2–7)

Nominal sample size for a population domain generally refers to the actual count of sample members in the domain (n_d), and the corresponding effective sample size ($n_{eff,d} = n_d/deff(\hat{p}) = n_d/meff_{\omega,d}$ for an unclustered sample) is the sample size required to achieve the same precision but with equal weights in the sample. The magnitude of the difference between n_d and

$n_{eff,d}$ is directly related to the amount of variation in weights, and since $meff_{o,d} \geq 1$, $n_{eff,d} \leq n_d$. Whereas the nominal sample size ratio for blacks measures the ability of oversampling to increase the number of blacks in the sample, the effective sample size ratios for blacks and the overall sample gauges the relative statistical strength of these samples when oversampling is used in this way. Observing these ratios as oversampling intensity (r) increases thus indicates not only how the count of those oversampled is affected but also how the statistical utility of the resulting samples is affected by the variable weights attributed to oversampling.

Consider, for example, a hypothetical oversampling of blacks in a school-based sample of students in grade 7 or above in U.S. public schools. Two strata are formed to select schools: one in which black enrollment is greater than 10% and a higher school sampling rate is used (stratum 1); and the other in which black enrollment is less than 10% and a lower school sampling rate is used (stratum 2). School selection probabilities are the same within but not between strata. All students in selected schools are sampled with equal probabilities. The overall probability of selection for any student equals the sampling rate for his or her school times the sampling rate for choosing the student once his or her school is chosen. Thus, the variation in student selection probabilities and sample weights is determined solely by the variation in sampling rates for the 2 school strata.

The strata in this hypothetical sample are mixtures of blacks and non-blacks. Using NCES data for 1999–2000 again (http://www.nces.ed.gov), we have $u = 16.126$ and $v = 1.643$ for the two strata, and we consider sample size effects for $1 \leq r \leq 21$ in this design (Fig. 2–1). The nominal sample size ratio for blacks (in Fig. 2–1) indicates that this oversampling approach can substantially increase the black student sample size, and that the sample size is double that from a proportionate design when $r = 8$, although nominal gains level off thereafter. The effective overall sample size ratio falls precipitously as r increases, dropping to less than 50% of nominal levels when $r \geq 6$. Although these losses in statistical effectiveness are sizable, the overall sample would be considerably greater than a straight sample of blacks, who constitute only about 18% of the middle and high school enrollment in U.S. public schools.

Notable in Figure 2–1 is the plot for the effective black student sample size, where the increase toward a maximum utility is approximately 1.47 at $r = 4$, at which point the effect of variable weights overtakes the nominal increase in sample size and statistical utility diminishes. A practical implication of this finding is that, to produce good estimates for blacks, one might best apply school sampling rates about 4 times greater in stratum 1 than in stratum 2. That level of oversampling would give the best possible estimates for blacks and incur only a modest loss in the effective overall sample size.

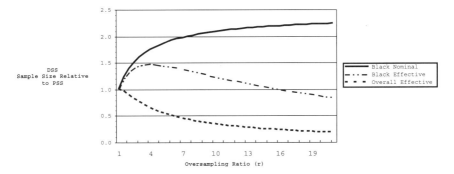

Figure 2–1 Effects of oversampling on sample sizes in a hypothetical school-based survey of students.

The Waksberg model does not assume cluster sampling. Thus, we can only conjecture from Eq. 2–2 how the findings in Figure 2–1 for effective sample sizes might be altered in such a case. To gain a sense of the effect of cluster sampling on effective sample sizes, recall that $n_{eff,\,d} = n_d/deff(\hat{p})$ and that the effect of cluster sampling on $deff(\hat{p})$ is $meff_{cs} = 1 + \rho(\bar{n} - 1)$, where $\bar{n} = n/m$ is the average sample cluster size and ρ is the intraclass correlation for school clusters when prevalence (p) is estimated. Because ρ would not be affected by the stratum allocation approach, we must focus on how $\bar{n}$ differs for the DSS and PSS allocation approaches. The ratio plot for the overall effective sample size would be unaffected because $\bar{n}$ would be the same for DSS and PSS for any value of r. The ratio plot for the effective sample size of blacks would be somewhat lower than that in Figure 2–1 because $ratio^{(nom)}_{n_{black}} > 1$ and thus $\bar{n}$, $meff_{cs}$, and $deff(\hat{p})$ would be greater for DSS than for PSS. Incorporating the effect of cluster sampling in our assessment of oversampling effects thus suggests even lower gains in the statistical strength of the sample of blacks than when unclustered sampling is assumed.

ISSUES OF DATA GATHERING

The challenges of monitoring people more likely to experience negative health attributes extend beyond subject selection. Those at higher risk may also present greater challenges to the process of data gathering than those at lower risk because of their relative inaccessibility, unwillingness to participate, or other social or cultural barriers. I now turn my attention to problems caused by nonresponse and measurement errors in surveillance systems. I explore the statistical implications of such errors and provide an overview of ways to deal with them.

Manifestation

Nonsampling error is present in the design and implementation of most surveillance systems. It contributes error to estimates generated by system data. Error from nonresponse in the sample occurs during the sample recruitment phase and is dealt with by developing strategies for finding sample members and persuading them to respond, and by adjusting for attrition. Measurement error appears during the data gathering and processing phases of the system and is dealt with primarily by effective questionnaire design and strategic monitoring of the data-gathering apparatus. The type and extent of both errors are determined mainly by the design of survey questionnaires and forms, the content and implementation of instructions for gathering or providing the data, and the process of preparing the data for analysis. Both types occur whether a respondent is at higher risk or not, although subgroups at higher risk can present extraordinary obstacles to preventing these errors. Many involved in data gathering may become circumstantial contributors to nonsampling error in surveillance systems. In the NYTS, for example, they include survey specialists who develop the plans for school and student recruitment; those who develop the content and format of self-administered questionnaires to measure tobacco use behavior; students who agree to complete the study questionnaire; field staff who schedule and oversee the in-school data-gathering sessions; and technicians and programmers who enter and edit the data.

Nonresponse and measurement lead to two types of statistical error in surveillance systems. Variable error presumes that the raw data from a sample are but one possible outcome of an underlying process that is inherently stochastic, or unpredictable in some sense. This presumption means that repeating the features that define the design of the system can result in other information outcomes; hence the notion that measurable outcomes may vary. For example, readministering an NYTS question on current smoking status to the same respondent, might produce a "yes" response on one occasion, a "no" response on another, or no response at all, depending on his or her physical, mental, and psychological state. The variation among these outcomes directly affects the quality of the estimates.

Survey error also may cause bias when estimates systematically drift away from the truth. For example, if nonrespondents to the NYTS questionnaire are more likely as a group to smoke than respondents, estimating smoking prevalence from respondent data alone will negatively bias the results and understate the prevalence of teenage smoking, unless adjustments are made for this nonresponse bias.

Nonresponse

Nonresponse exists in surveillance whenever participation in the data gathering process does not occur when it is sought. Under this definition, unit nonresponse exists whenever an organization or an individual sought for study does not participate, and item nonresponse exists when a (unit) respondent does not provide a usable response to an item (question) on the survey. Although both levels of nonresponse create data gaps and lead to the same statistical effects, the literature on methods for dealing with each problem is distinct (Lessler and Kalsbeek, 1992). Unless otherwise noted, nonresponse will be considered at the unit level here.

Nonresponse in surveillance is relevant whether formal sampling methods are used or not. In population-directed surveillance systems based on probability samples such as NYTS, nonresponse can compromise inferences from the sample to the population by biasing estimates. This bias can be expressed mathematically following the classical model for nonresponse first suggested by Hansen and Hurwitz (1946), in which each member of the population is either a respondent or nonrespondent with certainty. If the population prevalences are estimated as $p = \lambda_{nr}p_{nr} + (1 - \lambda_{nr})p_r$, where λ_{nr} is the proportion of the population who are nonrespondents, and p_r and p_{nr} are, respectively, the prevalence for the respondent and nonrespondent subgroups, then nonresponse bias for an unbiased estimate ($\hat{p}_r$) of p_r, but intended to estimate p, based solely on respondent data and making no adjustment for nonresponse, will be,

$$Bias(\hat{p}_r) = \lambda_{nr}(p_r - p_{nr}) \qquad (2–8)$$

Information from systems using less formal methods of subject selection may also be distorted if nonresponders are selectively different from responders. In both instances, the size of the effect is directly tied to the extent of nonresponse and the degree to which respondents and nonrespondents differ, as inferred from Eq. 2–8.

Although less clearly developed and understood, variable error in estimates can result from nonresponse (Lessler and Kalsbeek, 1992). Variable error requires a somewhat different perspective on nonresponse than the deterministic view assumed by the Hansen-Hurwitz model. Here, the response outcome (i.e., respond or not) is viewed as a stochastic event for each population members so that a response propensity (i.e., probability of responding) can be defined for each member. The extent of bias and variable error under this stochastic view of nonresponse depends on the levels of these propensities.

Unlike member-level sampling probabilities (π_i), which can be calculated in all probability samples, response propensities can only be estimated when they are needed to compensate for nonresponse in estimation. In some instances, these propensities may be estimated using subgroup response rates, where in general the response rate for any sample targeting a particular population is the percentage of those population members who respond. In unequal probability samples, this rate may be weighted by summing weights for sample members in the numerator and denominator. In any event, calculating these rates means that the denominators should exclude those sample members that are not members of the target population.

Dealing with nonresponse in surveillance involves some combination of the following three aspects: profiles of response status to identify correlates of response and thus important differences between respondents and nonrespondents, preventive strategies to maximize the likelihood of response among sample members, and statistical adjustment to reduce the bias of estimates caused by nonresponse. Much of my discussion on this topic is taken from several texts, which address all three aspects in the treatment of nonresponse (Groves, 1989; Lessler and Kalsbeek, 1992; Groves and Couper, 1998).

Profiling response status

One way to deal with nonresponse in a surveillance system is simply to examine the extent of it. Often this examination involves searching for patterns of subgroup response rates among sampled subjects to identify those factors that influence system participation. A multitude of interrelated factors characterizing the system design and its environment affect response outcomes, and patterns differ from one system to the next. The Groves and Couper (1998) model for making contact with the sample subject in interview surveys includes uncontrollable factors tied to the subject (social environment, physical impediments, availability, and personal attributes) and partially controllable system design factors (interviewer attributes, the timing and number of contact attempts). The interaction between subject and interviewer during the subject recruitment process is also important in determining the final response outcome.

Finding correlates of response outcomes that are also correlates of health risk is to discover the origins of nonresponse bias in surveillance systems. If, for example, response rates differ by race/ethnicity (or if respondents differ from nonrespondents in race/ethnicity) and race/ethnicity affects risk, then respondents and nonrespondents will also differ by health risk, and nonresponse bias will occur according to the Hansen-Hurwitz model. Understanding the likelihood of system participation in light of personal and environmental factors that are tied to sample members has thus been important in dealing with unit nonresponse. Gaining this understanding may involve something as simple as performing a descriptive search for differing patterns in response outcomes by factor (Groves, 1989) or fitting logistic models to discover what factors predict response outcomes (Groves and Couper, 1998).

In real terms for a system like the NYTS, such an understanding may be gained by comparing response rates for known determinants of tobacco use, such as race/ethnicity and school grade level, as seen in Table 2–3. Variation in student response rates among the schools groups reported there suggests a race/ethnicity effect on student participation, and thus the possibility of biased estimates in the direction of tobacco use rates of those groups with the higher response rates, unless steps are taken to attenuate this effect.

Nonresponse bias can be estimated directly from the Hansen-Hurwitz model of Eq. 2–8 if sample data are available to estimate prevalence for respondents (p_r) and nonrespondents (p_{nr}). Because respondent data are typically the only data available, special efforts may be needed to learn about nonrespondents. One long-standing approach is to sub-sample the nonrespondents in the sample and make extraordinary efforts to gather data from them (Lessler and Kalsbeek, 1992). In some longitudinal designs with a cohort sample, such as the Add Health Study, bias can be estimated by applying data from a prior round to respondents and nonre-

Table 2–3 Student response rates in Fall 1999 National Youth Tobacco Survey

	Rate (%)
MIDDLE SCHOOLS WITH	
High concentration of Blacks	95.7
(*Black%* > *Hispanic%* and *Black%* > *38*)	
High concentration of Hispanics	94.0
(*Hispanic%* > *Black%* and *Hispanic%* > *40*)	
Other	90.2
HIGH SCHOOLS WITH	
High concentration of Blacks	89.8
(*Black%* > *Hispanic%* and *Black%* > *38*)	
High concentration of Hispanics	92.7
(*Hispanic%* > *Black%* and *Hispanic%* > *40*)	
Other	92.8
Overall	93

Source: Fall 1999 NYTS student response counts by sampling stratum, as prepared by James Ross/William Robb at ORC MACRO, used with permission.

spondents in a given round (Kalsbeek et al., 2001). Bias estimated in this way is limited to nonresponse in the referent round.

Minimizing nonresponse

The logic of this class of remedies for survey nonparticipation is apparent from Eq. 2–8, where nonresponse bias is directly proportional to the expected rate of nonresponse (λ_{nr}) and thus inversely related to the expected response rate. Taking steps to increase the response rate reduces bias if the respondent–nonrespondent differences are not exacerbated in the process.

In interview surveys, the survey design and the capabilities of those handling subject recruitment affect subject participation (Groves and Couper, 1998). Design features that increase the likelihood of survey unit response are a salient but not overly penetrating survey topic, a relatively short questionnaire, and the strategic use of incentives. For example, in the Fall 1999 NYTS (CDC, 2000d), a $1000 incentive offered to selected schools, with the suggestion that it be used for tobacco use prevention curricula and other educational materials, resulted in a 90% school response rate. Sending an informational letter to potential respondents before the first contact may also improve response rates.

Sizing up the circumstances surrounding subject recruitment and effectively tailoring the solicitation strategy are essential for obtaining a response from subjects. Negative comments and higher refusal rates are more likely from males, in urban settings, in households with physical impediments to access, and in other higher risk groups (e.g., race/ethnic minorities). Lower response rates are more likely in telephone surveys than in in-person surveys. The larger number of negative comments and fewer questions expected from telephone respondents may explain this difference in rates.

Preparing subject recruiters to spot potential problems quickly and address them confidently minimizes refusals and increases response rates. The recruiter must get the respondent to voice concerns about participation and must quickly develop an appropriate response.

Soliciting survey participant among certain population subgroups of higher risk groups may present barriers to, or opportunities for, response. For example, Hispanics who are recent immigrants may have limited language skills or may not understand the purpose of survey participation. They may also be suspicious of strangers asking them questions. Those in the elderly population may have security concerns, but these fears may be offset by a greater availability, loneliness, and a desire for social contact. The parental consent required for survey participation by those less than 18 years of age presents a unique hurdle.

Adjusting the respondent data for nonresponse

Nonresponse invariably occurs, despite well-conceived efforts to control it and to examine its statistical impact. The remaining compensatory option for dealing with unit nonresponse in surveys is to adjust respondent data for the sample imbalance resulting from differential rates of nonparticipation (e.g., by race/ethnicity). This adjustment is typically a preliminary analysis step done after survey data have been gathered. It is accomplished by adjusting the probability sampling weight for each sample member (ω_i) to become, $\omega_i^* = a_i\omega_i$, where the adjustment (a_i) is computed in one or more steps appropriate to the sample design and the occurrence of nonresponse. A weighted Horvitz-Thompson estimate of a total is subsequently computed from respondent data, using the adjusted weights, as,

$$\hat{y}^*_{HT} = \sum_{i=1}^{n_r} \omega_i^* y_i \qquad (2\text{--}9)$$

where n_r is the respondent sample size.

Two adjustments often used to compute α_i are a nonresponse adjustment and a poststratification adjustment (Groves and Couper, 1998). A nonresponse adjustment, intended to deal with nonresponse in particular, is computed as 1 divided by the subjects' estimated probability of response, or response propensity. Estimates of the response propensity for a respondent might be the weighted response rates for similar members of the original sample, called the subject's weighting class, or the expected outcome from a fitted logistic model, with the 0–1 response outcome as the dependent variable and plausible sociodemographic predictors of the response outcome as independent variables. The nonresponse adjustment is thus the inverse of the estimated probability of response. The other adjustment, a poststratification adjustment, compensates for sample imbalance resulting from incomplete frame coverage, random selection, and any remaining imbalance from nonresponse and calibrates the weighted sample to known population subgroup frequencies. Calculating the final adjusted sample weight for the Fall 1999 NYTS involved separate weighting class adjustments for school- and student-level nonresponse and poststratification by grade and ethnicity to known national student enrollment data for the 1999–2000 school year (http://www.nces.ed.gov).

Survey Measurement and Data Quality

A surveillance system is only as good as the data it assembles to monitor its target population. Two components of system design impact the quality of the data. One is the nature of the requested information, which is determined primarily by the design of the survey questionnaires and forms. The other is the system's data acquisition apparatus, which consists of the plan, materials, and personnel that produce the data. People who contribute to the final outcome of the measurement process, include the interviewer and subject (respondent), as with nonresponse. Experts on the surveillance topic and survey specialists impact the design of survey instruments, and field staff supervisors and statisticians who oversee the gathering and processing of the survey data impact the data acquistion process.

Features of both components contribute so-called "response effects," or shifts in measurement that are attributable to these features. In combination, these effects ultimately determine values of individual data items for each respondent. Broadly focused texts by Lessler and Kalsbeek (1992), Lyberg (1997), and Tourangeau et al. (2000) summarize most existing contributions to meaurement and data quality in surveys, and much of the discussion in this section is drawn from these texts.

As with nonresponse, no universally held model exists for studying measurement outcomes and associated sources of survey error. Early models, contributed mostly by statisticians, provided a mathematical basis for understanding the statistical effects of measurement error on estimation and on estimates from specially designated studies to identify the components of measurement error (Lessler and Kalsbeek, 1992). Presuming the existence of a true value for individual measurements, these earlier measurement error models included various bias and variable error components of the mean squared error of estimates. Components appearing in these models depend on assumptions about the stochastic origin of measurement and about which response effects contribute to the measurement outcome (e.g., the interviewer). The main limitation of these models is their inability to incorporate the wide range of response effects that have been identified in the survey process.

More recently, psychologists and survey methodologists have contributed a number of models based less on the mathematical manifestations of error and more on the behavioral origins of the measurement process. This process view of measurement in the context of surveillance has led to the development of "cognitive models" that represent a broad range of process features contributing to the measurement outcome. Four steps in the surveillance process are common to these models: question comprehension (how the subject interprets the question), information retrieval (how the subject assembles the information to formulate a response to the question), judgment (how the subject formulates a response), and response (how the response is finally assembled by the respondent and checked by the investigator before analysis). Measurement error in these models may be viewed as the inability to achieve what the system intends, as opposed to the departure from truth presumed in earlier models. Regardless of orientation, both newer cognitive models and older mean squared error models provide a basis for identifying what can go wrong in the measurement process and insight on how to deal with response effects in surveillance data.

In the rest of this section several controllable features of a survey design that may impact the quality of surveillance data are considered. Each feature is connected to content and format of the survey questionnaire or to other aspects of data collection.

Improving the survey questionnaire

The survey questionnaire is the operational focal point of information exchange between investigator and respondent. In interview surveys the interviewer becomes the intermediary in this exchange, acting on behalf of the investigator to accomplish the aims of the survey. The presence or absence of an interviewer and the medium of the information exchange (usually in person or by telephone) defines the mode of data collection.

Several interconnected mode effects are related to measurement. Interview surveys often produce better factual data than surveys using self-administered questionnaires, because the interviewer is available to help with question comprehension. However, the absence of an interviewer may lead to more truthful reporting on sensitive topics, such as smoking, drinking, drug use, and other health behaviors with negative connotations. The medium of information exchange (audio or visual) can also affect the availability of measurement options (e.g., in the use of portion size indicators to gauge dietary intake), although mode effects between telephone and in-person interviewing have generally been modest.

In questionnaire design, question wording and format are both important sources of response effects. To minimize the size of effects tied to the questionnaire, a few general rules for crafting survey questions apply. Use:

1. *Understandable words.* The meaning of all key words should be known to all respondents.
2. *Clear time references.* Respondents should be given a clear time reference for all factual questions (e.g., within the past 30 days for a question on current use of tobacco products).
3. *Concise wording.* The sentence structure for questions should be kept as simple as possible to avoid confusing the question's intent and making information retrieval more difficult for the respondent.
4. *Controlled recall length.* Questions requesting factual information retroactively should limit the time reference.
5. *An objective tone.* Words in opinion questions should not influence respondents to answer in a particular way.

The understandability of questions is especially important in populations with considerable cultural diversity, where words may have different meanings. For example, differences in language and culture between recent immigrants and established farm workers in the National Agricultural Workers Survey may lead to differing interpretations of the phrase "access to health care." Understandability may also be an issue when children are interviewed, although growing evidence suggests that, if carefully done (e.g., consideration is given to the stages of child development), interviewing children about themselves is preferable to interviewing their primary caregivers.

Question formatting can be linked to other response effects. Format refers to the sequence of questions and to the content and order of responses to closed-ended questions, where a predetermined list of response options is offered. Question sequencing determines the context of a particular question and may lead to question order effects, determined by those questions that immediately precede the referent question. A few general rules on question formatting are to:

1. *Use buffer questions.* Including a number of unrelated (buffer) questions just before the referent question may reduce the effect of preceding related questions.
2. *Place sensitive questions strategically.* Leaving the most sensitive questions until the end reduces the chances that an interview will be aborted, but it may create vulnerability to respondent fatigue in a lengthy interview. Leading into sensitive questions with a series of less sensitive questions on the same topic may soften the effect of the sensitive topic.
3. *Be aware of response format effects.* The format of responses to questions with closed-ended responses can lead to certain tendencies. For example, respondents may avoid negative extremes of a rating scale, avoid extreme responses in any type of scale, or be influenced in their view of an object being rated by the range of responses offered.

Applying sound rules of questionnaire design is not the only key to devising an effective survey instrument. Subjecting an early draft of the survey instrument to a battery of so-called cognitive assessment tools is also helpful. For example, a question on frequency of teenage smoking might request that respondents to the cognitive interview articulate how they came up with their answers (think-alouds), restate the question in their own words (paraphrasing), or indicate how accurate they think their answer is (confidence rating). A group of teenagers might also be assembled to talk about participating in an interview on tobacco use (focus group). Cognitive testing is done to flag problems in the information exchange process and to find solutions before final pretesting and the main phase of data gathering.

Computer technology has increased the cost efficiency of survey data collection and now provides timely data assembly and reporting. It has also posed problems related to interviewer acceptance, lag time needed for preprogramming and testing, and hardware and software failures during the production phase. Computer-assisted data collection, whether by telephone, face to face, or self-administration, expands the capacity to gather and produce high-quality data. Documented reductions in subsequent data editing and the ability to construct more complex question formats provide compelling arguments for the use of this technology in surveys, although strong evidence that it markedly improves data quality is lacking. The use of technology improves the efficiency of scheduling and recording results of call attempts in interview surveys, but it has not been shown to improve the likelihood of response. Indeed, applying technology-based innovations should not substitute for applying sound principles of questionnaire design and survey practice.

Improving the data collection process

Although the questionnaire provides the template for information gathering, the actual data collection process is the heart of any surveillance system. Thus, a well-functioning operational system is required to generate good data. To assure that the data are the best possible, the system must be well designed and its operation carefully monitored.

Data quality assurance involves more than continuously monitoring a series of key process indicators by means of control charts or Pareto analysis, although these quality control activities are essential to the effective functioning of a data-gathering system. The set of indicators to be monitored depend on the design and information goals of the system. National Youth Tobacco Survey data are obtained from questionnaires self-administered by students chosen by classroom in a sample of schools. Recruitment and data collection are handled by a trained fieldworker whose work is overseen by a regional supervisor. For this system, a plausible set of indicators would be the schedule rate for recruiting the school, the school response rate, the student response rate, the item response rates on key smoking questions, and the fail-edit rate for completed questionnaires. Observing all these rates during data collection by supervisor region and by individual fieldwork coordinators provides a way to flag problem areas and performance difficulties with individual field staff. Monitoring of this type is facilitated by computerized data-gathering systems.

Although ongoing quality monitoring indicates how well a data-gathering system is functioning, it does not quantify the limitations of the system. Assessing these limitations in terms of measurement error may be accomplished by embedding field experimentation into the system design. Such experimentation is typically intended to gauge levels of individual bias or variable error components of the total mean squared error of system estimates. Two common experimental designs in health surveys are the record check study and the interviewer variance study.

The main purpose of a record check study design is to estimate the response bias of factual measurements, such as health care use and health behavior. An observed referent measurement is validated by a corresponding true measurement obtained from a presumably infallible record system, which gives the design its name. The "gold standard" in other types of validation studies might be obtained elsewhere (e.g., from the respondent's saliva to measure serum cotinine levels to validate self-reported cigarette smoking status; see Caraballo et al., 2001).

The goal of an interviewer variance study is to measure the within-interviewer correlation for measurements taken by the same interviewer, and thereby assess the effectiveness of training and its goal of standardizing data collection among all interviewers. Measuring this variance effect requires that sample respondents have been randomly assigned to interviewers, a situation more plausible in telephone interviewing operations than in systems employing in-person interviewing. Small values of interviewer variance indicate a data gathering operation with a high degree of standardization.

EVENT-RELATED SURVEILLANCE

Population-directed surveillance is occasionally needed in response to major world events with serious health implications, such as disease outbreaks, natural disasters, or social upheaval tied to warfare or terrorism. As with other forms of health surveillance, data in event-related surveillance studies are gathered through surveys and existing reporting systems. The need for rapid turnaround to enhance the timeliness of study findings typically leaves little opportunity to assemble substantial financial or organizational resources, nor does it allow the time for the more deliberate planning and careful execution that characterizes other types of surveillance systems.

The content of event-related surveillance goes beyond a focus on health risk because all populations are affected by the event and are thus presumed to be at higher risk. Indeed, objectives in event-related surveillance studies are often a combination of the following: quantitatively assessing the extent of adverse health outcomes from the event, providing a profile of the short-term response by the health care establishment to the consequences of the event, and studying the event's long-term implications for the public health infrastructure. The New York Health Department's response to the September 11, 2001 terrorist attacks on the World Trade Center (CDC, 2001c) points to the need for all three objectives. Retrospective epidemiologic assessments of specific health outcomes and active surveillance of noteworthy health effects tied to the event (e.g., injury to rescue workers, or sequelae of smoke inhalation by those in the impact area) gauge the immediate health impact on those most directly affected. Prospective studies of victims (e.g., those at "ground zero" and their rescue workers) indicate the effectiveness of care provided by the local health-care network. Resources profiles (e.g., of hospital staff capabilities or of available emergency room equipment to handle burn trauma) measure the ability of the health care delivery system to care for event victims. Ultimately, findings from these studies provide information needed for shaping subsequent public health system responses to the immediate event or to setting future health policy to prevent, or at least reduce, the adverse effects of similar catastrophic events.

Features related to the need for timeliness characterize event-related systems. The time available to collect, analyze, and report findings from system data is typically short and allows health officials to base subsequent responses to the event on relatively fresh findings. For example, results from several recent event-related surveillance studies conducted by the Centers for Disease Control were reported less than 1 year after the events (CDC, 2000b,c, 2001a,d).

The primary design implications of abbreviated timelines in these studies relate to subject selection and the data gathering process. Fairly basic methods of randomized sampling are used, and samples sizes are often limited. For example, the numbers of sample clusters might be limited to reduce travel costs for field interviewers (CDC, 2001b), and relatively simple quasi-random methods might be used for within-cluster sampling (e.g., interviewing neighboring households in the direction determined by a bottle spun in the center of the cluster). Stratification may also be basic or nonexistent. The scope of events, and thus the areas targeted by data gathering, tend to be relatively focused geographically. Studies tied to disastrous events are commonly aimed at cities (CDC, 2000c), substate areas (CDC, 2000a,b), or parts of countries (CDC, 2001a,b,d).

Time and resources limits make event-related surveillance studies vulnerable to potentially detrimental statistical errors. Study methods must be developed and implemented quickly, often leaving little time to evaluate methods for gathering data and generating findings or implementing methods to compensate for known study limitations. Sample coverage may be limited by the inaccessibility of parts of the target population (e.g., refugee camps with at least 1 month of mortality data; CDC 2001d) or to parts of existing reporting systems (e.g., to emergency departments in hospital surveillance; CDC, 2000b). Moreover, bias from nonresponse may affect findings when nonparticipants differ from participants (e.g., resident deaths in accessible versus inaccessible refugee camps; CDC, 2001d). Finally, limited opportunities to develop and test data collection instruments may also affect the quality of measurement (e.g., misclassification or recall bias in establishing the cause of death from famine, as determined by field interviewers, CDC, 2001a, or from storm-related death as determined by medical examiners, CDC, 2000a).

Event-based surveillance can help to provide health planners with rapidly obtained, strategically useful information that under other forms of surveillance would not be available in time to have an impact on public health. However, the scientific shortcuts that must often be taken in the interest of timeliness may require viewing the findings with some caution and as an important first look at public health outcomes of important catastrophic events.

CONCLUSION

In covering survey methods for health surveillance this chapter has focused on their use in identifying and examining groups at increased risk of adverse health outcomes. It has explored the statistical effects of sampling and nonsampling sources of survey error and the strategies of prevention, quantification, and adjustment aimed at curbing these errors. It has also described the challenges of oversampling to assure adequate precision for estimates derived from a sample. Challenges in soliciting survey participation and measuring the data gathered have been highlighted. Nonresponse is manifested primarily as bias, which is handled mainly through strategies to increase the likelihood of survey participation and through statistical adjustment to correct for sample imbalance. Problems with measurement error, on the other hand, occur as both variable error and bias, which can be handled by effective questionnaire design or strategic monitoring of the data-gathering apparatus and by specially planned experimental studies. Finally, the benefits and limitations of event-related surveillance for addressing the serious health implications of major world events have been noted. The need to quickly and effectively monitor the health of the public makes the survey method a plausible and useful surveillance tool for health professionals.

ACKNOWLEDGMENT

Work by Dr. Kalsbeek on this book was funded by the University of North Carolina Center for Health Statistics Research, as part of a grant from the CDC/National Center for Health Statistics. Dr. Kalsbeek also gratefully acknowledges the assistance of Juan Yang in the preparation of Tables 1–2 and 2–1.

REFERENCES

American Statistical Association (1998). What is a survey? *ASA Series*. http://www.amstat.org/sections/srms/brochures/survwhat.html.

Buehler, J.W. (1998). Surveillance. In Rothman, K.J. and Greenland S. (eds.) *Modern Epidemiology*. Philadelphia: Lippincott-Raven Publishers, pp. 435–457.

Carraballo, R.S., Giovino, G.A., Pechacek, T.F., and Mowery, P.D. (2001). Factors associated with discrepancies between self-reports on cigarette smoking and measured serum cotinine levels among persons aged 17 years and older. *American Journal of Epidemiology* **153,** 807–814.

Centers for Disease Control and Prevention (1988). *CDC Surveillance Update, January 1988*. Atlanta, GA.

Centers for Disease Control and Prevention (2000a). Storm-related mortality—central Texas, October 17–31, 1998. *Morbidity and Mortality Weekly Report* **49,** 133. http://www.cdc.gov/mmwr/PDF/wk/mm4907.pdf.

Centers for Disease Control and Prevention (2000b). Morbidity and mortality associated with hurricane Floyd—North Carolina, September–October, 1999. *Morbidity and Mortality Weekly Report* **49,** 369. http://www.cdc.gov/mmwr/PDF/wk/mm4917.pdf.

Centers for Disease Control and Prevention (2000c). Heat-related illness, deaths, and risk factors—Cincinnati and Dayton, Ohio, 1999, and United States, 1979–1997. *Morbidity and Mortality Weekly Report* **49,** 470. http://www.cdc.gov/mmwr/PDF/wk/mm4921.pdf.

Centers for Disease Control and Prevention (2000d). Youth tobacco surveillance: United States, 1998–1999. *Morbidity and Mortality Weekly Report, CDC Surveillance Summaries* **49,** SS 10.

Centers for Disease Control and Prevention (2001a). Outbreak of Ebola hemorrhagic fever—Uganda, August 2000–January 2001. *Morbidity and Mortality Weekly Report* **50,** 73. http://www.cdc.gov/mmwr/PDF/wk/mm5005.pdf.

Centers for Disease Control and Prevention (2001b). Mortality during a famine—Gode District, Ethiopia, July 2000. *Morbidity and Mortality Weekly Report* **50,** 285. http://www.cdc.gov/mmwr/PDF/wk/mm5015.pdf.

Centers for Disease Control and Prevention (2001c). New York City Department of Health response to terrorist attack, September 11, 2001. *Morbidity and Mortality Weekly Report* **50,** 821. http://www.cdc.gov/mmwr/PDF/wk/mm5038.pdf.

Centers for Disease Control and Prevention (2001d). Surveillance of mortality during refugee crisis—Guinea, January–May 2001. *Morbidity and Mortality Weekly Report* **50,** 1029. http://www.cdc.gov/mmwr/PDF/wk/mm5046.pdf.

Gabler, S., Haeder, S., and Lahiri, P. (1999). A model-based justification of Kish's formula for design effects for weighting and clustering. *Survey Methodology* **25,** 105–106.

Gordis, L. (2000) *Epidemiology*, 2nd edition. New York: W. B. Saunders, Company.

Groves, R.M. (1989). *Survey Errors and Survey Costs*. New York: Wiley.

Groves, R.M. and Couper, M. (1998). *Nonresponse in Household Interview Surveys*. New York: Wiley.

Hansen, M.H. and Hurwitz, W.N. (1946). The problem of nonresponse in sample surveys. *Journal of the American Statistical Association* **41,** 517–529.

Horvitz, D.G. and Thompson, D.J. (1952). A generalizaiton of sampling without replacement from a finite universe. *Journal of the American Statistical Association* **47,** 663–685.

Kalsbeek, W. and Heiss, G. (2000). Building bridges between populations and samples in epidemiological studies. *Annual Review of Public Health* **21,** 1–23.

Kalsbeek, W.D. (1988). Design strategies for nonsedentary populations, *Proceedings of the Section on Survey Research Methods*, American Statistical Association, 28–37.

Kalsbeek, W.D. (2003). Sampling minority groups in health surveys. *Statistics in Medicine*, **22**, 1527–1549.

Kalsbeek, W.D., Morris, C. B., and Vaughn, B.J. (2001). Effects of nonresponse on the mean squared error of estimates from a longitudinal study. *2001 Proceedings of the Joint Statistical Meetings*, (on CD-ROM), American Statistical Association, Alexandria, VA.

Kalton, G. (1991). Sampling flows of mobile human populations. *Survey Methodology* **17**, 183–194.

Kish, L. (1965). *Survey Sampling.* New York: Wiley.

Kish, L. (1987a). *Statistical Design for Research.* New York: Wiley.

Kish, L. (1987b). Weighting in Deft². *The Survey Statistician*, June 1987.

Lessler, J.T. and Kalsbeek, W.D. (1992). *Nonsampling Error in Surveys.* New York: Wiley.

Levy, P.S. and Lemeshow, S. (1991). *Sampling of Populations—Methods and Applications.* New York: Wiley.

Lohr, S. (1999). *Sampling: Design and Analysis.* Pacific Grove: Duxbury Press.

Lyberg, L. (1997). *Survey Measurement and Process Quality.* New York: Wiley.

Rothman, K.J. and Greenland, S. (1998). *Modern Epidemiology.* Philadelphia: Lippincott-Raven Publishers.

Stueve, A., O'Donnell, L.N., Duran, R., San Doval, A., and Blome, J. (2001). Methodological issues in time-space sampling in minority communities: Results with latino young men who have sex with men. *American Journal of Public Health* **17**, 922–926.

Thacker, S.B. (2000). Historical Development. In Teutsch, S.M., Churchill, R.E. (eds.) *Principles and Practice of Public Health Surveillance.* New York: Oxford University Press.

Tourangeau, R., Rips, L.J., and Rasinski, K.A. (2000). *The Psychology of Survey Response.* Cambridge: Cambridge University Press.

U.S. Department of Health and Human Services (1994). *Preventing Tobacco Use Among Young People: A Report of the Surgeon General.* Office of Smoking and Health, National Center for Chronic Disease Prevention and Promotion, CDC, July 1994. Washington, DC: U.S. Government Printing Office.

U.S. Department of Health and Human Services (2000). *Healthy People 2010: Understanding and Improving Health.* Washington, DC: U.S. Government Printing Office.

Waksberg, J. (1973). The effect of stratification with differential sampling rates on attributes of subsets of the population. *ASA Proceedings of the Section on Survey Research Methods*, American Statistical Association, 429–434.

3

Exploring Temporal and Spatial Patterns in Public Health Surveillance Data

OWEN DEVINE

The National Council on Vital and Health Statistics (NCVHS) recently published its recommendations for strengthening the public health information infrastructure in the United States (U.S. Department of Health and Human Services, 2001). These recommendations emphasize the importance of timely collection and assessment of disease incidence data to reduce the time between diagnosing a disease, or identifying specific symptoms of interest (Hutwagner et al., 1997), and communicating that information to public health officials. Timely acquisition of information is only the first step in implementing an efficient public health monitoring system. Ideally, data availability must be coupled with timely assessment. While complex examinations of these data (e.g., hierarchical modeling of potential associations) are an integral component of assessing disease etiology, ongoing preliminary examination of the data as they become available can lead to the timely identification of potentially important aberrations and trend shifts. Also, because exploratory analytic methods are not usually computationally difficult, they are useful for ongoing surveillance activities and may be more compatible with the analytic resources of local public health agencies. As a result, incorporating exploratory analytic techniques into health-monitoring systems is an integral step in achieving the NCVHS committee's goal of "real-time small-area analysis" of potential public health problems.

This chapter outlines a collection of easy-to-use, yet intuitively reasonable approaches for exploratory investigations of public health monitoring data. The focus is primarily on one- and two-dimensional smoothing methods for reducing the random variation expected in observable measures of disease and injury risk. The object of this variance reduction is to increase the signal-to-noise ratio and thus improve the assessment of potential patterns in the underlying risk. The preliminary nature of these types of approaches suggests their intended use as purely hypothesis-generating techniques. But when ease of use is considered, along with the fact that results of even highly sophisticated analyses of public health surveillance data are likely to be suggestive at best (Brookmeyer and Yasui, 1995; Gelman et al., 2001), the methods described in this chapter provide valuable tools for ongoing disease-surveillance activities.

SMOOTHING TECHNIQUES FOR TIME-REFERENCED HEALTH SURVEILLANCE DATA

Assume that a set of observable measures of disease risk, say y_k, each associated with a fixed point in time, t_k, where $k = 1, 2, 3 \ldots, N$ have been collected. For simplicity, also assume that the time points are equidistant. Figure 3–1 shows two examples of time-referenced information commonly collected in public health monitoring systems: the weekly number of pneumonia and influenza (P&I) deaths in the United States as reported to the Centers for Disease Control and Prevention (CDC) for 1999 and 2000 (CDC, 2002) (Fig. 3-1A) and the monthly number of motor vehicle crashes in the United States reported to the Fatal Accident Reporting System (FARS) from 1996 through 2000 (National Highway Traffic Safety Administration, 2002) (Fig. 3–1B).

Suppose the goal is to draw a line through the P&I mortality data that captures the clear seasonal pattern, yet also reduces the random variation among the observations. The difficulty in selecting such a line is that the observations represent some unknown combination of the true underlying risk and the random variability inherent in any observable measure of that risk. This duality can be reflected by the model

$$y_k = E_k + \varepsilon_k \qquad (3–1)$$

where E_k is the expected value of y_k based on the true risk at time t_k, and ε_k is the random component. Assume that the manner in which the E_k varies with time can be modeled by some unknown function, say, $f(t_k)$. Using $f(t_k)$, the model in Eq. 3–1 can be rewritten as

$$y_k = f(t_k) + \varepsilon_k \qquad (3–2)$$

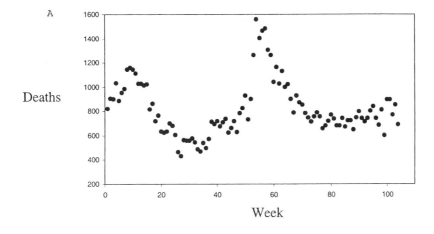

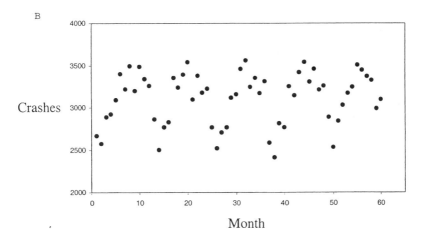

Figure 3–1 *A:* Number of pneumonia and influenza deaths in the United States reported to the CDC by week for 1999 and 2000. *B:* Motor vehicle crashes in the United States reported to the Fatal Accident Reporting System (FARS) by month from 1996 through 2000.

Knowing the structure of $f(t_k)$ and the magnitude of the ε_k's would simplify assessing trends and, perhaps more importantly, deviations from expected trends in the surveillance time series. Without this knowledge estimating the trend and the magnitude of the ε_k's must be based solely on the observations.

One approach to this problem is to postulate a specific model for the entire collection of E_k's and to fit that model to the observations using some model adequacy criterion. As the examples in Figure 3–1 illustrate, the postulated model for such a fit would most likely be quite complex (e.g., a high degree polynomial in t) making interpretation difficult. Also, we would likely have to make parametric assumptions about the distribution of the y_k's to produce the fitted line and it is unlikely that these assumptions could be adequately validated. Alternatively, we could use a collection of nonparametric smoothing methods for estimating $f(t_k)$ that do not require assumptions on the true form of $f(t_k)$ or on the distribution of the observed values. The focus is on estimators, which will be called $\hat{y}_k$, that are linear combinations of the observations such that

$$\hat{y}_k = \sum_{l=1}^{N} w_{kl} y_l \qquad (3\text{--}3)$$

where w_{kl} is a weight that reflects the contribution of the value observed at time t_l to $\hat{y}_k$. Given the form of the estimator in Eq. 3–3, the question becomes one of determining the weights to be used in estimating $f(t_k)$. In the following subsections, three approaches to deriving these weights: kernel smoothing, smoothing splines, and local polynomial regression are addressed.

Kernel Smoothing

In the kernel smoothing approach, the w_{kl} are defined by two attributes of the estimator: the kernel function, $K(\cdot)$, and the bandwidth, h. Again, consider the P&I mortality data in Figure 3–1A. Suppose that the goal is to obtain a smoothed estimate for $f(t_{13})$, that is, an estimate of the expected number of P&I deaths 13 weeks into the 2-year period. Suppose that this value is estimated by averaging the number of deaths observed in week 13 with the number of deaths observed 2 weeks before and 2 weeks after the 13th week. In other words, $f(t_{13})$ is estimated as

$$\hat{y}_{13} = \frac{y_{11} + y_{12} + y_{13} + y_{14} + y_{15}}{5}$$

This estimator can be written in the form of Eq. 3–3 by setting $k = 13$ and $w_{kl} = 1/5$, when $k = 13$ and $11 \le l \le 15$, and $w_{kl} = 0$ otherwise. Now suppose that this averaging process is repeated for all the observation times such that $f(t_k)$ is estimated by

$$\hat{y}_k = \frac{\sum_{l=k-2}^{k+2} y_l}{5} \qquad (3\text{--}4)$$

for $k = 1, \ldots, N$. Using Eq. 3–4, the expected value at a given point in time is estimated as the average of the five observations falling within a

5-week smoothing window centered at that point. Clearly, the estimate would be different if the smoothing window had a width of 11 weeks rather than 5. The dependence of the estimator on the width of the smoothing window reflects the importance of the selected bandwidth, and, thus, the impact of choosing a value for this parameter will be considered carefully.

Given a width of the smoothing window, say $h = 5$, the weights associated with observations within the window can be varied. For example, the estimator in Eq. 3–4 assigns a weight of 1/5 to all observations within the 5-week smoothing window and 0 to observations outside that interval. Alternatively, the weight on values observed close to t_{13} could be increased and the weight on values observed near the boundary of the smoothing window could be reduced. This type of differential weighting is applied by selecting an appropriate kernel function. Continuing with the example, a transformation of the time measure, which is called z_{kl}, is defined such that

$$z_{kl} = \frac{t_k - t_l}{5} \tag{3–5}$$

where z_{kl} specifies the location of the observations in time relative to t_k. Notice that $|z_{kl}| \leq 0.5$ only for those values observed within the specified smoothing window of t_k. Now consider the function

$$K(z_{kl}) = 1, \text{ if } |z_{kl}| \leq 0.5 \tag{3–6}$$
$$= 0, \text{ otherwise.}$$

Eq. 3–6, called the uniform kernel function, illustrates one potential weighting scheme that could be used in the estimator. Given any selection for h and $K(\cdot)$, the general form for the kernel smoother is given by

$$\hat{y}_k = \frac{\sum_{l=1}^{N} K\left(\frac{t_k - t_l}{h}\right) y_l}{\sum_{l=1}^{N} K\left(\frac{t_k - t_l}{h}\right)} \tag{3–7}$$

The kernel smoother in Eq. 3–7, sometimes referred to as the Nadarya-Watson (NW) kernel regression estimator (Sarda and Vieu, 2000), illustrates the weighted average form of the estimator, in which weights are determined by the combination of the kernel function and the bandwidth. Although kernel-based alternatives to the NW estimator have been proposed (Gasser and Muller, 1979), estimators of the type in Eg. 3–7 are the most common. Thus, focus will be on this type of kernel smoother.

Substituting the uniform kernel, Eq. 3–6, in Eq. 3–7 leads to the estimator in Eq. 3–4. Certainly, alternative forms for $K(\cdot)$ can be used in the smoothing process. Examples of commonly used kernel functions include the Gaussian

$$K(z_{kl}) = (\sqrt{2\pi})^{-1} \exp(-0.5 \, z_{kl}^2)$$

triangular

$$K(z_{kl}) = 1 - |z_{kl}|, \text{ if } |z_{kl}| \leq 1$$
$$= 0, \text{ } otherwise$$

and quadratic, or Epanechnikov,

$$K(z_{kl}) = 0.75(1 - z_{kl}^2), \text{ if } |z_{kl}| \leq 1$$
$$= 0, \text{ } otherwise$$

kernels, where

$$z_{kj} = \frac{t_k - t_l}{h}$$

Figure 3–2 illustrates the weighting functions that result from using each of the kernel functions above, centered at t = 13 with a bandwidth of $h = 5$. The w_{kl}'s are exactly zero for observation times further than

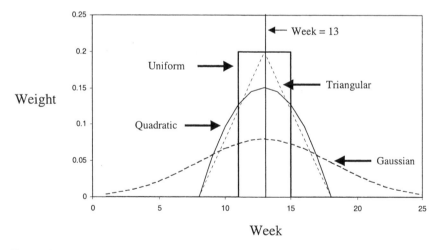

Figure 3–2 Weights associated with the uniform, Gaussian, triangular, and quadratic kernel functions, centered on week 13 of the pneumonia and influenza mortality data with bandwidth $h = 5$.

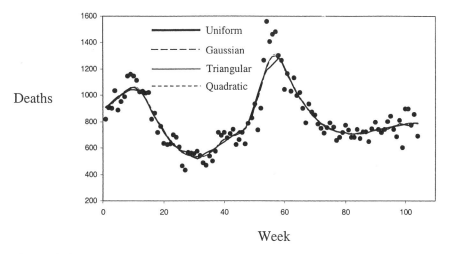

Figure 3–3 Smoothes produced using 4 kernel functions with comparable bandwidths for the pneumonia and influenza mortality data.

$(h - 1)/2$ from the center of the smoothing window only for the uniform kernel. Thus, h does not, in general, specify the exact number of neighboring observations to be included in the smoothing widow but instead provides a scale for the relative weighting of nearby observations.

Figure 3–3 shows the observed values for the weekly P&I mortality data and the smoothed estimates for each of the kernel functions listed above. The bandwidths for each kernel were selected to provide approximately equal weights in each of the estimators. The smoothed estimates indicate little difference resulting from the choice of a particular kernel function. Although there is no rule of thumb for selecting a kernel function, theoretical arguments might favor selecting the quadratic kernel (Epanechnikov, 1969; Hart, 1997). In general, however, differences in the estimated values attributable to the form of the kernel function are outweighed by the influence of the selection of h.

Figure 3–4 shows the observed values for the FARS crash data as in Figure 3–1B. Also shown are two collections of smoothed estimates developed using a Gaussian kernel: one with a bandwidth of $h = 0.5$, and the other with $h = 3.0$. As expected, comparing the estimates indicates that increasing the bandwidth produces a smoother estimate of the time trend. Viewed in this light, selecting a particular value for h represents an implied trade-off between the fidelity of the estimator to the observed values and a reduction in random variation. Selecting an optimal bandwidth to achieve this balance is an integral question when kernel smothers, or for that matter, smoothers in general, are used. To determine the optimal bandwidth,

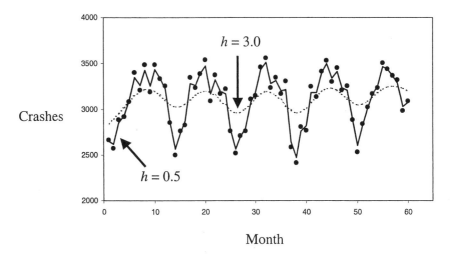

Figure 3–4 Smoothes produced using a Gaussian kernel with bandwidths of $h = 0.5$ and $h = 3.0$ for the FARS crash data.

a criteria for the optimum balance between smoothness and variance reduction must be defined. Clearly, the smoothed line should be close to the E_k's. As a result, one measure of a desirable bandwidth is minimization of bias. Alternatively, because smoothing is meant to reduce the random variation among the observed values, the chosen bandwidth should provide a collection of estimates that reduces the variation among the observed values. In addition, balancing, these potentially opposing minimization goals, small variance versus small bias, must be based only on the information provided by the observed values. Given this limitation, a reasonable criterion for selecting an optimum bandwidth might be the mean squared error (MSE) associated with the estimator, where

$$MSE(h) = \frac{\sum_{k=i}^{N} (\hat{y}_k^h - y_k)^2}{N} \qquad (3\text{–}8)$$

and y_k^h is the smoothed estimate for y_k, based on a bandwidth of size h. However, using Eq. 3–8 to select an optimal bandwidth implies that the optimal estimator is the collection of observed values such that $\hat{y}_i^h = y_i$, and, thus, we are no better off than where we started. However, because the expectation for *MSE(h)* has both variance and bias components, Eq. 3–8 may still be considered as a starting point for defining a optimal value of h.

Using MSE(h) to balance bias and variance in bandwidth selection generally follows 1 of 2 types of approaches (Herrmann, 2000). Approaches of the first type focus on minimizing a penalized version of Eq. 3–8 where the penalty corresponds to the amount of roughness remaining in the smoothed estimates. Generalized cross validation (GCV) is the most common method of this type. Approaches of the second type, sometimes called plug-in methods, derive an optimal bandwidth based on the asymptotic properties of funtionals of *MSE(h)*. Plug-in approaches generally require estimating the variance of the observations (Dette et al., 1998) and, more importantly, the integrated second derivative of $f(t_k), f''(t_k)$. Various methods have been proposed for estimating $f''(t_k)$ that usually involve selecting an alternative kernel function and bandwidth having certain conditions. Although plug-in methods do well relative to simpler GCV-type criteria in some instances (Jones et al., 1996), potentially they can lead to oversmoothing in others (Park and Turlach 1992). Also, because they depend on estimating $f''(t_k)$, plug-in optimal values for h can be difficult to compute. The focus in this chapter is on GCV-based approaches because they are the most commonly used in available smoothing software. However, a variety of references are available on the use of plug-in methods for estimating optimal bandwidths (Herrmann, 2000; Hart, 1997).

The GCV approach for selecting a bandwidth is based on replacing *MSE(h)* in Eq. 3–8 with the leave-one-out cross validation (CV) sum of squared errors given by

$$CV(h) = \frac{\sum_{k=1}^{N} (\tilde{y}_k^h - y_k)^2}{N}$$

where $\tilde{y}_k^h$ is a smoothed estimate for $f(t_k)$ based on a bandwidth of h but omits y_k from the smoothing process. Using the notation of Eq. 3–3, a computationally convenient version of CV(h) is given by

$$CV(h) = \frac{1}{N} \sum_{k=1}^{N} \left(\frac{\tilde{y}_k^h - y_k}{1 - w_{kk}} \right)^2$$

GCV (Craven and Wahba, 1979) builds on the leave-one-out CV(h) approach and is based on the modified criteria given by

$$GCV(h) = N \sum_{k=1}^{N} \left(\frac{\hat{y}_k^h - y_k}{N - \sum_{k=1}^{N} w_{kk}} \right)^2 \qquad (3\text{–}9)$$

To illustrate the concept behind GCV(h), consider a kernel smoother of the type given in Eq. 3–7 that is based on a uniform kernel with bandwidth h. In this case $w_{kk} = 1/h$ and, therefore,

$$N - \sum_{k=1}^{N} w_{kk} = \frac{N(h-1)}{h}$$

indicating that Eq. 3–9 can be written as

$$GCV(h) = \frac{1}{N} \left(\frac{h}{h-1} \right)^2 \sum_{k=1}^{N} (\hat{y}_k^h - y_k)^2$$

$$= \frac{1}{N} \left(\frac{h}{h-1} \right)^2 s_h^2$$

In this form, it is easy to see that, as h approaches N, that is as $\hat{y}_k^h$ approaches $\bar{y}$, s_h^2 will approach the presumably large value defined by the sums of squared errors of the observations about their mean, whereas $h/(h-1)$ approaches 1. Alternatively, as h approaches 1, that is as the level of smoothing decreases, s_h^2 will go to zero, but $h/((h-1)$ will increase. Thus, the GCV criteria function tends to increase for both large (large bias) and small (large variance) values of h.

The FARS crash data from Figure 3–1B can be used to illustrate selecting an optimal bandwidth using the GCV criteria. In this example, a Gaussian kernel function is used and a direct search is conducted over a specified range of possible values for h to identify an optimal bandwidth under the criterion in Eq. 3–9. Notice, that the w_{kk} in Eq. 3–9 correspond to the value of the kernel function at $z_{kl} = 0$. Figure 3–5 illustrates a portion of the search showing the GCV(h) values for the subset of candidate values that contain the minimizing value of $h = 1.048$. The smooth that results from using this bandwidth in a Gaussian kernel, and its relation to the observed crash counts is shown in Figure 3–6.

Although the GCV approach is computationally and intuitively pleasing, it should not be viewed as the ultimate method in data-driven bandwidth selection. In fact, several alternative approaches based on penalized forms of the MSE have been suggested (Hurvich et al., 1998). Also, when criteria that require a search for a minimizing value of h are used, care should be taken to assure that the search range is wide enough to preclude selecting local minima. In addition, empirical evidence suggests that bandwidths selected on the basis of criteria similar to those in Eq. 3–9 are sub-

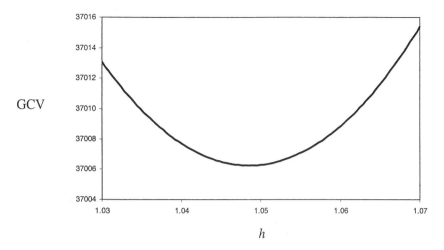

Figure 3–5 Search for the optimum bandwidth (h) based on the generalized cross validation (GCV) criterion for a Gaussian kernel smooth of the FARS crash data. Optimal bandwidth is $h = 1.048$.

ject to large sampling variability (Herrmann, 2000). The plug-in estimators mentioned earlier are an alternative approach to addressing this variability concern. Alternative methods have also been proposed for bootstrap-driven selection of optimal smoothing bandwidths (Faraway, 1990, Hardle and Bowman, 1988).

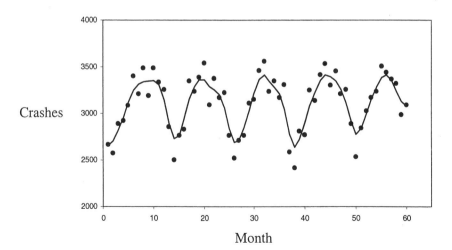

Figure 3–6 Observed and smoothed values for the FARS crash data using a Gaussian kernel with bandwidth $h = 1.048$.

Two implied assumptions inherent in with using these types of data-driven bandwidth selection procedures are that observations that fall near the ends of the series are not exerting undue influence on the selection of h and that the residual errors associated with the smoothed values are independent. While boundary effects are addressed in more detail, one approach for reducing the effect of boundary points is to use a weighted version of the GCV given by

$$GCV(h) = N \sum_{k=1}^{N} \left(\frac{G_k(\hat{y}_k^h - y_k)}{N - \sum_{k=1}^{N} G_k w_{kk}} \right)^2 \qquad (3\text{--}10)$$

where the weights, G_k, are selected to increase the relative emphasis on time periods in the interior of the series and to reduce the emphasis on points close to the boundary. With regard to the assumption of independence, concerns about the impact of autocorrelation, which could be based, for example, on lag plotting of the residuals, can be addressed by repeating the bandwidth selection process using modified criteria that address lack of independence among the ε_k's (Buhlmann and Kunsch, 1999; Buhlmann 1998; Hardle et al., 1997). In addition, focus is only on selecting globally optimum bandwidths for kernel regression. Alternative methods for selecting locally optimum values for this parameter have been presented by others (Herrmann, 1997; Sain and Scott, 1996; Schucany, 1995). Finally, only bandwidth selection criteria that focus on minimizing various manipulations of the MSE are addressed. Alternative criteria for defining the optimum bandwidth have been suggested. For example, Marron and Tsybakov (1995) developed criteria that emphasize capturing important characteristics of the true trend, as opposed to minimizing average squared differences. Alternatively, Chaudhuri and Marron (1999) suggest examining the validity of trend features by simultaneously assessing the smooth across a range of possible values for h.

Although the idea of totally data-driven bandwidth selection is appealing, especially when these types of smoothers are integrated into ongoing surveillance activities, those involved in public health surveillance monitoring should probably not rely entirely on these methods. Bandwidth selection procedures can be viewed as a process for deriving a starting point for evaluating smoothing results, but analysts should combine this with interpretations based on their subject matter knowledge and expereince to determine the adequacy of the fit.

Smoothing Splines

In the kernel smoothing approach, the weights used in the linear estimator are determined by the selection of the kernel function and the bandwidth. Alternatively, suppose the kernel selection problem is removed from the process and, instead, the weights are selected solely by determining an optimal balance between fidelity to the observed data and minimizing bias. A general approach to selecting such an estimator is to minimize

$$\sum_{k=1}^{N} (\hat{f}(t_k) - y_k)^2 + \lambda \int f''(t)^2 dt \qquad (3\text{--}11)$$

where $\hat{f}(t_k) = \hat{y}_k$ is an estimator as defined in Eq.3, $f''(\cdot)$ is the second derivative of $f(t_k)$ and λ is a parameter that controls the level of smoothing in the estimates. By minimizing Eq. 3–11, a penalized sum of squared errors criterion similar to that in Eq. 3–9 is used. The smoothing penalty in this approach, represented by the integrated second derivative, increases with the roughness of the estimate. The estimator resulting from minimizing this specific penalized sum of squared errors criterion, at a specified value for λ, is called the smoothing, or cubic, spline (Wahba, 1990). Like the kernel smoother, the smoothing spline estimator is a linear combination of the observed values. In the case of equidistant t_k, the smoothing spline estimates can be derived as (Lange, 1999)

$$\hat{\mathbf{Y}}^{\lambda} = \mathbf{H\,Y}$$

where $\hat{\mathbf{Y}}^{\lambda}$ is a N-dimensional vector containing the smoothing spline estimates, $\mathbf{Y}$ is the vetor of observed values, and

$$\mathbf{H} = [\mathbf{I} - \lambda\ \mathbf{Q'}\ \mathbf{R}\ \mathbf{Q}]^{-1} \qquad (3\text{--}12)$$

In Eq. 3–12, $\mathbf{R}$ is the $(N - 2)$ by $(N - 2)$ matrix given by

$$\mathbf{R} = \left(\frac{1}{6}\right)
\begin{bmatrix}
1 & 4 & 1 & 0 & & 0 & 0 & 0 & 0 \\
0 & 1 & 4 & 1 & \cdots & 0 & 0 & 0 & 0 \\
0 & 0 & 1 & 4 & & 0 & 0 & 0 & 0 \\
0 & 0 & 0 & 1 & & 0 & 0 & 0 & 0 \\
 & & & & \cdot & & & & \\
 & & & & \cdot & & & & \\
0 & 0 & 0 & 0 & & 1 & 4 & 1 & 0 \\
0 & 0 & 0 & 0 & \cdots & 0 & 1 & 4 & 1 \\
0 & 0 & 0 & 0 & & 0 & 0 & 1 & 4 \\
0 & 0 & 0 & 0 & & 0 & 0 & 0 & 1 \\
\end{bmatrix}$$

and Q is the $(N - 2)$ by N matrix defined as

$$
\mathbf{Q} =
\begin{bmatrix}
1 & -2 & 1 & 0 & & 0 & 0 & 0 & 0 \\
0 & 1 & -2 & 1 & \cdots\cdots & 0 & 0 & 0 & 0 \\
0 & 0 & 1 & -2 & & 0 & 0 & 0 & 0 \\
0 & 0 & 0 & 1 & & 0 & 0 & 0 & 0 \\
 & & & & \cdot & & & & \\
 & & & & \cdot & & & & \\
0 & 0 & 0 & 0 & & 1 & 0 & 0 & 0 \\
0 & 0 & 0 & 0 & \cdots\cdots & -2 & 1 & 0 & 0 \\
0 & 0 & 0 & 0 & & 1 & -2 & 1 & 0 \\
0 & 0 & 0 & 0 & & 0 & 1 & -2 & 1
\end{bmatrix}
$$

These matrices provide all that is needed to derive the smoothing spline estimates with the exception of a value for λ. As in kernel smoothing, a level of smoothing is desired that, somehow, best balances variability and bias. Because the goal is similar to that in kernel smoothing, the GCV criterion is also commonly used in data-driven derivations of an optimal value for λ. The definition of the GCV(λ)criterion in Eq. 3–9 can be used. In this case, h is replaced by λ, and a direct search can be conducted across a range of possible values for λ with the optimum defined as that value yielding the minimum GCV value. In the smoothing spline approach, however, the w_{kk}'s are defined by the diagonal elements of the **H** matrix given in Eq. 3–12.

Figure 3–7 illustrates a search for an optimal GCV-based λ value based on the FARS crash data, and Figure 3–8 shows the smooth produced using the a value of $\lambda = 0.177$ selected on the basis of a direct search.

Based on the fact that both kernel smoothers and smoothing can be represented using Eq. 3–3, it is clear that both estimators are linear combinations of the observed data. In this light, smoothing splines may be viewed as a kernel smoothing approach with the difference being only the choice of the kernel function. In fact, Silverman (1984) has shown that using a smoothing spline is asymptotically equivalent to kernel smoothing based on the kernel function

$$
K(z_{kl}) = 0.5 \exp(- \sqrt{2}\, z_{kl}) \sin\left(\frac{|z_{kl}|}{\sqrt{2}} + \frac{\pi}{4}\right)
$$

Local Polynomial Estimation

The discussion of smoothing techniques began with the suggestion that attempting to model the entire collection of observations simultaneously is not likely to be fruitful because of the complexity of any reasonably de-

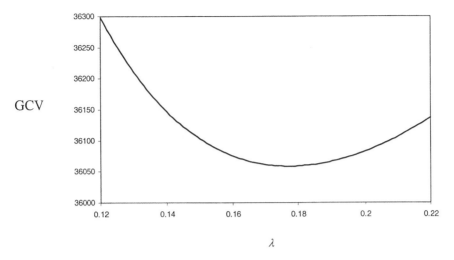

λ

Figure 3–7 Search for the optimum smoothing parameter (λ) based on the generalized cross validation (GCV) criterion for a smoothing spline fit to the FARS crash data. Optimum value is $\lambda = 0.177$.

scriptive model. As an alternative to fitting one model to the entire data set, the observations could be partitioned into overlapping subsets, as in kernel smoothing, and simpler models could then be fit successively within each of the windows. This type of moving regression modeling is the ba-

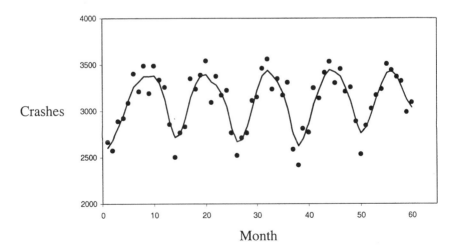

Month

Figure 3–8 Observed and smoothed values for the Fatal Accident Reporting System (FARS) crash data based on a smoothing spline with smoothing parameter $\lambda = 0.177$.

sic idea behind smoothing by local polynomials. To illustrate this concept, consider the local linear estimator given by

$$\hat{y}_k = \beta_{0k} + \beta_{1k}\, t_l^k \tag{3–13}$$

where β_{0k} and β_{1k} are unknown constants, and t_l^k takes value t_l for all observation times in a specified period surrounding t_k. Using least squares, the unknown coefficients in Eq. 3–13 can be estimated by minimizing

$$\sum_{l=1}^{N}(y_l - \beta_{0l} - \beta_{1l}\, t_l)^2\; I\left(\frac{|t_k - t_l|}{h} \leq C\right)$$

where C is a user-specified constant and $I(z)$ takes value one if z is true and zero otherwise. Thus, the linear regression model is simply fit to the subset of the observations that fall within the specified bandwidth. This local fitting idea can be improved by using locally weighted regression, in which the data points (t_l, y_l) are weighted based on their proximity to t_k such that points falling closer to t_k receive greater weight in estimating the regression coefficients. The kernel functions discussed earlier are good candidates for such a weighting scheme. In addition, as the name suggests, linear models are not the only ones that can be used. Higher-order polynomials can also be used in the local fits. The complexity of the model, however, does depend on the magnitude of h, although in most cases the order used in local polynomial fitting rarely exceeds 2.

To fit a local polynomial of order p, the kth row of the hat matrix, $\mathbf{H}$, is given by

$$\mathbf{H'_k} = \mathbf{T'_k}[\mathbf{T'KWT}]^{-1}\,\mathbf{TKW} \tag{3–14}$$

where

$$\mathbf{T'_K} = (1, t_k, \ldots\ldots, t_k^p)$$

and

$$\mathbf{T} = \begin{bmatrix} 1 & t_1 & \ldots & t_1^p \\ 1 & t_2 & \ldots & t_2^p \\ . & . & & . \\ . & . & & . \\ 1 & t_N & \ldots & t_N^p \end{bmatrix}$$

In Eq. 3–14, $\mathbf{KW}$ is an $N \times N$ matrix, with off diagonal elements equal to zero and diagonal elements given by

$$KW_{ll} = K\left(\frac{t_k - t_l}{h}\right)$$

where $K(\cdot)$ is the selected kernel function. The complete hat matrix, $\mathbf{H}$, is constructed by combining the $\mathbf{H}'_k$ from Eq. 3–14 for $k = 1, 2, \ldots, N$. Once completed, $\mathbf{H}$ is used to obtain the local polynomial regression estimate of

$$\hat{y}^h_k = \mathbf{H}\,\mathbf{Y}.$$

As in kernel smoothing, fitting local polynomial regression models requires selecting a bandwidth, h. Again, minimizing the GCV statistic is a common criterion for deciding on an acceptable value for h. Eq. 3–9 can be used to obtain a data-driven optimal bandwidth based on the GCV criteria with the w_{kk}'s now defined by the kth diagonal element of $\mathbf{H}$. Variations of local polynomial smoothing algorithms are available in a wide variety of statistical software packages. One approach, called loess (Cleveland and Devlin 1988), allows for the selection of locally, as opposed to globally, optimum bandwidths. In addition, a modification of the approach, based on iteratively reweighted regression, can be used to build in resistance to potential outliers (Fox, 2000).

Figure 3–9 shows the search for an optimum GCV-based bandwidth for a local linear regression fit to the FARS crash data. The resulting smooth, with $h = 1.06$, is shown in Figure 3–10.

Moving Median Smoothers

All of the smoothers discussed thus far are constructed using linear combinations of the form given in Eq 3–3. A simple nonlinear smoother can

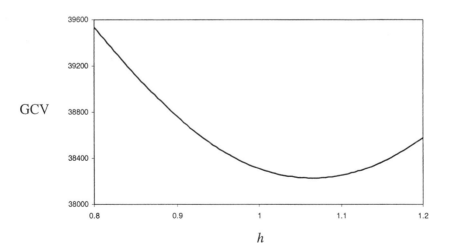

Figure 3–9 Search for the optimum bandwidth (h) based on the generalized cross validation (GCV) criterion for a local linear regression with a Gaussian kernel. Optimal bandwidth $h = 1.06$.

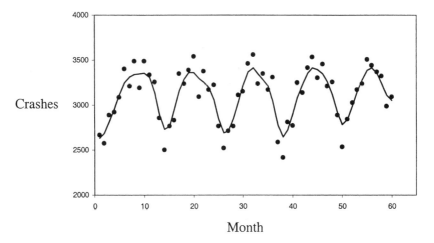

Figure 3-10 Observed and smoothed values for the Fatal Accident Reporting System (FARS) crash data based on a local linear regression, using a Gaussian kernel with bandwidth $h = 1.06$.

be obtained by constructing a smoothing window using the uniform kernel and replacing the central value with the median of all observations that fall within the window. The advantage of this approach is the resistance of the estimate to highly unusual observations that may occur at time points close to the one being smoothed. In Figure 3-11, a uniform kernel smooth of the weekly P&I data is compared to the moving median smoother. Both

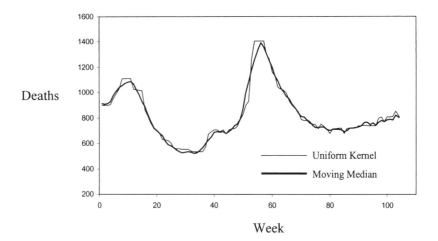

Figure 3-11 Smoothed estimates for the P&I mortality data based on uniform kernel and moving median smoothers both using a bandwidth of $h = 5$.

smoothes in this example are based on a bandwidth of $h = 5$. In this example, the median smoother appears to provide a somewhat smoother fit to the data than does kernel estimator. This result illustrates the increased resistance of the median-based approach to variations among observations in the smoothing window. Although this resistance lends robustness to the fit, potentially important observations in terms of disease surveillance, for example aberrations reflecting outbreak of an infectious disease, might be down weighted when using the median smother.

Confidence Intervals for One-Dimensional Smoothers

Although an apparent contradiction to the exploratory motivation underlying these types of smoothers, constructing confidence intervals for the smoothed fit may sometimes be informative. For example, observations that fall outside some measure of the random variation expected among the fitted values may be of interest. Several approaches for producing both pointwise and simultaneous confidence intervals for linear smoothers have been developed. For example, Wahba (1983) suggests pointwise confidence intervals for smoothing splines of the form

$$\hat{y}_k \pm z_{\alpha/2} \sqrt{\hat{\sigma}^2 \, w_{kk}}$$

where $z_{\alpha/2}$ is the appropriate percentile of the standard normal distribution, $\hat{\sigma}^2$ is an estimator of the residual variance, and w_{kk} is the kth diagonal component of the $\mathbf{H}$ matrix in Eq. 3–12. Similarly, a general asymptotic confidence interval for the linear smoothers is given by

$$\hat{y}_k \pm z_{\alpha/2} \sqrt{\hat{\sigma}^2 \sum_{l=1}^{N} w_{kl}^2} \tag{3–15}$$

where w_{kl} is the element in the kth row and 1th column of the weight matrix. Although empirical evidence indicates that intervals based on Eq. 3–15 provide adequate average coverage, their performance is likely to be highly nonuniform across the range of the observations (Cummins et al., 2001; Eubank and Speckman, 1993). Alternative approaches that pose greater computational challenges but yield improved pointwise performance include estimating a localized residual variance (Cummins et al. 2001), correcting for the bias in the linear smoother (Xia, 1998; Eubank and Spekman, 1993) and a wide range of bootstrap methods (Choi and Hall, 2000; Faraway, 1990). A simultaneous version of the interval Eq. 3–15 can be derived using a Bonferroni adjustment on the standard deviate. Limited simulation experiments indicate that the resulting intervals have acceptable average simultaneous coverage and are fairly uniform, at least in the interior of the data. Alternatively, Eubank and Speckman (1993) suggest a simple simultaneous confidence interval for kernel smoothers given by

$$\hat{y}_k \pm \frac{\hat{\sigma}^2 \, V \, z_{\alpha/2N}}{\sqrt{h}}$$

where

$$V = \sqrt{\int K(t)^2 \, dt}$$

The remaining issue in constructing confidence bounds is selecting an estimator for $\hat{\sigma}^2$. Wahba (1983) suggests an estimator similar to the GCV criterion given by

$$\hat{\sigma}^2 = \frac{\sum\limits_{k=1}^{N} (\hat{y}_k - y_k)^2}{N - \sum\limits_{k=1}^{N} w_{kk}}$$

Gasser et al.(1986) suggest an estimator based on differences in the observed values, as opposed to a measure of the selected fit. Their variance estimate, given by

$$\hat{\sigma}^2 = \frac{1}{N-2} \sum\limits_{k=1}^{N-2} \frac{y_k}{2} - y_{k+1} + \frac{y_{k+2}}{2}$$

appears to perform quite well based on empirical investigations (Dette et al., 1998).

Boundary Effects

The smoothers described here require subdividing the collection of observations into successive partitions based on the selection of the particular value for the smoothing parameter. Near the boundaries of the data, the information available to construct the smoothed estimates becomes more and more limited until the point, at the first and last observations, where only information from one side of the point of interest is available. The bias introduced by this boundary effect may be substantial (Fox, 2000) and is especially troubling in public health surveillance because observations from the recent past are likely to be of particular interest. Methods for adjusting smoothing procedures to account for boundary effects include using modified kernel functions near the boundary (Muller and Stadt-muller, 1999) and generating pseudodata to append to the observations (Zhang et al., 1999). A point favoring the use of the local linear smoother is that bias near the endpoints in this approach is less than that in comparable kernel smoothing methods (Fox, 2000). In most applications, it is probably advisable to reduce the influence of a portion of the earliest and most recent observations when using data-driven methods for selecting the smoothing parameter. This reduction can be accomplished, for example, using the weighted version of the GCV criterion given in Eq. 3–10.

SMOOTHING TECHNIQUES FOR SPATIALLY-REFERENCED HEALTH SURVEILLANCE DATA

I now focus on nonparametric smoothing approaches that can be useful for increasing the signal-to-noise ratio in maps of aggregated public health surveillance data. A thematic map of the reported incidence rates of primary and secondary (P&S) syphilis for the year 2000 among counties in North Carolina illustrates the type of data to which these approaches can be applied (Fig. 3–12). Easy to use mapping software has made the use of this type of map extremely common, both in the epidemiologic investigations and in public health surveillance reporting (CDC, 2001). Unfortunately, thematic maps suffer from the same interpretation difficulties as do the temporally reference data in that the observed rate in a given area reflects an unknown combination of the effect of the true underlying risk and the random variation in the observable measure of that risk. Interpreting public health maps is hindered by the fact that different areas across the map may have strikingly different population sizes and, as a result, substantial differences in the stability of the observed rate estimates (Devine et al., 1994).

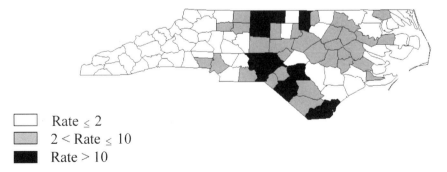

☐ Rate ≤ 2
▨ 2 < Rate ≤ 10
■ Rate > 10

Figure 3–12 Primary and secondary syphilis rates per 100,000 population by county in North Carolina, 2000.

In the following subsections, a collection of easy to use nonparametric approaches for exploratory visualization of potential geographic trends in aggregated public health surveillance data is reviewed. Research on methods for assessing the geographic attributes of disease risk has been, and remains, quite active (Lawson, 2001; Elliott et al., 2000). Focus is on purely exploratory approaches: more intensive methods for evaluating potential geographic trends in disease and injury risk (e.g., hierarchical spatial temporal modeling) are discussed in Chapters 7, 10, and 11.

Smoothing Neighborhoods

Creating two-dimensional smoothing neighborhoods surrounding the area of interest is a natural extension of the moving window techniques used for temporally referenced data. The spatial smoother for the value observed in area j, y_j, is again constructed as a linear combination of the observed values, such that

$$\hat{y}_j = \frac{\sum_{l=1}^{N} w_{jl} y_l I(y_l \in \eta_j)}{\sum_{l=1}^{N} w_{jl} I(y_l \in \eta_j)} \tag{3-16}$$

where w_{jl} are user-assigned weights and $I(y_l \in \eta_j)$ takes value one if area l is contained in the specified neighborhood, η_j, of area j, and zero otherwise. As with the temporal smoothers, criteria must be established to define each area's membership in the collection smoothing neighborhoods.

I consider two approaches to defining membership in η_j: distance and adjacency. For the distance based criteria, members of the smoothing neighborhood are defined as all areas having an identified geographic attribute (e.g., the area centroid or the closest point on the area boundary) within a specified distance of a geographic location associated with area j. Alternatively, η_j could be defined by adjacency such that all areas sharing a common boundary with area j are included in the smoothing neighborhood. An advantage of the adjacency definition is that distances that define the smoothing neighborhood do not need to be determined. However, the adjacency approach can be troublesome if the areas differ substantially in size so that some areas share boundaries with only a few neighbors.

An alternative to distance and adjacency criteria is to focus on creating smoothing neighborhoods with comparable population sizes. When this neighborhood definition is used, each area surrounding area j is evaluated for membership in η_j, in order of distance from area j, until a fixed population size is attained within the neighborhood.

Smoothers for Spatial Data

Once the smoothing neighborhood is defined, several options are available for obtaining $\hat{y}_j$. For example, any of the kernel functions discussed earlier in this chapter could be used in Eq. 3–15 to define the w_{jl}'s based on relative distances within the smoothing neighborhood. Alternatively, because areas with large populations are likely to have more stable observed rates, a reasonable approach is the population-weighted smoother

$$\hat{y}_k = \frac{\sum_{l=1}^{N} p_l y_l \, I(y_l \in \eta_j)}{\sum_{l=1}^{N} p_l \, I(y_l \in \eta_j)} \tag{3–17}$$

where p_l is the population size in area l. A smoother with increase resistance to extreme values can be obtained by setting $\hat{y}_j$ equal to the median of the area-specific values observed in the smoothing neighborhood. A resmoothing approach in which the median smoothing process is carried out twice has also been suggested (Kafadar, 1994). Although the median smoother has the appeal of resistance to exceptionally high or low observed rates, especially if the smoothing neighborhood contains only a few areas, it does not take advantage of information on the relative population sizes of area j's neighbors. This information can be included in a resistant estimator by using a weighted median smoother (Cressie, 1991). In this approach, $\hat{y}_j$ is set equal to the rate observed in the area within the smoothing neighborhood that has a population size closest to the median population of all areas within η_j.

In Figure 3–13, the average, population-weighted average, median, and population-weighted median smoothes for the county P&S syphilis rates in North Carolina are compared using a distance-based neighborhood definition of 50 miles between county centroids. All the smoothed maps highlight the middle section of the state as an area of potentially elevated P&S syphilis risk more clearly than does the map of the observed rates in Figure 3–12. In this example, the maximum amount of smoothing is produced using the median estimator.

As with the one-dimensional smoothers, the size of the smoothing neighborhood has a much greater effect on the resulting level of smoothing than does the use of a particular smoothing approach. Direct extensions of kernel and smoothing spline approaches to two-dimensional smoothing are available (Gu, 2000; Hardle and Muller, 2000) enabling data-driven evaluation of smoothing parameters. A similar approach could be used in selecting the bandwidth for multivariate versions of local polynomial regres-

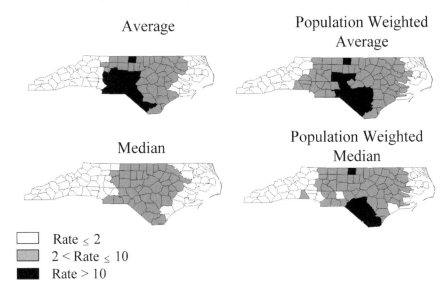

Average

Population Weighted
Average

Median

Population Weighted
Median

☐ Rate ≤ 2
▨ 2 < Rate ≤ 10
■ Rate > 10

Figure 3–13 Smoothed primary and secondary syphilis rates per 100,000 population by county in North Carolina, 2000, using different smoothers.

sion (Cleveland and Devlin, 1988). Again, a knowledgeable analyst should couple data-driven neighborhood size determination with an assessment of the adequacy of the smooth.

As an alternative to the spatial smoothers discussed thus far, Iterative Random Partitioning (IRP) uses a different approach to define the smoothing neighborhoods. In IRP, the user does not select the neighborhood size per se, but instead selects the number of neighborhoods. An IRP smooth is accomplished by the following steps:

1. Select a number $n \leq N$, where N is the total number of areas being mapped.
2. Randomly select n areas, called pivotal areas, from the N candidates.
3. Construct neighborhoods surrounding the pivotal areas by assigning each area to the neighborhood containing the nearest pivotal area.
4. Replace the observed rates for all members of each neighborhood by that neighborhood's population-weighted average rate.
5. Store results and return to step 1.

Steps 1 through 5 are repeated K times. The result is a collection of K possible smoothed values of the rate for each area, each of which is based on a random partitioning of the entire region. The smoothed rate for area j is then defined as the median of the K-iterated smoothed values. Figure 3–14 shows an IRP smooth for the North Carolina P&I syphilis rates based on using 20 pivotal counties and $K = 1000$. This approach also highlights the

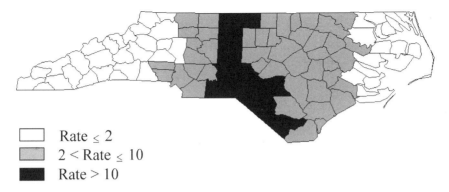

Rate ≤ 2
2 < Rate ≤ 10
Rate > 10

Figure 3–14 Primary and secondary syphilis rates per 100,000 population by county in North Carolina, 2000, smoothed using Iterative Random Partitioning (IRP).

center region of the state as one of potentially elevated risk. Although the IRP approach alters the parameter that controls the amount of smoothing by changing the size of the smoothing neighborhoods in each iteration, the number of pivotal areas still needs to be specified with a smaller value of n/N leading to smoother IRP maps.

Contour Maps

Several methods can be used to create continuous representations of potential trends in risk based on spatial interpolations of observed disease burden measures. For example, multivariate extensions of kernel smoothing and smoothing splines are available in some software packages. Alternative interpolation methods, for example, kriging (Carrat and Valleron, 1992), median polish (Cressie, 1991), and headbanging (Hansen, 1991), have been used to create continuous estimators of geographic trends in disease risk from area-specific observed measures.

SOFTWARE

Various proprietary software packages (e.g., Xplore, SAS, and S-Plus) have built in functionality to perform some or all of the smoothing approaches described in this chapter. A particularly appealing feature in some packages is the ability to visually assess the effect of altering the smoothing parameter on the fit. In addition, many free software packages (e.g., CRIME-STAT and R) have either built in capability to perform these types of smoothing procedures or have the functionality available using download-able code. Many packages, both proprietary and free, also seamlessly interface with GIS software. In many cases exploratory temporal and spatial assessments can be integrated into ongoing GIS-based surveillance activities (Wall and Devine, 2000). Additional information on software can be obtained at http://www.healthgis- li.com/researchers /software.htm and http://socserv2.socsci.mcmaster.ca/jfox/Books/Nonparametric-Regression/computing.html.

REFERENCES

Brookmeyer, R. and Yasui, Y. (1995). Statistical analysis of passive disease registry data. *Biometrics* **51,** 831–842.

Buhlmann, P. (1998). Sieve bootstrap for smoothing in nonstationary time series. *The Annals of Statistics* **26,** 48–83.

Buhlmann, P. and Kunsch, H. (1999). Block length selection in the bootstrap for time series. *Computational Statistics & Data Analysis* **31,** 295–310.

Carrat, F. and Valleron, A. (1992). Epidemiologic mapping using the kriging method: Application to an influenza-like illness epidemic in France. *American Journal of Epidemiology* **135,** 1293–300.

Centers for Disease Control and Prevention. (2001). *Sexually Transmitted Disease Surveillance, 2000.* Atlanta: U.S. Department of Health and Human Services.

Centers for Disease Control and Prevention. (2002). Morbidity and Mortality Weekly Report Mortality Tables. http://wonder.cdc.gov/mmwr.

Chaudhuri, P. and Marron, J. (1999). Sizer for exploration of structures in curves. *Journal of the American Statistical Association* **94,** 807–823.

Choi, E. and Hall, P. (2000). Bootstrap confidence regions computed from auto-regressions of arbitrary order. *Journal of the Royal Statistical Society Series B* **62,** 461–477.

Cleveland, W. and Devlin, S. (1988). Locally weighted regression: An approach to regression by local fitting. *Journal of the American Statistical Association* **83,** 596–610.

Craven, P. and Wahba, G. (1979). Smoothing noisy data with spline functions. *Numerical Mathematics* **31,** 377–403.

Cressie, N. (1991). *Statistics for Spatial Data.* New York: Wiley.

Cummins, D., Filloon, T., and Nychka, D. (2001). Confidence intervals for non-parametric curve estimates: Toward more uniform pointwise coverage. *Journal of the American Statistical Association* **96,** 233–246.

Dette, H., Munk, A., and Wagner, T. (1998). Estimating the variance in nonparametric regression—what is a reasonable choice? *Journal of the Royal Statistical Society Series B* **60,** 751–764.

Devine, O., Louis, T.A., and Halloran, M.E. (1994). Empirical Bayes methods for stabilizing incidence rates before mapping. *Epidemiology* **5,** 622–630.

Elliott, P., Wakefield, J., Best, N., and Briggs, D. (2000). *Spatial Epidemiology: Methods and Applications.* Oxford: Oxford University Press.

Epanechnikov, V. (1969). Nonparametric estimation of a multivariate probability density. *Theory of Probability and Its Applications* **14**, 153–158.

Eubank, R. and Speckman, P. (1993). Confidence bands in nonparametric regression. *Journal of the American Statistical Society* **88**, 1287–1301.

Faraway, J. (1990). Bootstrap selection of bandwidth and confidence bands for nonparametric regression. *Journal of Statistical Computation and Simulation* **37**, 37–44.

Fox, J. (2000). *Nonparametric Simple Regression: Smoothing Scatterplots*. Thousand Oaks: Sage Publications.

Gasser, T. and Muller, H.G. (1979). Kernel estimation of regression functions. In Gasser, T. and Rosenblatt, M., eds. *Smoothing Techniques for Curve Estimation*. Heidelberg: Springer-Verlag, pp. 23–68.

Gasser, T., Sroka, L., and Jennen-Steinmertz, C. (1986). Residual variance and residual pattern in nonlinear regression. *Biometrika* **73**, 625–633.

Gelman, A., Park, D., Ansolabehere, S., Price, P., and Minnite, L. (2001). Models, assumptions and model checking in ecological regression. *Journal of the Royal Statistical Society Series A* **164**, 101–118.

Gu, C. (2000). Multivariate spline regression. In Schimek, M., ed. *Smoothing and Regression: Approaches, Computation and Application*. New York: Wiley.

Hansen, K. (1991). Headbanging: Robust smoothing in the plane. *IEEE Transactions on Geoscience and Remote Sensing* **29**, 369–378.

Hardle, W. and Bowman, A. (1988). Bootstrapping in nonparametric regression: Local adaptive smoothing and confidence bands. *Journal of the American Statistical Society* **83**, 102–110.

Hardle, W., Lutkepohl, H., and Chen, R. (1997). A review of nonparametric time series analysis. *International Statistical Review* **65**, 49–72.

Hardle, W. and Muller, M. (2000). Multivariate and semiparametric kernel regression. In Schimek, M. ed. *Smoothing and Regression: Approaches, Computation and Application*. New York: Wiley, pp. 357–392.

Hart, J. (1997). *Nonparametric Smoothing and Lack of Fit Tests*. New York: Springer-Verlag.

Herrmann, E. (1997). Local bandwidth choice in kernel regression estimation. *Journal of Computational and Graphical Statistics* **6**, 35–54.

Herrmann, E (2000). Variance estimation and bandwidth selection for kernel regression. In Schimek, M. ed. *Smoothing and Regression: Approaches, Computation and Application*. New York: Wiley, pp. 71–108.

Hurvich, C., Simonoff, J., and Tsai, C. (1998). Smoothing parameter selection in nonparametric regression using an improved Akaike information criterion. *Journal of the Royal Statistical Society Series B* **60**, 271–293.

Hutwagner, L., Maloney, E., Bean, N., Slutsker, L., and Martin, S. (1997). Using laboratory-based surveillance data for prevention: An algorithm for detecting *Salmonella* outbreaks. *Emerging Infectious Diseases* **3**, 395–400.

Jones, M., Marron, J., and Sheather, S. (1996). A brief survey of bandwidth selection for density estimation. *Journal of the American Statistical Society* **91**, 401–407.

Kafadar, K. (1994). Choosing among two-dimensional smoothers in practice. *Computational Statistics and Data Analysis* **18**, 419–439.

Lange, K. (1999). *Numerical Analysis for Statisticians*. New York: Springer-Verlag.

Lawson, A. (2001). *Statistical Methods in Spatial Epidemiology*. New York: Wiley.

Marron, J. and Tsybakov, A. (1995). Visual error criteria for qualitative smoothing. *Journal of the American Statistical Association* **90**, 499–507.

Muller, H., and Stadtmuller, U. (1999). Multivariate boundary kernels and a continuous least squares principle. *Journal of the Royal Statistical Society Series B* **61**, 439–458.

National Highway Traffic Safety Administration. (2002). Fatal Accident Reporting System (FARS). http://www-fars.nhtsa.dot.gov.

Park, B., and Turlach, B. (1992). Practical performance of several data driven bandwidth selectors. *Computational Statistics* **7**, 251–270.

Sain, S. and Scott, D. (1996). On locally adaptive density estimation. *Journal of the American Statistical Association* **91**, 1525–1534.

Sarda, P. and Vieu, P. (2000). Kernel regression. In Schimek, M. ed. *Smoothing and Regression: Approaches, Computation and Application.* New York: Wiley, pp. 43–70.

Schucany, W. (1995). Adaptive bandwidth choice for kernel regression. *Journal of the American Statistical Association* **90**, 535–540.

Silverman, B.W. (1984). Spline smoothing: The equivalent variable kernel method. *Annals of Statistics* **12**, 898–916.

U.S. Department of Health and Human Services, National Committee on Vital and Health Statistics. (2001). *Information for Health, A Strategy for Building the National Health Information Infrastructure.* Washington: U.S. Department of Health and Human Services.

Wahba, G. (1983). Bayesian confidence intervals for the cross-validated smoothing spline. *Journal of the Royal Statistical Society Series B* **45**, 133–150.

Wahba, G. (1990). *Spline Models for Observational Data.* Philadelphia: SIAM.

Wall, P. and Devine, O. (2000). Interactive analysis of the spatial distribution of disease using a geographic information system. *Geographical Systems* **2**, 243–256.

Xia, Y. (1998). Bias-corrected confidence bands in nonparametric regression. *Journal of the Royal Statistical Society Series B* **60**, 797–811.

Zhang, S., Karunamuni, R., and Jones, M. (1999). An improved estimator of the density function at the boundary. *Journal of the American Statistical Society* **94**, 1231–1241.

4

Temporal Factors in Public Health Surveillance: Sorting Out Age, Period, and Cohort Effects

THEODORE R. HOLFORD

Temporal patterns are an important aspect of public health surveillance. Time can enter into the analysis of disease trends in a variety of ways. Age is a critical risk factor for most diseases; however, in public health surveillance, other temporal trends, especially those attributed to calendar time or to year of birth are often of more interest.

A common problem in analyzing trends over time is removing the effect of age, so that the true effect associated with chronological time can be observed in the data. For example, in a group that is relatively old in comparison to a referent population, we would expect the incidence rate for stroke to be higher due to the relatively higher risk of the group as a whole. The task of controlling for age is often accomplished by using direct or indirect methods of standardizing rates. Although simple, this approach is limited. For example, details that are important for understanding time trends for disease are lost in the averaging process for generating a summary rate.

Initial approaches to analyzing time trends in detail rely on presenting graphically age-specific rates and considering whether the resulting age patterns are consistent with knowledge about the biology of a disease. Although a visual analysis of time trends is important, a more formal analysis that includes temporal effects is also necessary. More formal modeling requires understanding the limitations in the results that arise from the relationships among the concepts of time used by epidemiologists.

This chapter considers three temporal perspectives used by epidemiologists and the inherent redundancy that develops from these perspectives. Next, it explores graphical methods that provide good preliminary analyses of time trends. Finally, formal statistical methods that summarize temporal trends by fitting statistical models to the data are discussed. Each method is applied to data on either lung or breast cancer incidence.

TEMPORAL COMPONENTS OF DISEASE

Age, which is labeled t_A, is an important cause of most diseases. For example, older persons are often more vulnerable to disease because aging has degenerative effects on health. Thus, age must be controlled for in any analysis of temporal trends. Age is usually not the primary interest in public health surveillance but is rather a nuisance factor that can mislead interpretations if it is not taken into account. For example, in most parts of the world, the average age is increasing, so the crude incidence rate for a degenerative disease should also increase with calendar time, even in the absence of temporal trends for important risk factors.

Of more immediate interest are the effects associated with calendar time, because sudden increases in rates can prompt concern for the public health of a population. For example, identifying a change in the populationwide exposure to an important risk factor may motivate strategies for controlling disease by reducing that exposure. Similarly, decreases in rates can suggest that something is "going right" with disease control. Period, which is labeled t_P, is time associated with the date of occurrence of disease. Unfortunately, observational data recorded by vital statistics registries are sometimes affected by artifacts that change the estimates of disease rates but do not affect the true underlying disease burden. For example, increased knowledge about the pathology of a disease can cause coders who record the cause of death or the diagnosis of disease to change the case definition. Such a change can result in a period change in the rates under study, because all age groups may be similarly affected. In a similar way, changes in medical technology (e.g., a more sensitive screening test) can cause cases to be diagnosed that would otherwise be missed, thus artificially inflating the incidence and prevalence of the disease.

The weakness of trying to draw conclusions about temporal trends by limiting the analysis to considering changes in period summary rates is that the population changes dynamically over time. Yet another analytic perspective arises from analyzing the follow-up experience of the same generation of individuals as they age. It is convenient to refer to these groups by the year in which they were born and to refer to the temporal pattern as a birth cohort effect, sometimes known simply as a cohort effect, which is labeled t_C. The relationship among these temporal factors is shown in the Lexis diagram in Figure 4–1 (Keiding, 1998).

Biological factors that can affect a cohort trend may well be associated with birth itself. For example, diethylstilbesterol was once used during pregnancy to lower the risk of spontaneous abortion in women with such a history, even though little scientific evidence supported this therapy. Young women whose mothers had used the drug while they were in utero were found to have a greatly increased risk of vaginal cancer. Thus, a sudden increase in vaginal cancer rates might be expected for a birth cohort that had a substantial history of diethylstilbesterol exposure before birth. Detecting

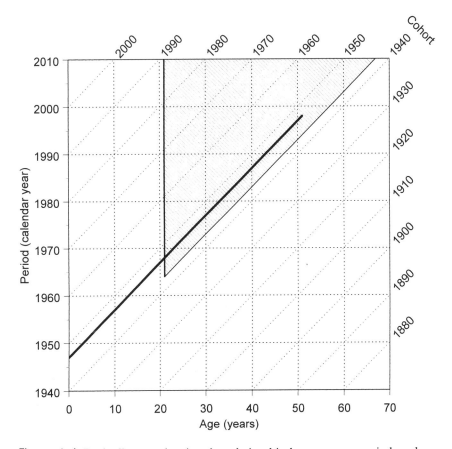

Figure 4–1 Lexis diagram showing the relationship between age, period, and cohort. The hatched triangle represents the cohort exposed over time to a factor introduced to 22-year-olds in 1964 and in subsequent years.

such an effect through surveillance would require looking for a more sub-
tle temporal change than would be seen for a period effect (e.g., the effect
would first be apparent only among young women). If this exposure contributed to most of the temporal trend, the most effective approach to the
analysis would be to track birth cohort changes over time, instead of limiting the analysis to period trends.

Factors that influence cohort effects are not limited to exposures related to birth, but include exposures that primarily affect the cohort and
not the population as a whole. For example, efforts to increase cigarette
smoking have been most effective when advertisers focus on young adults.
Among American men, an increased rate accompanied the practice of giving free cigarettes to new recruits during World War II. Among American
women, the first sharp increase occurred some years later, as a result of a
cynical advertising campaign that equated smoking with women's libera-
tion. Both of these campaigns primarily affected certain generations; hence,
their effects on subsequent smoking rates would gradually unfold if trends
were monitored from the perspective of period (Fig. 4–1). Monitoring the
effect of such campaigns would be far more effective if time were considered not just from the period perspective but from the cohort perspective
as well.

AGE, PERIOD, AND COHORT TRENDS

The temporal effects of age, period, and cohort have useful epidemiologic
interpretations with respect to the types of variables that might affect disease surveillance. However, simultaneously considering these factors has
limitations because the factors are not independent. In the two-dimensional
Lexis diagram, Fig. 4–1, all possible combinations of age, period, and cohort can be identified, rendering unnecessary the third dimension that
would typically be needed to represent these three factors. This rendering
implies that these factors are uniquely interrelated. In addition, we shall
see that the typical way in which time is categorized to tabulate data for
constructing rates does not necessarily result in unique categories.

Relationship between Age, Period and Cohort

If any two temporal factors are known, the third can be derived. For example, the diagnosis of cancer on the 53rd birthday of a person born in
1944 would be recorded in 1997. A linear relationship among temporal
effects can be expressed more generally using the algebraic expression
$t_P = t_C + t_A$. This interrelationship is exact and has nothing to do with the

categorization of time when constructing tables of rates. As is shown in the following section, the loss of temporal detail from grouping time into intervals further lowers precision when all three temporal factors are considered.

Interval Overlap

When population-based data are tabulated for calculating age-specific rates, time must be grouped into intervals. Data are commonly presented in 5- or 10-year intervals for age and period. I will consider primarily the use of the same interval widths; because the use of unequal intervals raises still further issues in data analysis (see Unequal Intervals, below).

A typical display of rates is shown in Table 4–1, in which 5-year age and period categories were used to construct incidence rates for breast cancer in women. The rows represent age groups, the columns represent periods, and individual cohorts may be followed down the diagonals. Because the age and period intervals are somewhat crude measures for these times,

Table 4–1 Breast cancer incidence data from the surveillance, epidemiology and end results (SEER) program for premenopausal* women from 1973 to 1997

Age (Years)	Period (Calendar year)				
	1973–1977	1978–1982	1983–1987	1988–1992	1993–1997
	Number of cases				
25–29	359	437	460	419	413
30–34	937	1275	1466	1507	1484
35–39	1718	2298	3230	3686	3756
40–44	3095	3289	4954	6761	7439
45–49	5357	4687	5944	8263	10,801
	Person years				
25–29	4,072,026	4,894,238	5,267,236	5,106,372	4,667,668
30–34	3,388,205	4,467,657	5,010,563	5,407,370	5,328,697
35–39	2,724,326	3,507,789	4,362,147	5,011,399	5,517,088
40–44	2,596,365	2,861,964	3,511,195	4,477,439	5,157,005
45–49	2,738,703	2,678,223	2,810,580	3,430,255	4,328,342
	Rate per 100,000 person years				
25–29	8.82	8.93	8.73	8.21	8.85
30–34	27.65	28.54	29.26	27.87	27.85
35–39	63.06	65.51	74.05	73.55	68.08
40–44	119.21	114.92	141.09	151.00	144.25
45–49	195.60	175.00	211.49	240.89	249.54

Women under 50 years of age.

Source: (http://seer.cancer.gov/seerstat/).

the cohorts identified along the diagonals suffer further ambiguity. For example, a woman aged 30 to 34 years when diagnosed with cancer during the 1993–1997 period might have been born as early as 1958 or as late as the end of 1967, that is, during the period 1958–1967. Similarly, a 35- to 39-year-old woman would have been born in the period 1963–1972. Short-term cohort changes over time are more difficult to identify because the intervals are twice as wide, 10 instead of 5 years; and, they overlap.

Disease registries often record date of birth, which permits the numerators to be tabulated by fixing the width of the cohort intervals. However, if the data are tabulated by age using equal cohort intervals, a similar interval overlap issue occurs for period. Likewise, there would be overlap for age intervals for a period by cohort tabulation. Robertson and Boyle (1986) considered an approach that avoids the problem of interval overlap, but its practical benefit is limited (Clayton and Schifflers, 1987b; Tango, 1988; Osmond and Gardner, 1989).

A more effective approach for reducing the masking of short-term changes in trend is to refine the tabulation of data by using shorter time intervals. For example, Tarone et al. (1997) use 2-year age and period intervals that gave rise to 4-year overlapping cohort intervals. If the number of cases in the cells of such a table is large enough to provide accurate estimates of the rates, discerning sudden changes in the rates should be possible. The approach often works well for analyzing national mortality rates or tabulating data on diseases with relatively high rates, but it can perform poorly for an uncommon disease or a rate based on a small population.

Effect of Dependence on Linear Trends

The interpretational difficulty that arises from the linear dependence among the temporal factors can be illustrated by a hypothetical model in which the log rates are linearly related to these factors:

$$\log \lambda(t_A, t_P, t_C) = \mu + \beta_A t_A + \beta_P t_P + \beta_C t_C \tag{4-1}$$

I have already noted that $t_P = t_C + t_A$, so

$$\log \lambda(t_A, t_P, t_C) = \mu + \beta_A t_A + \beta_P(t_C + t_A) + \beta_C t_C \tag{4-2}$$

$$= \mu + (\beta_A + \beta_P)t_A + (\beta_C + \beta_P)t_C$$

Although the model started with three regression parameters, one for each temporal variable, the linear dependence implies that only two combinations of these parameters can be identified. This limitation, called the identifiability problem, is inherent in statistical models used to analyze the effects of age, period, and cohort.

The implications of the identifiability problem are that, for a particular set of data, any combination of regression parameters that gives rise to identical values of $(\beta_A + \beta_P)$ and $(\beta_C + \beta_P)$ provides identical values for the log rate. The idea may also be expressed in the context of the true value of the parameter, which is signified by an asterisk. A particular value of the parameter that would be estimated by fitting the model to the data would, on average, be related to the true value by

$$\beta_A = \beta_A^* + v$$

$$\beta_P = \beta_P^* - v \qquad (4\text{--}3)$$

$$\beta_C = \beta_C^* + v$$

where v is an arbitrary constant. Because v is arbitrary, the parameters in the model can take any value. However, this same constant biases each parameter, thus certain combinations allow one to get rid of the constant altogether; for example, $(\beta_A + \beta_P) = (\beta_A^* + \beta_P^*)$

GRAPHICAL DISPLAYS

An early approach for recognizing cohort effects was to use graphical displays of age trends in which different line styles connected the rates for each period and cohort. Figure 4–2 shows such a relationship using data on lung cancer in Connecticut women. Solid lines connect the age-specific rates for the identical periods, and the broken lines, for specific cohorts. The effect of age from a period perspective tends to plateau, or even decline, for the oldest ages, where the rates increase steadily for individual cohorts. The rate increase offers a biologically more plausible pattern that is consistent with what is generally known about carcinogenesis. Therefore, the graph suggests that generational changes in exposure are more likely to be affecting temporal trends for lung cancer in women. This interpretation is also consistent with the view that most lung cancer is caused by cigarette smoking, a habit that tends to be fixed when a generation is approximately 20 years of age.

In Figure 4–2, age so dominates the temporal trends that some subtler features that might arise from the effects of period or cohort are difficult to see. An alternative approach is to plot age-specific rates against period

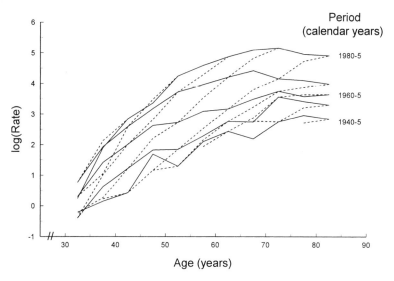

Figure 4–2 Period (solid lines) and cohort (broken lines) trends by age for lung cancer in Connecticut women. *Source:* Holford, T.R. (1998). Age-period-cohort analysis. In Armitage, P. and Colton, T., eds. *Encyclopedia of Biostatistic*, pp. 82–99.

or cohort (Fig. 4–3). Such displays can be helpful in monitoring temporal trends, and they can suggest potentially useful models. Lines that are more nearly parallel for one temporal effect suggest that this effect had the potential to offer a more parsimonious description of the age-specific rates.

In displays that attempt to distinguish period and cohort effects, adopting the same scale in each case is often helpful (Fig. 4–3). In general, when default dimensions are used in constructing a graph, more cohorts are represented in a typical set of data, and the periods are more spread out than the cohorts. The visual impression is a straightening of the curves (Fig. 4–4) which hinders comparing the effects of period and cohort.

Weinkam and Sterling (1991) have described an interesting way of displaying contours for rates that incorporates the concept of the Lexis diagram and also equal density of time scales for all three temporal axes; an idea that Keiding (1998) attributes to Lexis. This approach uses a triangular grid as the basis for the plot (Fig. 4–5). In a contour plot, the trend is steep when the lines are close together and flat when they are far apart. Hence, in Figure 4–5, a plateau for age is reached along the period axis, which is especially apparent for 1980. The continually crossing lines along the cohort axis imply that the rates are always increasing with age.

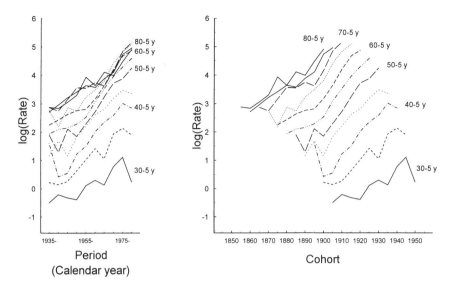

Figure 4–3 Age trends by period and cohort for lung cancer incidence rates in Connecticut women. *Source:* Holford, T.R. (1998). Age-period-cohort analysis. In Armitage, P. and Colton, T., eds. *Encyclopedia of Biostatistic*, pp. 82–99.

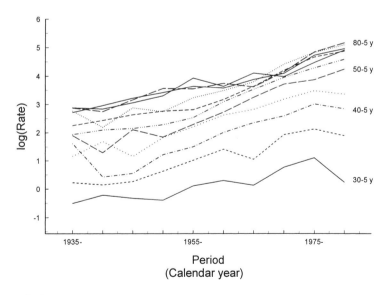

Figure 4–4 Alternative spread for abscissa; age trends by period for lung cancer incidence in Connecticut women. *Source:* Holford, T.R. (1998). Age-period-cohort analysis. In Armitage, P. and Colton, T., eds. *Encyclopedia of Biostatistic*, pp. 82–99.

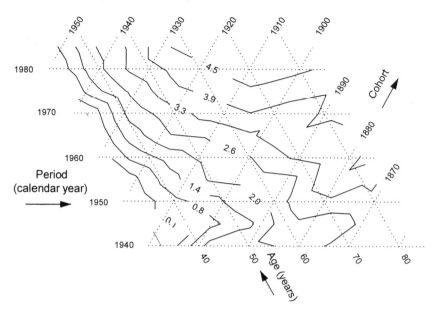

Figure 4–5 Contour plot of age, period, and cohort trends in lung cancer incidence for Connecticut women using a triangular grid. *Source:* Holford, T.R. (1998). Age-period-cohort analysis. In Armitage, P. and Colton, T., eds. *Encyclopedia of Biostatistic*, pp. 82–99.

MODEL FITTING FOR TEMPORAL TRENDS

Now a more formal approach to analyzing temporal trends is considered. A model with equal interval widths for age and period will be fitted to tabulated data. Let $t_A(=1, \ldots, T_A)$ represent an index for the age groups, and $t_P(=1, \ldots, T_P)$ and $t_C(=1, \ldots, T_C = T_A + T_P - 1)$ represent the corresponding indices for period and cohort. For the data in Table 4–1, t_A identifies the rows of the tables, t_P identifies the columns, and $t_C = t_P - t_A + T_A$ identifies the upper-left to lower-right diagonals, beginning with the cell in the lower-left corner of the table. A log-linear, age-period-cohort model for the disease rate may be expressed as

$$\log \lambda (t_A, t_P, t_C) = \mu + \alpha(t_A) + \pi(t_P) + \gamma(t_C) \qquad (4\text{–}4)$$

where μ is an intercept, $\alpha(t_A)$ the effect of age, $\pi(t_P)$ the effect of period, and $\gamma(t_C)$ the effect of cohort. This equation has the same general form as an analysis of variance model with only main effects. Thus, an additional constraint must be used, such as $\alpha(T_A) = \pi(T_P) = \gamma(T_C) = 0$, or the so-called "usual constraints" in which $\sum \alpha(t_A) = \sum \pi(t_P) = \sum \gamma(t_C) = 0$. Unfortunately, these constraints do not solve the uniqueness problem, and a further constraint is necessary. The source of this problem is the linear relationship between these indices, which have already been noted.

The numerator will be used for the rate (i.e., the number of new cases of disease for incidence, or the number of deaths from a specified cause for mortality), as the response variable, $Y(t_A, t_P, t_C)$. This response is assumed to have a Poisson distribution with mean $\lambda(t_A, t_P, t_C) n(t_A, t_P, t_C)$. Using the log-linear model for the rates shown in Eq. 4–4, a corresponding model is obtained for the mean numerator,

$$\log E[Y(t_A, t_P, t_C)] = \mu + \alpha(t_A) + \pi(t_P) + \gamma(t_C) + \log n(t_A, t_P, t_C) \quad (4\text{–}5)$$

where $\log n(t_A, t_P, t_C)$ is an offset term. This model is a generalized linear model, which can be fitted by software available in a variety of statistical packages.

Many statistical software packages allow for the possibility of linear dependence among covariates, either by using generalized inverses or by setting arbitrary constraints on the parameters. The results from the various approaches can be very different, depending on the program used, and even depending on the order in which the temporal effects are presented to the model. To better understand the need for additional constraints, the trend for a particular temporal factor can be represented in the framework of simple linear regression, which identifies the overall trend or slope, as well as the departure from that trend, including any curvature. In the case of the usual constraints, this trend can be represented by a linear-curvature partition of effects in which $\alpha(t_A) = i_A \beta_A + \breve{\alpha}(t_A)$, where $i_A = t_A - \bar{t}_A$ and $\breve{\alpha}(t_A)$ is the curvature or residuals about the line. If period and cohort effects are similarly partitioned, the model presented in Eq. 4–4 can be represented as

$$\log \lambda(t_A, t_P, t_C) = \mu + [i_A \beta_A + \breve{\alpha}(t_A)] + [i_P \beta_P + \breve{\pi}(t_P)] + [i_C \beta_C + \breve{\gamma}(t_C)]$$

$$= \mu + i_A(\beta_A + \beta_P) + i_C(\beta_C + \beta_P) + \breve{\alpha}(t_A) + \breve{\pi}(t_P) + \breve{\gamma}(t_C)$$

$$(4\text{–}6)$$

because $i_P = i_A + i_C$. All curvature effects, $\breve{\alpha}(\cdot)$, $\breve{\pi}(\cdot)$, and $\breve{\gamma}(\cdot)$, can be estimated, which means that they are unique and not changed by arbitrary constraints that may be decided by the statistical software. However, the individual slopes, β_A, β_P, and β_C, cannot be estimated, and can actually take any value, but they each have in common an unidentifiable constant as shown in Eq. 4–3 (Holford, 1983). Many implications flow from these basic results that profoundly affect the ability to interpret the results of model fitting. These implications are explained in the following subsection.

Significance Testing

The goal of analyzing multiple factors is to examine the effect of one factor in the presence of the others. If age, period, and cohort are included as nominal variables, these effects can be partitioned equivalently in terms of linear and curvature trends. For example, it can be determined whether removing period from a model with all three factors significantly worsens the fit. However, Eq. 3–6 shows that the only effect for period that can be removed is period curvature. Therefore, the test of period in the presence of age and cohort is a test of period curvature, with degrees of freedom, $df = T_P - 2$. By including the effect of age and cohort in the model, it is unavoidable to also include a linear period component, and the three linear terms are so hopelessly entangled that they cannot be separated. Likewise, the effect of cohort in the presence of age and period, and age in the presence of period and cohort can only determine curvature components, and not the linear term.

The inability to determine the overall linear component of trend is a serious limitation for any analyses that attempt to consider all three factors simultaneously, because the component determines the overall direction of the particular temporal trend. The fact that it cannot be determined whether the period effects are increasing or decreasing with time has led some authors to dismiss the formal analysis of these factors altogether (Rogers, 1982; Kupper et al., 1985; Moolgavkar et al., 1998). However, several interesting quantities remain as effects that are not affected by the identifiability problem, so will continue to be pursued, albeit with considerable care. Ways of doing the calculations for these quantities will be demonstrated with a numerical example.

Curvature Hypotheses

We have seen that the curvature component in the partition of temporal effects is estimable, and we will now explore the implications of that fact in greater detail. Curvature means any departure from a linear trend. This departure has been effectively used in several ways:

1. *Second differences.* These are differences in the trends for two adjacent times, for example, for period we might consider

$$[\pi(t_P + 2) - \pi(t_P + 1)] - [\pi(t_P + 1) - \pi(t_P)] =$$
$$\pi(t_P + 2) - 2\pi(t_P + 1) + \pi(t_P)$$

which is estimable (Tango and Kurashina, 1987).

2. *Change in slope.* Second differences represent the change in trend in two adjacent time points, but this idea can be extended to trend changes over longer periods (Tarone and Chu, 1996).

3. *Polynomial trends.* Temporal effects are represented by including integer powers, t^p; but the coefficient for the first order term, $p = 1$, is not estimable whereas all higher order terms are (Holford, 1983, 1985).
4. *Splines.* Spline functions are sometimes preferred for representing curves, but it is useful to first remove the linear component by constructing variables that are orthogonal to linear trend.

The change in slope may be estimated through the use of contrasts. If c_k represents a series of specified constants, the contrast estimate for a series of estimated regression parameters is given by $\hat{C} = \sum_k c_k \hat{\theta}_k$. For the slope, or the change in slope, the set of constants that will yield the estimate of interest must be determined. To estimate the slope among a set of K regression parameters, we can find

$$\hat{C} = \frac{\sum_k \dot{k} \hat{\theta}_k}{\sum_k \dot{k}^2} = \sum_k \left[\frac{\dot{k}}{\sum_k \dot{k}^2} \right] \hat{\theta}_k \qquad (4\text{–}7)$$

which indicates that the needed constants are $c_i = \dot{k} / \sum_k \dot{k}^2$, where $\dot{k} = k - \bar{k}$; and these can be given in a row vector, $\mathbf{C} = (c_1, c_2, c_3, \ldots)$. If $\mathbf{C}_1$ represents the constants needed to determine the slope in one span of time, and $\mathbf{C}_2$ for the second, the constants required for determining the change in slope will be $\mathbf{C} = \mathbf{C}_2 - \mathbf{C}_1$.

For example, suppose that we have eight cohorts and wish to estimate the change in trend among the first five compared with the last four cohorts. For the first five, $(\dot{k}) = (-2, -1, 0, 1, 2)$ and $\sum_k \dot{k}^2 = 10$. Therefore, the vector of constants for slope in the first five cohorts will be $\mathbf{C}_1 = (-0.2, -0.1, 0, 0.1, 0.2, 0, 0, 0)$. Similarly, for the last four cohorts, $(\dot{k}) = (-1.5, -0.5, 0.5, 1.5)$ and $\sum_k \dot{k}^2 = 5$, yielding $\mathbf{C}_2 = (0, 0, 0, 0, -0.3, -0.1, 0.1, 0.3)$. Therefore, the contrast vector for the difference in slopes is

$$\mathbf{C} = \mathbf{C}_2 - \mathbf{C}_1 = (0.2, 0.1, 0, -0.1, -0.5, -0.1, 0.1, 0.3) \qquad (4\text{–}8)$$

Drift

When the age-period-cohort model is expressed in terms of the partitioned effects shown in Eq. 4–6, the sum of the overall slopes for period and cohort, $\beta_C + \beta_P$, can be estimated. Clayton and Schifflers (1987a,b) refer to this estimated sum as the net drift, and suggest its use as an overall indication of the direction of trend. To see how this quantity can be helpful in appreciating the overall direction for a set of rates, suppose that we are interested in the experience of individuals in a specified age group. As calendar time passes, the periods will increase along with the cohorts; in fact, it would be impossible to hold one period fixed while changing the other. Therefore, the net change will necessarily be determined by the combined effect of these two temporal effects (i.e., the net drift). If the net drift is to be determined using contrasts, the contrast vectors must be defined for period and cohort slopes.

Epochal Drift

If the effect of a temporal variable is not adequately represented by a straight line, a disadvantage of using net drift as a summary of trend is that curvature implies a change in direction over time. For example, if a set of rates had historically increased with period for a long time but had recently reached a plateau, that fact would not be reflected by the net drift. Instead, the current overall direction would be much more relevant for the purposes of disease surveillance. For current drift, the current period slope would be estimated using the most recent periods, $\tilde{\beta}_P$, and similarly, the recent slope for cohort, $\tilde{\beta}_C$, would be obtained. Individually, these parameters cannot be estimated, so the specific values depend on the arbitrary constraints used by the software to obtain a particular set of estimates. However, their sum, $\tilde{\beta}_P + \tilde{\beta}_C$, is estimable and would be referred to as *recent drift*.

This approach can be extended to epochs other than the extremes, which would also be estimable. However, for the results to be interpretable, the choice of period and cohort epochs must make sense. For example, if the drift for a given set of periods is of interest, cohorts that are represented in those periods should be chosen.

Epochal Constraints

An early approach for dealing with the identifiability problem involved an assumption that two adjacent temporal effects were identical, because there was no reason to believe that any change had occurred to the population that would have caused such an effect on the rates. For example, it might be assumed that the first two period effects were identical, $\pi(1) = \pi(2)$ (Barrett, 1973, 1978). The advantage of such an approach is that it yields a unique set of parameter estimates, thus offering a potential solution to the identifiability problem. However, such an approach must be adopted with care, because equating two effects may not have a sound basis. If the rationale is that "If there is no reason to expect a change during these years, then the effects will be assumed to be equal," a similar argument could be made for other periods.

Equating two effects is equivalent to assuming that the trend between two points has a slope of zero. In the framework described above, this could be accomplished by setting one of the slopes to zero (e.g., $\beta_P = 0$) in the case of period slope. This approach was adopted by Roush et al. (1985, 1987) in a comprehensive analysis of the incidence rates for major cancer sites, using data from the Connecticut Tumor Registry. To apply this approach, the overall trend for one temporal factor is estimated using the concepts that underlie simple linear regression. Once one of the overall slopes is set to zero, or to any other value, the remaining slopes would be identified, and a unique set of parameters could be estimated.

An alternative approach for estimating overall trend is to use the mean of the first differences for a temporal factor (Clayton and Schifflers, 1987b). In the case of period this becomes

$$\overline{\beta}_P = \frac{\sum_{t_P=1}^{T_P-1}[\pi(t_P + 1) - \pi(t_P)]}{T_P - 1} = \frac{\pi(T_P) - \pi(1)}{T_P - 1} \qquad (4\text{--}9)$$

This estimator depends only on the first and last period instead of all intermediate values, as is the case for the usual regression estimator. Thus, the mean of the first differences usually has a much larger standard error than that of the overall slope. This difference is especially true for cohort trends, because the first and last cohort effects depend on a single rate. In addition, the last cohort effect is only observed in the youngest age group, which typically has the smallest numerator and thus the largest standard error of the estimated log rate. Therefore, a regression-like estimator is preferred.

We have considered constraining trends based on the extremes (i.e., adjacent times or the entire time span for which data are available). An intermediate approach would be to apply this constraint during a limited epoch only. For example, suppose that an aggressive screening program was introduced on a specified date, which would be expected to influence period trend. In addition, we are confident that no artifactual or etiological changes have resulted in change with period before that date. Hence, it might make sense to constrain the period slope to be zero only during the epoch before the date when aggressive screening began. The validity of this assumption depends entirely on the accuracy of the assumption, because the identifiability problem implies that the assumption cannot be assessed by using the data themselves.

Projections

The problem of forecasting trends is one that is difficult, because assumptions must be made that cannot be verified. For example, the assumption might be made that the trends of the past will continue into the future, a strong assumption that may be unwarranted in a particular instance (Kupper et al., 1983). Nevertheless, this assumption is commonly made in other contexts and it seems reasonable in the absence of contradictory information. If a linear extrapolation is made for all three time parameters, the resulting projected rates are identifiable (Holford, 1985; Osmond, 1985). This property can be demonstrated by using a model that includes only linear terms. (Remember that more complicated models that include curvature terms present no new problems, because the curvature parameters are estimable.) If one wishes to extrapolate the rate for age t_A to the next period, $T_P + 1 = t_A + T_C + 1$, the calculation will involve an extrapolation to the next cohort; that is

$$\log \lambda(t_A, T_P + 1, T_C + 1) = \mu + \beta_A t_A + \beta_P(T_P + 1) + \beta_C(T_C + 1) \quad (4\text{--}10)$$

$$= \mu + (\beta_A + \beta_P)t_A + (\beta_C + \beta_P)(T_C + 1)$$

which is an estimable function of the slopes, as has been shown.

EXAMPLE

The data in Table 4–1 on breast cancer incidence among premenopausal women provide a numerical example of the methods that have been described for modeling trends in surveillance data. The data were collected by the SEER program of the National Cancer Institute and tabulated using SEER*Stat which can be obtained at no charge from the SEER Web site (http://seer.cancer.gov/seerstat/). Five-year intervals have been used for age and period. The five intervals for age and period give rise to nine cohorts. The data have been stored as a SAS dataset that includes indices for age (beginning at 1 for the 25- to 29-year-old age group) and period (beginning at 1 for the 1973–1978 group), along with the number of cases and the denominator for the rate.

The SAS program for conducting the analyses described is listed in the Appendix. In the data step, the cohort index is created, along with the offset, the crude estimate of the rate, and midinterval identifiers for age, period, and cohort. The model is fitted using "proc genmod," assuming that the numerator has a Poisson distribution (dist = p) and the specified offset variable. By including the temporal indices (a, p, and c) in a "classes" statement, they are treated as nominal categories, which essentially places no constraints on the resulting pattern for trend. This procedure uses an algorithm that tries to estimate a parameter for each level of a nominal variable, until it recognizes the impossibility of doing so and is forced to take a value of zero. Therefore, the last level for each temporal factor is necessarily zero. In addition, the program encounters the identifiability problem before it reaches the last cohort, so it constrains the penultimate level to be zero as well. This additional constraint was applied to the cohorts simply because of the order in which they were presented in the model statement. Had either "a" or "p" appeared last, those penultimate levels would have been similarly constrained to be zero, thus giving rise to very different temporal patterns, which is the essence of the problem with these models.

The output produced by this program is also presented in the Appendix, and the results that have been produced thus far are explored. After initially describing the model to be fitted, one finds that deviance = 11.4747, df = 9, and Pearson chi-square statistic = 11.4872, df = 9. These tests can be interpreted as tests of goodness of fit. In this instance, they are both less than the 10% critical value of 14.68, which suggests the absence of strong evidence of a lack of fit. The parameter estimates that arise from the constraints adopted by the software are also in the Appendix. The values for cohorts 8 and 9 are set to 0.0000. In general, one ought not try to interpret these parameters, unless one is really comfortable with an assumption that constrained the equality of these final cohorts.

The type 3 analysis provides a likelihood ratio test of each temporal factor in the presence of the others. Because of the identifiability problem, these analyses are essentially tests of curvature; thus, they have 2 fewer degrees of freedom than the number of levels. In each case, evidence of a contribution to the model is strong; that is, no simple linear trend exists for any of these factors.

Now some estimable functions of the parameters are considered by using a series of estimate statements. In this case, evaluating the magnitude of the estimate is of interest, but if one were interested only in a significance test for one or more of these functions, one would similarly use a contrast statement. The specific estimates that will be considered are overall trend, change in trend, and drift.

First, consider an overall estimate of trend, which would be obtained in a way that is similar to estimating the slope of a line, as described in Eq. 4–7. If period is used as the specific factor to illustrate the approach, a slope estimate can be obtained by using

$$\mathbf{C} = (-2 \ -1 \ 0 \ 1 \ 2)/[(-2)^2 + (-1)^2 + 0^2 + 1^2 + 2^2]$$

$$= (-0.2 \ -0.1 \ 0.0 \ 0.1 \ 0.2)$$

This calculation is described to the SAS program by the first estimate statement. However, "Non-est" in the corresponding output indicates that this function of the period effects is not estimable, thus confirming my earlier abstract discussion.

More aggressive screening for breast cancer began in earnest around 1983. Screening would be expected to occur to some extent in all age groups, possibly changing the period trend. To estimate this change, the difference in slope would be calculated for periods 2 through 5 and the first two periods. This estimate can be formed by taking the difference between the two slopes estimated in a manner similar to that described in the previous paragraph for overall period trend; that is,

$$\mathbf{C} = (0 \;\; -0.3 \;\; -0.1 \;\; 0.1 \;\; 0.3) - (-1 \;\; 1 \;\; 0 \;\; 0 \;\; 0)$$
$$= (1.0 \;\; -1.3 \;\; -0.1 \;\; 0.1 \;\; 0.3)$$

The command is initiated through the second estimate statement in the program, and the results are given in the output. In this case, the result is estimable and is one type of curvature that was specified earlier as an identifiable quantity. These results indicate that the period change in trend for the log rate is 0.1194 per unit change in the period index (i.e., 5 years). The corresponding chi-square statistic shows that this change in trend is significant

Finally, consider an estimate of drift for two different epochs. After the beginning of aggressive screening (i.e., the second and third periods covering the years 1978–1987), all cohorts represented during those years (i.e., cohorts 2–7 in which the middle year of birth is 1933–1963) are included. This estimate, called screen drift in the program, gives rise to an estimate of 0.1227 for the change per 5 years. Along with the corresponding significance test, this estimate suggests strong evidence of increasing drift for breast cancer incidence during this time. The final estimate is the corresponding drift for the most recent periods, which shows a marginally significant decline, with a slope of -0.0240 per 5 years.

A final calculation is an approach for partitioning the estimates of temporal effects into their corresponding linear and curvature components. This approach can be accomplished readily by performing simple linear regression on the parameters. First create a SAS data set using the "make" statement, which is the last statement in the "proc genmod" step. Then break the file into smaller files, each containing the parameters for one of the temporal effects. This division is illustrated for the age parameters. In the next "data" step, create a file for just the age parameters. The various levels of "a" are numbers stored as characters, so they must be converted to numbers by performing the seemingly redundant operation of adding 0 to "Level 1." The partitioned effects are calculated by regression using "proc reg," which produces the corresponding slope (0.77297), and the residuals provide an estimate of curvature.

Similar calculations provide an estimate of period (0.05283) and cohort (-0.01996) slope, along with their curvature components. Were this process to be repeated using an alternative model statement in "proc genmod," the curvatures would remain the same, but the slopes would be quite different. However, $\hat{\beta}_A + \hat{\beta}_P = 0.82580$ and $\hat{\beta}_C + \hat{\beta}_P = 0.03287$ are estimable functions and remain constant. As noted, disentangling these quantities is impossible using only the data at hand, but some plausible values can be explored. Suppose, for example, that β_P plausibly lies between -0.1 and 0.1. Figure 4–6 shows a series of plots based on alternative values for period slope, $\beta_P = -0.1(0.05)0.1$. This plausible range includes no trend for the first 2 periods, followed by a steady increase, which is consistent with the screening hypothesis (thin broken line). However, the corresponding cohort trend is fairly flat until the 1953 cohort, after which it declines steadily. In general, as the period slope increases, the period effects are rotated clockwise, and the corresponding age and cohort slopes decrease, resulting in a counterclockwise rotation of the effects. The fact that these variables are linked means that accepting the parameters for any one temporal effect implies a corresponding set of estimates for the others.

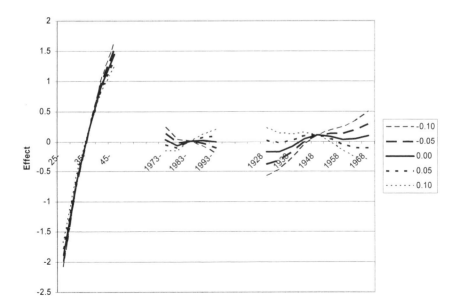

Figure 4–6 Equivalent age, period, and cohort effects for the data in Table 4–1.

SPECIAL PROBLEMS

Here extensions to approaches that have been presented are considered. First consider the fact that the distributional assumptions may not adequately describe the data, thus resulting in extra-Poisson variation. Next, consider the results of using data in which the age and period intervals differ, as well as the possibility of introducing interaction terms into the model.

Extra-Poisson Variation

For the Poisson distribution, the mean and the variance are equal, a fact important in the formulas for obtaining variance estimates and significance tests. However, data from vital statistics registries often violate this assumption by exhibiting a variance that is greater than the mean. An example is a population of people with a mixture of risks because of susceptibility to disease or exposure to causative agents. If the assumptions of the Poisson distribution are violated, the resulting standard errors and p-values are too small.

The form of over-dispersion that is analytically most convenient to deal with occurs when the variance is proportional to the mean;

$$Var(Y) = \phi \cdot E[Y]$$

where ϕ is an unknown scale parameter. In the case of the Poisson distribution, the scale parameter is assumed to be 1, but in other instances it would need to be estimated. An estimate that works well in many instances is the ratio of the Pearson chi-square goodness-of-fit statistic to its degrees of freedom;

$$\tilde{\phi} = \frac{X^2}{df}$$

where X^2 is the Pearson chi-square goodness of fit statistic and df is the corresponding degrees of freedom (McCullagh and Nelder, 1989). This estimate is reminiscent of the estimate of the error variance in ordinary least-squares regression; indeed, the same distributional assumptions would be used for inferences based on a model in which the scale parameter was estimated. For example, confidence limits and tests for individual parameters would make use of the t-distribution instead of the normal distribution, z. The likelihood ratio tests would also be modified, using

$$F_{\Delta df, df} = \frac{\Delta G^2 / \Delta df}{\tilde{\phi}}$$

where Δdf is the number of regressor variables dropped from a nested set of models, and that is then compared to an F-distribution. A variance that is proportional to the mean is just one of many possible candidate models for the relationship between the mean and the variance. Other models of potential interest are discussed by McCullagh and Nelder (1989).

Unequal Intervals

The problem of temporal modeling of disease trends when the rates are specified for equal age and period intervals has been discussed. When the intervals are unequal, further identifiability problems arise (Fienberg and Mason, 1978; Holford, 1983). Tabulations that use unequal intervals for age and period can arise from annual (1-year) reports of rates expressed in terms of 5-year age intervals, that is, 1- and 5-year intervals. Sometimes reporting annual data raises confidentiality concerns, especially for relatively small geographic regions. The temptation is to try to maintain as much detail as possible, but this approach may not be worthwhile because it brings additional identifiability problems.

One source of the identifiability problem is associated with a phenomenon that is similar to the confounding of the overall linear trends for age, period, and cohort. The additional identifiability problems can be associated with short-term or micro trends, which can introduce cyclical patterns into the temporal trends that are entirely attributable to arbitrary constraints used to obtain parameter estimates. The period of these cycles is equal to the least common multiple of the age and period widths, and these can affect all 3 temporal effects. Suppose that the data have been tabulated using 5-year age and 3-year period intervals. The least common multiple is 15 years; therefore, the micro identifiability problem can induce a 15-year cycle into the parameters for age, period, and cohort.

The cyclical nature of the additional identifiability problem for the unequal interval case can give especially misleading results. Epidemiologists are used to seeing cycles in the incidence rates for infectious diseases, which result from the ebb and flow of epidemics. When such a pattern emerges for a chronic disease such as cancer, it can be very tempting to conclude that a viral cause may be involved—a putative risk factor that has long been suspected for some cancers, but one that has often been difficult to prove. Cycles in data with unequal interval widths must be very carefully analyzed, especially if the periodicity is close to the least common multiple of the period and cohort interval widths. In this instance, disentangling the identifiability problem from what may be a real cyclical pattern may be impossible.

An investigator who wishes to pursue short-term cyclical patterns within the age-period-cohort framework, should use equal intervals that are sufficiently narrow to allow the cycle to emerge. Tarone et al. (1997) used 2-year age and period intervals, which provided a greater opportunity for cycles to be observed. However, setting up the more detailed tabulations that are required cannot always be arranged.

Spline regression is one approach for eliminating short-term fluctuations caused by the identifiability problem, and it also enables estimates of the unidentifiable pieces to be removed. Essentially, this removal amounts to assuming that the unidentifiable contribution is zero, which cannot be known for sure. In fact, another arbitrary assumption could have been made that would have forced the cyclical pattern to be arbitrarily large, but instead the pattern was dampened as much as possible. The danger of this damping approach is that it could remove a cycle that is really present. Interpreting results from such an analysis must account for this possibility. This damping approach is conservative in that cycles that remain will tend to be real.

Interactions

The models considered above assume that the trend for each time factor does not depend on other factors, that is, that the factors do not interact. A problem with considering interactions between these temporal variables is that incorporating an interaction in any two-factor model results in a saturated model. For example, if only age and period are considered, the model becomes

$$\log \lambda(t_{A}, t_{P}, t_{C}) = \mu + \alpha(t_{A}) + \pi(t_{P}) + \alpha\pi(t_{A}, t_{P}) \qquad (4\text{--}11)$$

where $\alpha(t_{A})$ and $\pi(t_{P})$ are main effects, and $\alpha\pi(t_{A}, t_{P})$ is the interaction. The difference between the model in Eq. 4–11 and that in Eq. 4–4 is that the latter shows a cohort effect, $\gamma(t_{C})$, in place of the age $\times$ period interaction. Because the interactions saturate the model, the cohort effect might be interpreted as a particular type of age $\times$ period interaction (Kupper et al., 1983). Similarly, the period effect could be described as a particular type of age $\times$ cohort interaction. Fienberg and Mason (1985) studied polynomial models for the three time factors and indicated the interactions that can be identified. Interpreting interactions of higher-order polynomial models is difficult under the best circumstances, without further complications from the identifiability problem. Therefore, special care is needed when interactions are introduced into these models.

An alternative to polynomial interactions among the temporal factors is to split the times into groups, as in the comparison of cohort trends in breast cancer among women younger and older than 50 years (Holford et al., 1991). This division arose because of a suggestion that breast cancer trends may differ between pre- and postmenopausal women (Avila and Walker, 1987). In examining an interaction between cohort and these two age groups (i.e., a difference in the cohort trend for pre- and postmenopausal women), considerable care must be taken to obtain a sensible representation of the results (Holford et al., 1991).

CONCLUSION

The problem of modeling simultaneously the temporal effects of age, period, and cohort on disease rates have been explored and the limitations of the identifiability problem on the ability to interpret the resulting parameter estimates have been demonstrated. Data analysts were forced to recognize this difficulty when they adopted a formal modeling approach over the simpler graphical display of trends. The problem arises from the attempt to extract three separate temporal elements from what are inherently only two temporal dimensions, as described by the Lexis diagram. Numerical difficulties are picked up during the regression calculations in a modeling approach, whereas no such difficulties are apparent in a graphical approach. Nevertheless, the extent to which the separate contribution of these factors can be evaluated, is even limited in a graphical display, so such data must always be approached with considerable care.

All three temporal factors in the analysis are used persistently because the interpretational implications of these factors are important to people who conduct public health surveillance. Despite the inherent limitations of this approach, interesting aspects of the three temporal trends can still be separately identified. These aspects have been described and approaches for obtaining them using numerical examples are indicated.

Finally, when unequal interval widths are used for age and period, the identifiability problem not only persists but causes further interpretational problems. These problems can produce especially misleading results because they induce cycles into the fitted estimates of trend, which can mistakenly lead to an etiologic interpretation that a contagion is involved.

REFERENCES

Avila, M.H. and Walker, A.M. (1987). Age dependence of cohort phenomena in breast cancer mortality in the United States. *American Journal of Epidemiology* **126,** 377–384.

Barrett, J.C. (1973). Age, time, and cohort factors in mortality from cancer of the cervix. *Journal of Hygiene* **71,** 253–259.

Barrett, J.C. (1978). The redundant factor method and bladder cancer mortality. *Journal of Epidemiology and Community Health* **32**, 314–316.

Clayton, D. and Schifflers, E. (1987a). Models for temporal variation in cancer rates. I: Age-period and age-cohort models. *Statistics in Medicine* **6**, 449–467.

Clayton, D. and Schifflers, E. (1987b). Models for temporal variation in cancer rates. II: Age-period-cohort models. *Statistics in Medicine* **6**, 469–481.

Fienberg, S.E. and Mason, W.M. (1978). Identification and estimation of age-period-cohort models in the analysis of discrete archival data. *Sociological Methodology* **1979**, 1–67.

Fienberg, S.E. and Mason, W.M. (1985). *Specification and Implementation of Age, Period and Cohort Models*. New York: Springer-Verlag.

Holford, T.R. (1983). The estimation of age, period and cohort effects for vital rates. *Biometrics* **39**, 311–324.

Holford, T.R. (1985). An alternative approach to statistical age-period-cohort analysis. *Journal of Clinical Epidemiology* **38**, 831–836.

Holford, T.R. (1998). Age-period-cohort analysis. *Encyclopedia of Biostatistic*. In Armitage P. and Colton T. Chichester: John Wiley and Sons, pp. 82–99.

Holford, T.R., Roush, G.C., and McKay, L.A. (1991). Trends in female breast cancer in Connecticut and the United States. *Journal of Clinical Epidemiology* **44**, 29–39.

Keiding, N. (1998). Lexis diagram. *Encyclopedia of Biostatistics*. P. Armitage and T. Colton. Chichester: Wiley. **3**, 2232–2234.

Kupper, L.L., Janis, J.M., Karmous, A., and Greenberg, B.G. (1985). Statistical age-period-cohort analysis: a review and critique. *Journal of Chronic Diseases* **38**, 811–830.

Kupper, L.L., Janis, J.M., Salama, I.A., Yoshizawa, C.N., and Greenberg, B.G. (1983). Age-period-cohort analysis: an illustration of the problems in assessing interaction in one observation per cell data. *Communication in Statistics-Theory and Methods* **12**, 2779–2807.

McCullagh, P. and Nelder, J.A. (1989). *Generalized Linear Models*. London: Chapman and Hall.

Moolgavkar, S.H., Lee, J.A.H., and Stevens, R.G. (1998). Analysis of vital statistics data. In Rothman, K.J. and Greenland S., eds. *Modern Epidemiology*. Philadelphia: Lippincott-Raven Publishers, pp. 481–497.

Osmond, C. (1985). Using age, period and cohort models to estimate future mortality rates. *International Journal of Epidemiology* **14**, 124–129.

Osmond, C. and Gardner, M.J. (1989). Age, period, and cohort models: Non-overlapping cohorts don't resolve the identification problem. *American Journal of Epidemiology* **129**, 31–35.

Robertson, C. and Boyle, P. (1986). Age, period and cohort models: The use of individual records. *Statistics in Medicine* **5**, 527–538.

Rogers, W.L. (1982). Estimable functions of age, period, and cohort effects. *American Sociological Review* **47**, 774–796.

Roush, G.C., Schymura, M.J., Holford, T.R., White, C., and Flannery, J.T. (1985). Time period compared to birth cohort in Connecticut incidence rates for twenty-five malignant neoplasms. *Journal of the National Cancer Institute* **74**, 779–788.

Roush, G.D., Holford, T.R., Schymura, M.J., and White, C. (1987). *Cancer Risk and Incidence Trends: The Connecticut Perspective*. New York: Hemisphere Publishing Corp.

Tango, T. (1988). RE: Statistical modelling of lung cancer and laryngeal cancer incidence in Scotland, 1960–1979. *American Journal of Epidemiology* **128,** 677–678.

Tango, T. and Kurashina, S. (1987). Age, period and cohort analysis of trends in mortality from major diseases in Japan, 1955 to 1979: Peculiarity of the cohort born in the early Showa Era. *Statistics in Medicine* **6,** 709–726.

Tarone, R. and Chu, K. (1996). Evaluation of birth cohort patterns in population disease rates. *American Journal of Epidemiology* **143,** 85–91.

Tarone, R.E., Chu, K.C., and Gaudette, L.A. (1997). Birth cohort and calendar period trends in breast cancer mortality in the United States. *Journal of the National Cancer Institute* **80,** 43–51.

Weinkam, J.J. and Sterling, T.D. (1991). A graphical approach to the interpretation of age-period-cohort data. *Epidemiology* **2,** 133–137.

APPENDIX

The following is a listing of a SAS program designed to fit an age-period-cohort model to the SEER data on breast cancer incidence in premenopausal women.

```
options nocenter;
libname out 'folder_name';

*--------------------------------------------------------------------;
*                                                                    ;
* Setup data for analysis using the following input variables:       ;
*         a = age index                                              ;
*         p = period index                                           ;
*         n = numerator                                              ;
*         d = denominator                                            ;
* The created variable are:                                          ;
*         c = cohort index                                           ;
*         log_d = log of the denominator                             ;
*         rate = age-specific rate                                   ;
*         age, period and cohort = interval midpoints                ;
*                                                                    ;
*--------------------------------------------------------------------;

data rates; set out.dsname;
c = p-a+5;                          *Create cohort index;
log_d = log(d);                     *OFFSET is the log of the denominator;
rate = 100000*n/d;                  *Estimate the rate;
age = 22.5 + 5*a;                   *Midpoint of AGE intervals;
period = 1970 + 5*p;                *Midpoint of PERIOD intervals;
cohort = period - age;              *Midpoint of COHORT intervals;

title 'Results from GENMOD';
proc genmod data=rates; classes a p c;
model n = a p c / dist=p offset=log_d type3; *Specify model to be fitted;
```

```
*-----------------------------------------------------------------------;
*                                                                       ;
* Estimable functions of the model parameters.                         ;
*                                                                       ;
*-----------------------------------------------------------------------;


estimate 'Period trend' p -0.2 -0.1 0.0 0.1 0.2;
estimate 'Period change' p 1 -1.3 -.1 .1 .3;
estimate 'Screen drift' p 0 -1 1 0 0
     c 0 -0.142857 -0.085714 -0.028571 0.028571 0.085714 0.142857 0 0;
estimate 'Recent drift' p 0 0 21 1
     c 0 0 0 -0.142857 -0.085714 -0.028571 0.028571 0.085714 0.142857;


*-----------------------------------------------------------------------;
*                                                                       ;
* Create a dataset consisting of the parameters, which will be used to  ;
* estimate the slope and curvature                                      ;
*                                                                       ;
*-----------------------------------------------------------------------;
make ParameterEstimates out=parms;
run;


*-----------------------------------------------------------------------;
*                                                                       ;
* Estimate the slope and curvature for the AGE effects                  ;
*                                                                       ;
*-----------------------------------------------------------------------;


title 'AGE slope and curvature effects';
data age(keep=a est); set parms;
if (Parameter = 'a');
a = Level1 + 0;
est = Estimate;


proc reg data=age outest=age_parm;
     model est = a;
     output out+age_c r=a_curv;
     run;
proc print data=age_c;   run;    *Print out the age curvature effects;
```

Output from the SAS program listed above is as follows:


```
Results from GENMOD

The GENMOD Procedure

        Class Level Information

Class      Levels     Values

a             5        1 2 3 4 5
p             5        1 2 3 4 5
c             9        1 2 3 4 5 6 7 8 9
```

```
          Criteria For Assessing Goodness Of Fit

Criterion                DF        Value   Value/DF

Deviance                  9      11.4747    1.2750
Scaled Deviance           9      11.4747    1.2750
Pearson Chi-Square        9      11.4872    1.2764
Scaled Pearson X2         9      11.4872    1.2764
Log Likelihood                 626225.1380

Algorithm converged.
```

```
                   Analysis Of Parameter Estimates

                              Standard    Wald 95%         Chi-
Parameter      DF  Estimate     Error  Confidence Limits  Square   Pr > ChiSq

Intercept       1   -6.2217    0.1855  -6.5852  -5.8582  1125.37    <.0001
a         1     1   -3.1110    0.2266  -3.5552  -2.6669   188.50    <.0001
a         2     1   -1.9777    0.1775  -2.3256  -1.6299   124.17    <.0001
a         3     1   -1.1197    0.1171  -1.3493  -0.8901    91.38    <.0001
a         4     1   -0.4701    0.0590  -0.5858  -0.3545    63.47    <.0001
a         5     0    0.0000    0.0000   0.0000   0.0000      .         .
p         1     1   -0.1700    0.2334  -0.6274   0.2875     0.53    0.4665
p         2     1   -0.2181    0.1751  -0.5612   0.1250     1.55    0.2129
p         3     1   -0.0881    0.1168  -0.3171   0.1408     0.57    0.4504
p         4     1   -0.0297    0.0586  -0.1446   0.0852     0.26    0.6123
p         5     0    0.0000    0.0000   0.0000   0.0000      .         .
c         1     1    0.1548    0.4180  -0.6644   0.9740     0.14    0.7111
c         2     1    0.1066    0.3596  -0.5982   0.8114     0.09    0.7669
c         3     1    0.1468    0.3014  -0.4439   0.7374     0.24    0.6263
c         4     1    0.2190    0.2430  -0.2572   0.6952     0.81    0.3674
c         5     1    0.2271    0.1853  -0.1360   0.5903     1.50    0.2203
c         6     1    0.1546    0.1279  -0.0960   0.4052     1.46    0.2267
c         7     1    0.0498    0.0722  -0.0918   0.1913     0.48    0.4906
c         8     0    0.0000    0.0000   0.0000   0.0000      .         .
c         9     0    0.0000    0.0000   0.0000   0.0000      .         .
Scale           0    1.0000    0.0000   1.0000   1.0000
```

NOTE: The scale parameter was held fixed.

```
LR Statistics For Type 3 Analysis

                  Chi-
Source    DF    Square   Pr > ChiSq

a          3   1202.31    <.0001
p          3     61.49    <.0001
c          7    230.39    <.0001
```

```
                   Contrast Estimate Results

                    Standard          Confidence    Chi-
Label      Estimate   Error  Alpha      Limits      Square  Pr > ChiSq

Period trend  Non-est     .      .      .       .        .        .
Period change  0.1194  0.0179  0.05  0.0843  0.1544   44.60   <.0001
Screen drift   0.1227  0.0128  0.05  0.0976  0.1478   91.56   <.0001
Recent drift  -0.0240  0.0122  0.05 -0.0479 -0.0002    3.89    0.0485
```

AGE slope and curvature effects

The REG Procedure
Model: MODEL1
Dependent Variable: est

Parameter Estimates

Variable	DF	Parameter Estimate	Standard Error	t Value	Pr > |t|
Intercept	1	-3.65462	0.24907	-14.67	0.0007
a	1	0.77297	0.07510	10.29	0.0020

Obs	a	est	a_curv
1	1	-3.11103	-0.22938
2	2	-1.97772	0.13096
3	3	-1.11973	0.21599
4	4	-0.47010	0.09264
5	5	0.00000	-0.21022

5

Temporal Factors in Epidemics: The Role of the Incubation Period

RON BROOKMEYER

The quantitative study of the rise and fall of epidemics dates back to the pioneering work of William Farr (Eyler, 1979). This chapter reviews factors that affect the temporal evolution of epidemics, particularly epidemics of infectious origin. Time trends in disease incidence (new cases of disease per unit time) are difficult to interpret from public health surveillance data because of a number of critical questions. For example, does a slowing in the growth of disease incidence necessarily indicate that an epidemic is waning? Can one reliably forecast the future growth of an epidemic from surveillance data?

Time trends in disease incidence determined from public health surveillance data arise from a complex interaction of factors. These factors include the transmission dynamics and epidemiology of the disease, the incubation period of the disease, the introduction of public health interventions and control programs that reduce morbidity and mortality, changes in public awareness and behavior, and reporting characteristics of the public health surveillance system. The following sections review the quantitative effect of these factors on patterns of infectious disease incidence over time, focusing on the unique role of the incubation period.

Epidemics or outbreaks of three diseases are used to illustrate many points throughout this chapter: the HIV/AIDS epidemic in the United States, the Bovine spongiform encephalopathy (BSE) and variant Creutzfeldt-Jakob disease (vCJD) epidemics in the United Kingdom, and anthrax outbreaks in Sverdlovsk, Russia, in 1979 and the United States in 2001. These three diseases differ widely in their incubation periods and their modes and dynamics of transmission. Understanding the temporal pattern of epidemic curves for these diseases requires careful evaluation of the underlying epidemiology, natural history, and transmission dynamics of each disease.

The first AIDS cases were reported in 1981. The cause of AIDS, the human immunodeficiency virus (HIV), is transmitted through sexual contact, the exchange of blood and blood products (such as through sharing of contaminated needles among intravenous drug users), and perinatal transmission. Most countries have reporting and surveillance systems for AIDS cases, and some countries have developed systems for monitoring HIV infections. The World Health Organization has developed a global AIDS surveillance system. The Centers for Disease Control and Prevention (CDC) in the United States maintains a national AIDS surveillance system. AIDS cases in the 50 states are reported to a central registry using a standardized case definition. The annual U.S. AIDS incidence reported to the national surveillance system from 1981 through 2000 is shown in Figure 5–1.

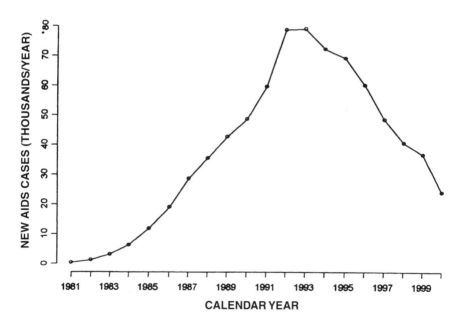

Figure 5–1 Reported annual AIDS incidence in the United States from 1981 through 2000. Data are unadjusted for reporting delays. *Source*: www.cdc.gov.

Bovine spongiform encephalopathy, or mad cow disease, was first reported in cattle in the United Kingdom in 1986. The disease appears to spread through feeding the carcasses of affected animals to other animals. The number of new clinical cases of BSE annually in cattle in the United Kingdom from 1986 to 2000 is shown in Figure 5–2. The BSE epidemic in cattle appears to have spawned the subsequent epidemic in humans, which apparently spread through human consumption of contaminated beef products from BSE-affected cattle. The first case of vCJF surfaced in 1995, and approximately 100 vCJD cases were confirmed in the United Kingdom between 1995 and 2001 (Fig. 5–2). The pattern of disease incidence of vCJD reflects a complex interaction of meat consumption, public health control measures, and incubation periods of BSE and vCJD.

Anthrax is caused by the bacterium *Bacillus anthracis* and occurs in three forms. Cutaneous anthrax is transmitted through broken skin; gastrointestinal anthrax typically occurs from ingesting contaminated meat; and inhalational anthrax is acquired from breathing anthrax spores into the lungs. An outbreak of inhalational anthrax occurred in Sverdlosvsk, Russia on April 2, 1979 when people inhaled spores that were accidentally released from a military microbiology facility. The number of lethal cases by

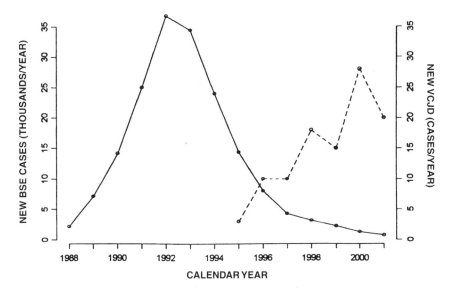

Figure 5–2 Annual number of new clinical cases of BSE in the United Kingdom from 1986 through 2000 (solid line). Annual number of confirmed cases of vCJD from 1995 through 2001 (dotted line). *Source*: Brown, P., Will, R.G., Bradley, R., Asher, D., and Detwilder, L. (2001). Bovine spongiform encephalopathy and variant Creutzfeldt-Jakob disease: Background, evolution and current concerns. *Emerging Infectious Diseases* **7**, 6–16.

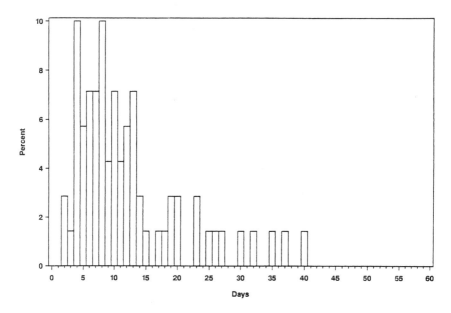

Figure 5–3 Distribution of lethal cases in anthrax outbreaks in Sverdlovsk, Russia by day of onset of symptoms from release of the anthrax spores on April 2, 1979. *Source*: Brookmeyer, R., Blades, N., Hugh-Jones, M., and Henderson, D.A. (2001). The statistical analysis of truncated data: application to the Sverdlovsk, Russia outbreak. *Biostatistics* **2**, 233–247, used with permission.

date of onset of symptoms is shown in Figure 5–3. An outbreak of inhalational anthrax occurred in the United States in the fall of 2001 from the intentional dissemination of anthrax spores.

In the section Temporal Factors, some factors are identified that can affect time trends in surveillance data, using the three diseases as examples. In the section The Incubation Period Distribution, the incubation period distribution is discussed. In the sections The Common Source Epidemic and Continuous Exposure Epidemics, quantitative methods of monitoring common source and continuous exposure epidemics are described. In the section Epidemic Transmission Models, simple mathematical models for describing the transmission of diseases that are spread from person to person are presented.

TEMPORAL FACTORS

Several factors affect the temporal evolution of epidemics. One factor is the reporting characteristics of the surveillance system, such as reporting delays, changes in the surveillance definition of a disease, and changes in the proportion of unreported cases. Accurate monitoring of disease trends requires adjusting for delays in disease reporting. The delay in disease reporting is the lag from the onset of disease to the reporting of cases to the surveillance system (Brookmeyer and Gail, 1994). Without such adjustments, reporting delays can produce false declines in disease incidence in the most recent calendar periods, when reporting of diagnosed cases is the least complete.

For example, in the United States, AIDS cases are first reported to state health departments, which then report them to the national AIDS surveillance system at the CDC. In order to accurately monitor disease trends, one must adjust for delays in disease reporting (Brookmeyer and Gail, 1994). The data for AIDS incidence in the United States shown in Figure 5–1 have not been adjusted for reporting delays, and the sharp decline in incidence in the most recent year is mainly from incomplete reporting of the most recently diagnosed cases. Specialized statistical methods are required to adjust for reporting delays. Naively calculating the usual sample mean of the reporting delays of cases (i.e., the lags from onset of disease to report to the surveillance system) tends to underestimate the true mean reporting delay, because reporting delays based on cases reported to the surveillance system are a right-truncated, or biased sample. With long reporting delays, new cases may not yet be included in the surveillance data. Thus, naïve calculations based only on simple means of the reporting delays of cases in the surveillance database tend to underestimate the mean reporting delay. Specialized statistical methods have been developed to estimate the reporting delay without bias and to adjust the disease incidence data appropriately (Zeger et al., 1989; Brookmeyer and Liao, 1990).

Altering the case surveillance definition of a disease can also affect temporal trends. For example, the surveillance definition of AIDS was revised several times during the epidemic, typically by broadening the case criteria or, for some cases, accelerating the time of diagnosis. The effect of some changes was an abrupt increase in the incidence of AIDS. Changes in the proportion of cases that are never reported, perhaps as public awareness of an epidemic rises and wanes, can also affect temporal trends.

A second factor that affects trends in surveillance data is the transmission dynamics of the epidemic, which are driven by the sources of exposure and the way in which the epidemic propagates within a population. For example, simple epidemic models of transmission can explain the early exponential rise in AIDS incidence seen in Figure 5–1. Reductions in high-risk behaviors in a population, or reductions in the number of people who are susceptible to the infection (sometimes called saturation effect) can slow the epidemic to subexponential growth. The transmission dynamics for BSE in cattle are entirely different because the disease spreads solely by rendering and recycling contaminated carcasses as livestock feed. In contrast to the BSE and AIDS epidemics, the outbreak of inhalational anthrax in Sverdlovsk, Russia was a common source outbreak, that is, all affected persons were infected at about the same time; they were exposed to anthrax spores immediately after the spores were released into the air, a period believed to have lasted 1 day at most.

A third factor is the incubation period distribution of the disease. Typically surveillance systems track new cases of disease by the onset of clinical or symptomatic disease rather than by onset of exposure to the infectious agent or infection. For example, the incidence curves for AIDS, BSE, and anthrax in Figures 5–1, 5–2, and 5–3, respectively, indicate the onset of symptomatic disease, rather than the onset of exposure to the infectious agent or infection. Thus, these curves describe the epidemic curve of clinical disease, which lags the underlying epidemic curve of infections. The lag is determined by the incubation period distribution.

A fourth factor that affects temporal trends is the instituting of public health interventions and control measures that can interrupt the natural course of an epidemic. For example, in 1988 the United Kingdom banned all ruminant protein in ruminant feed to control the BSE epidemic. The decline in BSE cases became apparent several years later and the lag undoubtedly reflected the incubation period of the disease (Fig. 5–2). A decline in AIDS incidence from 1993 to 2000 was related to a decrease in high-risk behaviors as people became aware of the risks of HIV infection and also to new therapies that lengthened the incubation period (Gail et al., 1990) (Fig. 5–1). The incidence of inhalational anthrax in the Sverdlovsk outbreak of April 2, 1979 may have decreased because in mid-April prophylactic antibiotics and vaccines were distributed widely after public health officials became aware of the outbreak (Fig. 5–3).

THE INCUBATION PERIOD DISTRIBUTION

The incubation period is broadly defined as the time from exposure to an infectious agent to the onset of disease. To avoid ambiguity, exposure and onset of disease must be clearly defined. The incubation period of AIDS illustrates the potential for confusion. In AIDS studies, onset of disease can be defined as either the time that a person's condition first meets the surveillance definition of AIDS, or the time of onset of one or more clinical symptoms. The use of the surveillance definition requires care because it has changed several times during the epidemic.

The exposure date can also be ambiguous. Typically, the exposure date is the time that individuals are exposed to the disease-causing microbes. The earliest study on the incubation period of AIDS was based on AIDS cases associated with transfusions, in which the time of exposure was taken to be the date of transfusion of contaminated blood or blood products. However, the date of exposure cannot be determined in most people who have AIDS, so instead, the date of exposure is estimated from the time that a positive result is obtained from a serologic or virologic test for evidence of infection. Most studies of the incubation period of AIDS have been cohort studies in which HIV antibody tests are given at each follow-up visit. The date of infection is assumed to fall between the last antibody test with a negative result and the first antibody test with a positive result and is typically approximated by the midpoint of the interval. However, exposure could have occurred earlier because several weeks or months can elapse between exposure to the microbe and the production of antibodies that could be detected. As HIV antibody tests have become more sensitive and infection is detected sooner, the presumed start of the incubation period has become earlier. However, estimates of HIV incubation periods are not greatly affected by different diagnostic approaches for estimating exposure dates and disease onset dates because the incubation period is vastly longer (median of about 10 years) than the time interval that could be affected by using different diagnostic approaches for estimating the data of exposure or infection. Nevertheless, these issues underscore the importance of having established and consistent criteria for defining the start point (exposure) and endpoint (disease onset) of the incubation period, especially if incubation periods are to be compared across studies.

The incubation period distribution $F(t)$ is the probability that an infected individual will develop disease within t time units after being exposed to the infectious agent. If the random variable T represents the incubation period, then $F(t) = P(T < t)$.

Various functional or mathematical forms of the parametric model for the incubation period distribution $F(t)$ have been applied to infectious diseases. Sartwell (1950) pioneered the use of the lognormal distribution which assumes that the logarithm of the incubation period follows a normal distribution, with mean μ and standard deviation σ. The distribution is right-skewed. The median incubation period is $m = exp(\mu)$. Sartwell defined the dispersion as $\delta = exp(\sigma)$, as which, like the standard deviation (σ), is a measure of the spread or variability among incubation periods. One interpretation of the dispersion factor (δ) is that approximately 68% of incubation periods will fall in the interval defined by m/δ to $m \times \delta$. Approximately 95% of incubation periods will fall in the interval m/δ^2 to $m \times \delta^2$. Sartwell applied the lognormal distribution to a wide range of infectious diseases, including measles, poliomyelitis, and salmonelliosis. Although the median incubation periods for these very different diseases varied widely, Sartwell found that the dispersion factors (δ) were broadly consistent across the diseases and ranged from approximately 1.1 to 2.1. If heterogeneity increases because of such factors such as dose of exposure, it is reasonable to suspect that the dispersion factor would become higher. For example, Brookmeyer et al. (2001) estimated a dispersion $\delta - 2.04$ for the incubation periods of inhalational anthrax in Sverdlovsk. Variability in doses of inhaled spores among individuals may have caused more variability in incubation periods, which could explain the higher δ.

The Weibull distribution has also been used to describe the incubation period distribution. The incubation period for the Weibull model has the form $F(t) = 1 - exp(-\lambda t^\gamma)$. The hazard function of this model refers to the risk of disease onset at time t, given that the person does not have disease just before time t. This function increases monotonically if $\gamma > 1$, decreases monotonically if $\gamma < 1$, and is constant (called the exponential model) if $\gamma = 1$. The model has been used to study the incubation period of HIV infection (Brookmeyer and Goedert, 1989; Darby et al., 1990; Medley et al., 1987). A key assumption of the Weibull distribution is that the hazard is proportional to a power of time and is monotonically increasing, decreasing, or constant. Other functional forms for the incubation period have been used that relax that assumption, including the gamma model, the log-logistic and the piecewise exponential model.

Another model for the incubation period distribution is a mixture model. Suppose a proportion of the population p has an incubation period distribution $F_1(t)$, and the remaining proportion $(1 - p)$ has an incubation period distribution $F_2(t)$. The incubation period distribution in the population of exposed persons is then

$$F(t) = pF_1(t) + (1 - p)\, F_2(t)$$

A mixture model for the incubation period may be a sensible model for some applications, such as the incubation period of inhalational anthrax. For example, persons close to the release of anthrax spores may have a shorter incubation period distribution than persons who were not in the immediate vicinity.

Thus far, I have assumed that exposure to an infectious agent automatically leads to disease. However, exposure may not lead to infection or to clinical disease. For example, nasal swab tests with positive results document exposure to anthrax spores. A person who has been exposed may never develop disease if the spores are not deposited deep in the lungs or do not germinate. Thus, the incubation period distribution $F(t)$ may not be a proper distribution, that is, 100% of exposed persons may never develop disease. Mixture models can be used to describe this situation. Suppose only a proportion p of exposed persons will develop clinical disease, and the remaining fraction $(1 - p)$ of exposed persons will never develop disease. The incubation period distribution among the fraction of exposed persons (p) who will develop disease is called $F_c(t)$. The incubation period distribution in the population of exposed persons is then

$$F(t) = pF_c(t)$$

The incubation period distribution among persons who eventually develop disease, $F_c(t)$, is called the *case incubation period distribution* to distinguish it from the incubation period distribution $F(t)$ among all exposed persons. The case incubation period distribution $F_c(t)$ is necessarily a proper distribution function (i.e., it eventually approaches 1 as t increases). On the other hand, $F(t)$ is an improper distribution function if $p < 1$ (i.e., not all exposed persons develop disease). The Sverdlovsk anthrax outbreak illustrates these concepts. Thousands of persons living in Sverdlovsk were undoubtedly exposed to spores that were released into the atmosphere, but fewer than 100 cases of inhalational anthrax were reported. The incubation period distribution estimated from these 100 cases is the case incubation period distribution $F_c(t)$ and not the distribution $F(t)$ of incubation periods among *all* exposed persons.

THE COMMON SOURCE EPIDEMIC

A common source epidemic is defined as one in which the exposure source is the same for all cases. In this section, a common source epidemic is defined as one in which both the time and the location of the exposure to the infectious agent is the same for all affected cases. The Sverdlovsk anthrax outbreak of 1979 could be reasonably assumed to be a common source outbreak because spores were released into the atmosphere on a single day and remained in the atmosphere for probably no more than 1 day before they fell to the ground. Spores on the ground were considered not likely to have reaerosolized because resuspension of spores requires considerable energy.

If all persons are exposed at exactly the same time, then the temporal evolution of the epidemic curve of cases of disease is determined solely by the case incubation period distribution, $F_c(t)$. Figure 5–3 is a histogram of case incidence and incubation times. Suppose C is the total number of cases of disease that would ultimately surface in a common source epidemic. The expected number of cumulative cases of disease at or before t time units after exposure, called $N(t)$, is

$$N(t) = C \times F_c(t) \qquad (5\text{--}1)$$

If E is the total number of exposed persons in a common source outbreak, including persons who do and do not develop disease, then,

$$N(t) = E \times F(t) \tag{5–2}$$

Eq. 5–2 is analogous to Eq. 5–1 except that the case incubation period distribution $F_c(t)$ in Eq. 5–1 is replaced by the incubation period distribution $F(t)$. In the midst of an outbreak, Eq. 5–1 can be used to estimate the total size of a common source outbreak, if an estimate of the incubation period is available. For example, suppose $N(t) = n$ cumulative cases of disease at or before t time units after the exposure has been observed. The total number of persons C in whom clinical disease would eventually develop from this exposure can be estimated by

$$\hat{C} = n/F_c(t)$$

The intuition for this equation is that the observed number of cases n is only a fraction of the total number of cases C that will occur and that fraction is given by $F_c(t)$. These n cases have incubation periods shorter than t.

Such calculations for a lognormal incubation distribution with median $m = 15.8$ days and dispersion factor $\delta = 1.7$ are illustrated. This distribution implies that the log of the incubation periods is approximately normally distributed with a mean $\mu = ln(15.8) = 2.76$ and a standard deviation $= ln(1.7) = 0.53$. Table 5–1 gives the estimated value of C for different values of n and t, where n is the cumulative number of cases that occurred within t days of exposure. For example, if 50 cumulative cases occurred within 10 days of exposure, then the total number of cases that would ultimately surface from this common source outbreak (in the absence of any public health intervention to prevent disease) is estimated to be $\hat{C} = 255$, because $F(10) = 0.196$, and $50/.196 = 255$. On the other hand, if 50 cases occurred within 5 days of exposure, the size of the epidemic is estimated to be much larger; $\hat{C} = 3221$ cases.

Assuming the probability model that n is binomially distributed with sample size C and probability $F_c(t)$, then the standard error for $ln(\hat{C})$ is approximately $((1 - F_c(t))/n)^{1/2}$, if n is sufficiently large. This standard error formula could be used to obtain an approximate confidence interval for C by first obtaining a confidence interval for $ln(C)$ and then taking the antilogs of the end points of that confidence interval. However, a better method for obtaining a confidence interval for C that does not rely on normal approximation to the sampling distribution (especially if n is small) is to invert a hypothesis test as follows. A $(1 - \alpha) \times 100\%$ confidence interval for C is given by the set of all values of C_0, where the null hypothesis,

Table 5–1 Estimated total numbers of cases from an outbreak C if a cumulative number of n cases are observed within t days of the common source exposure, $C = n/F_c(t)$.

Number of cases (n)	Days (t)			
	5	10	15	20
5	322	26	11	7
10	644	51	22	15
20	1289	102	43	30
30	1933	153	65	45
40	2577	204	87	60
50	3221	255	108	74
60	3866	306	130	89
70	4510	357	151	104
80	5154	408	173	119
90	5798	459	195	134
100	6443	510	216	149

Calculations are Based on a Lognormal Distribution for $F_c(t)$ with Median $\exp(\mu) = 15.8$ and Dispersion Factor $\exp(\sigma) = 1.7$.

H_0: $C = C_0$, is not rejected at level α by a two-sided test. This hypothesis test can be performed by using the exact binomial distribution for calculating the probability of observing such an extreme result as $X = n$ successes where X is binomially distributed with sample size C_0 and success probability $F(t)$.

A generalization of the common source outbreak is the multicommon source outbreak, which comprises several distinct common source outbreaks that may be separated both in time and place and each resulting in clusters of cases. The outbreak of inhalational anthrax in the United States in fall 2001 was a multicommon source outbreak (Fig. 5–4) (Brookmeyer and Blades, 2002). Three clusters of cases were detected among employees of a media publishing company in Florida, postal workers in New Jersey and postal workers in the District of Columbia. The sources of exposure were believed to be letters contaminated with anthrax spores. After the outbreak was recognized, public health officials distributed prophylaxis antimicrobials to persons presumptively exposed including employees of the Florida media company and postal workers in New Jersey and the District of Columbia (Fig. 5–4). Using methods similar to those outlined in this section, Brookmeyer and Blades (2002), estimated the total number of cases that would have occurred without the use of antibiotics and thus the number of cases that were prevented. A complication was that the date of exposure for the Florida outbreak could not be determined because the contaminated letter was not identified. Brookmeyer and Blades (2002) generalized the methods to allow for an unknown date of exposure using maximum likelihood methods.

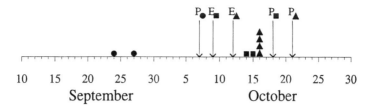

Figure 5–4 Disease onset dates for 3 clusters of cases of inhalational anthrax in the United States outbreak of 2001 among employees of a media publishing company in Florida (●), New Jersey postal workers (■) and District of Columbia postal workers (▲). Each symbol indicates 1 case. Dates of exposure and distribution of antimicrobial prophylaxis in year 2001 indicated by E and P, respectively. The date of exposure for Florida media company employees is not established. *Source*: Brookmeyer, R. and Blades, N. (2002). Prevention of inhalational anthrax in the United States outbreak. *Science* **295**, 1861, used with permission.

CONTINUOUS EXPOSURE EPIDEMICS

A common source outbreak assumes that exposure for all cases occurs at a single point in time, and a multicommon source outbreak assumes that exposures occur at a relatively few distinct points in time. More typically, exposure to a microbe can occur continuously in time as in the case of the AIDS, BSE, and vCJD epidemics. Such epidemics are called continuous exposure epidemics.

Let $g(s)$ represent the exposure (or infection) rate that is a continuous function of calendar time; that is, the numbers of new exposures to the microbe per unit time at calendar time s. In this formulation, there is no distinction made between exposure to the microbe and actual infection that could be detected by a diagnostic test. Either definition can be used as long as the incubation period distribution is defined accordingly. The expected cumulative number of cases with disease onset up to calendar time t, $N(t)$, is given by the convolution equation

$$N(t) = \int_0^t g(s)F(t - s)ds \qquad (5–3)$$

This equation is justified by the fact that if an individual has disease onset by calendar time t, he or she must have been exposed at a previous time s, and the incubation period must be less than $(t - s)$. Eq. 5–3 reveals that the epidemic curve of incident (new) cases of clinical disease lags the epidemic curve of incident exposures. The AIDS epidemic in San Francisco illustrates this concept (Fig. 5–5). The epidemic curve of infections peaks years before the epidemic curve of clinical disease. The incubation period

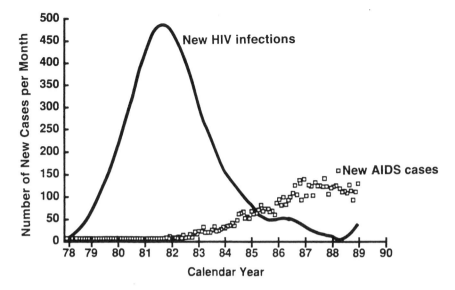

Figure 5–5 The monthly HIV infection rate (solid line) and monthly AIDS incidence (squares) in San Francisco, as estimated by Bacchetti (1990). *Source:* Bacchetti, P. (1990). Estimating the incubation period of AIDS by comparing population infection and diagnosis patterns. *Journal of the American Statistical Association* **85,** 1002–1008, used with permission.

distribution transforms the epidemic curves of infections to the epidemic curve of onset of clinical disease through the convolution Eq. 5–3.

If the case-incubation period distribution $F_c(t)$ is used in place of F(t) in Eq. 5–3, $g(s)$ is replaced by $g_c(t)$, which represents the number of persons newly exposed to the microbe per unit time at calendar time s that will eventually develop disease:

$$N(t) = \int_0^t g_c(s)F_c(t - s)\,ds \qquad (5\text{–}4)$$

Back-Calculation Methods

Public health surveillance systems collect data on incident (new) cases of disease. Thus, an estimate of $N(t)$ can be obtained from surveillance data. If the incubation period distribution F(t) or the case incubation period distribution $F_c(t)$ are known then either Eq. 5–3 or 5–4 can be used to estimate $g(s)$ or $g_c(s)$ through deconvolution. This method, known as back-calculation, uses number of cases of disease, as reported to a public health surveillance system, together with the incubation period distribution to reconstruct the number of exposures (or infections) that must have occurred in the past to give rise to the observed pattern of cases of disease (Brookmeyer, 1991; Brookmeyer and Gail, 1986; Rosenberg, 1995).

The statistical methodology and computational issues for performing back-calculation along with its strengths and weaknesses have been reviewed extensively by Brookmeyer and Gail (1994). Back-calculation has been applied successfully to the AIDS epidemic. Brookmeyer (1991) reconstructed the underlying epidemic curve of incident HIV infections in the United States using AIDS surveillance data. The analyses showed that infections grew rapidly from 1978 to 1981, began to slow, peaked in about 1984, and then markedly declined.

Back-calculation methods have also been applied to the BSE and vCJD epidemics. However, both $g(s)$ and $F(t)$ are uncertain in these epidemics. Different parametric models have been applied to help resolve the inherent uncertainty, such as the assumption that the hazard of infection with vCJD is proportional to the incidence of BSE. However, in the absence of a reliable estimate of the incubation period, such deconvolution methods produce wide ranges for the extent of the resulting epidemics (Donnelly and Ferguson, 2000; Huillard d'Aignaux et al., 2001; Medley, 2001).

Even when the incubation period distribution is known, the back-calculation method has its limitations because little information can be gleaned from disease surveillance data regarding the recent numbers of incident infections, especially if the incubation period is long. For example, little statistical information is available from AIDS surveillance systems about the numbers of persons infected the past year because the median AIDS incubation period is about 10 years, and thus very recent infections are not yet reflected in AIDS cases. An approach for estimating the incidence rate of infections is to conduct a cohort study of uninfected individuals who are followed to identify new infections. However, cohort studies are limited because they require considerable time to and are prone to follow-up bias. Follow-up bias occurs when persons who return for follow-up have different risks of infection than persons who do not return for follow-up. Follow-up bias can seriously distort estimates of incidence rates. An alternative approach for estimating incidence rates, that is not prone to follow-up bias, called snapshot estimators, is discussed in the next section.

Snapshot Estimators

Relatively new surveillance methods termed snapshot estimators have been developed to circumvent the problems of cohort studies for estimating recent infection rates. A biological marker is used to determine whether persons have been recently infected, and a random sample is drawn from the target population to determine the number of people who have the biological marker. The key epidemiologic relationships among incidence, prevalence, and duration are used to convert that number into an incidence rate.

The methodology was first proposed by Brookmeyer and Quinn (1995) to estimate the recent HIV incidence rate based on two different diagnostic tests. One test (P24 antigen) gives positive results for some period following exposure before the second test (HIV enzyme-immunoassay antibody test), and the mean duration of this period is d. A positive result on the first diagnostic test and a negative on the second diagnostic test indicate that the person has been infected recently and is in the window period of recent infection. Thus, the key idea is to use dual diagnostic tests for infection where one test becomes positive before the other. If an individual is positive on the first test, but negative on the second, then the individual is said to be in the "window" period. Brookmeyer and Quinn (1995) applied the method to persons attending a sexually transmitted disease clinic in India. Of 1241 persons whose tests were negative for antibodies, 15 were in the window period of recent infection. The key epidemiologic relationship is then used:

$$\text{Prevalence} = \text{incidence} \times \text{mean duration} \qquad (5\text{--}5)$$

Although this equation is typically used in steady-state situations, its use in an epidemic can be justified if the mean duration (d) is relatively short (Brookmeyer, 1997). The mean duration d of the window period of recent infection for the P24 antigen/HIV antibody markers was approximately 22.5 days (or 0.0616 years). Thus, Eq. 5–5 shows that the incidence rate of new infection is $(15/1241)/(.0616) \times 100 = 19.6\%$ per year. Confidence interval procedures could be obtained using Poisson data methods. Brookmeyer (1997) generalized the confidence interval procedures to account for uncertainty in the mean duration of the window period (d).

If the mean duration d is short (as in the example above), then few persons will be detected in the window period of recent infection, and accordingly the statistical estimate of the incidence rate will be imprecise. To address that concern, the CDC developed a detuned EIA system that involves two antibody tests that increased the mean duration d of the window period; one EIA test is more sensitive and gives positive results about 4 months earlier than the other, less sensitive, test (Janssen et al., 1998). This method can produce statistically reliable estimates of HIV incidence for a range of situations because more persons can be found in the window period of recent infection. The statistical theory underlying the use of snapshot estimators is given by Kaplan and Brookmeyer (1999).

EPIDEMIC TRANSMISSION MODELS

Mathematical models for transmission of epidemics can provide insight into, and explanations for, temporal trends in surveillance data on epidemics. The theory and application of transmission models have been described extensively and reviewed by Anderson and May (1991). Here, only the simplest, most rudimentary of these models to provide insight into their use is described.

The simplest model for a disease that is transmitted from person to person is a two compartmental model in which persons are either uninfected (susceptible) or infected. Such models can be formulated as differential equations or as difference equations, which can be propagated through time. For example, the number of infected persons in the population at time $t + \Delta t$, called $I(t + \Delta t)$, is the number of persons infected at time t plus the number of persons newly infected in the time interval $(t, t + \Delta t)$, called $n(t)$, minus the number of infected persons that may have been removed from the population in the interval (e.g., because of death), called $r(t)$:

$$I(t + \Delta t) = I(t) + n(t) - r(t)$$

To derive expressions for $n(t)$ and $r(t)$, critical assumptions are then made about the rates at which infected persons interact with susceptible persons, the probability of infection transmission when persons do interact, and the rate that persons are removed from the population.

A simple assumption is that of homogenous mixing, sometimes called the law of mass action, which states that a person who has a contact with another person is equally likely to have that contact with any person in the population. Under this assumption, the number of newly infected persons in a population in a time interval $(t, t + \Delta t)$ is proportional to the product of the number of infected persons in the population and the numbers of susceptible persons $(S(t))$ in the population at time t; that is, $n(t) = \theta I(t) \cdot S(t)$, where the proportionality constant θ is the product of two other parameters: the rate that new contacts (or interactions) are formed between two members of the population per unit time, and the probability of transmission of infection per contact. Under the simple assumption that the proportionality constant θ does not vary with time and that the only infected persons removed from the population are those who die, then a mathematical derivation shows that the fraction of the population that is infected follows a logistic curve over time. These equations predict that the number of new infections per unit time grows exponentially, and then slows to subexponential growth because of saturation effects, ultimately peaks, and decreases to zero. As the susceptible population of uninfected persons becomes depleted, saturation occurs and the number of new contacts between susceptible and infected persons eventually decreases.

While simple epidemic models of the sort described above can provide insight into the temporal trends in epidemics, they must be interpreted and applied with caution to surveillance data. For example, the simple model described above made numerous assumptions including (*1*) a two compartmental model, (*2*) homogeneous mixing, (*3*) infected persons are infectious, (*4*) the degree of infectiousness is constant until removal from the population, and (*5*) only infected persons are removed from the population because of death. Such a model predicts a simple rise and fall of an epidemic. However, epidemics can be considerably more complex if for example, the population is composed of different subgroups with different initial prevalences of infections and different contact rates within and between subgroups. For example, the epidemic curve can appear to fall off as one subgroup saturates but then rise again as the epidemic ignites in another subgroup. Thus, extrapolations with such a curve just as it begins its temporary decline can be misleading. Furthermore, the parameters and proportionality constants in the transmission models may vary over time. For example, the rate of formation of new contacts between two members of the population per unit time may decrease when a population becomes aware of behaviors that carry a high risk of disease transmission.

Surveillance data typically refer to incident cases of clinical (symptomatic) onset of disease rather than new incident infections. The epidemic curve for new infections may follow a bell-shaped curve, but may not resemble the epidemic curve of incident clinical disease (Fig. 5–5) because of the lag due to incubation periods. Epidemic transmission models provide insight into the curve of new incident infections. The convolution equation, Eq. 5–3 must be used to relate the epidemic curve of new incident infections to the epidemic curve of incident cases of clinical disease that is typically available from public health surveillance data.

DISCUSSION

This chapter reviews key factors in interpreting time trends in surveillance data from epidemics: the reporting characteristics of the surveillance system, the transmission dynamics of the epidemic, the incubation period distribution of the disease, and the introduction of public health interventions and control measures that can interrupt the natural course of the epidemic. Correctly interpreting trends in surveillance data requires accounting for and adjusting the data for incomplete reporting and reporting delays.

The incubation period distribution plays a central role in the interpretation of time trends in an epidemic. The epidemic curve of disease incidence lags the epidemic curve of infection or exposure. The lag is determined by the incubation period distribution. The observed cases of disease are only a fraction of the total cases that have been infected as the other cases may still be incubating; and, that fraction is determined by the incubation period distribution. If the incubation period is known, it is possible to estimate the underlying size of the infected population by deconvolution and back-calculation methods.

However, when the incubation period is long, alternative models, such as snapshot estimators based on biological markers of recent infection, may be useful for monitoring current trends in incident infections. Mathematical models for transmission dynamics can provide qualitative insight into the propagation of epidemics and the temporal evolution of the underlying epidemic curves. However, such models often rely on assumptions that should be critically evaluated.

Tracking, understanding, and forecasting temporal trends in epidemics from surveillance data require a variety of methodologies, models, and techniques. These methods and models must take into account the unique epidemiology, transmission dynamics, and natural history of the infectious agents under study.

REFERENCES

Anderson, R.M. and May, R.M. (1991). *Infectious Diseases of Humans: Dynamics and Control*. Oxford: Oxford University Press.

Bacchetti, P. (1990). Estimating the incubation period of AIDS by comparing population infection and diagnosis patterns. *Journal of the American Statistical Association* **85,** 1002–1008.

Brookmeyer, R. (1991). Reconstruction and future trends of the AIDS epidemic in the United States, *Science* **253,** 37–42.

Brookmeyer, R. (1997). Accounting for follow-up bias in estimation of HIV incidence rates. *Journal of the Royal Statistical Society Series A* **160,** 127–140.

Brookmeyer, R. and Blades, N. (2002). Prevention of inhalational anthrax in the U.S. outbreak. *Science* 295, 1861.

Brookmeyer, R., Blades, N., Hugh-Jones, M., and Henderson, D.A. (2001). The statistical analysis of truncated data: Application to the Sverdlovsk anthrax outbreak. *Biostatistics* **2,** 233–247.

Brookmeyer, R. and Gail, M.H. (1986). The minimum size of the AIDS epidemic in the United States. *Lancet* **2,** 320–322.

Brookmeyer, R. and Gail, M.H. (1994). *AIDS Epidemiology: A Quantitative Approach*. Oxford: Oxford University Press.

Brookmeyer, R. and Goedert, J.J. (1989). Censoring in an epidemic with an application to hemophilia-associated AIDS. *Biometrics* **45,** 325–336.

Brookmeyer, R. and Liao, J. (1990). The Analysis of delays in disease reporting. *American Journal of Epidemiology* **132**, 355–365.

Brookmeyer, R. and Quinn, T. (1995). Estimation of current HIV incidence rates from a cross-sectional survey using early diagnostic tests. *American Journal of Epidemiology* **141**, 166–172.

Brown, P., Will, R.G., Bradley, R., Asher, D., and Detwiler, L. (2001). Bovine spongiform encephalopathy and variant Creutzfeldt-Jakob disease: Background, evolution and current concerns. *Emerging Infectious Diseases* **7**, 6–16.

Darby, S.C., Doll, R., Thakrar, B., Rizza, C.R., and Cox, D.R. (1990). Time from infection with HIV to onset of AIDS in patients with hemophilia in the U.K. *Statistics in Medicine* **9**, 681–689.

Donnelly, C.A. and Ferguson, N.M. (2000). *Statistical Aspects of BSE and vCJD: Models for Epidemics*. New York: Chapman and Hall/CRC. Monographs on Statistics and Applied Probability 84.

Eyler, J.M. (1979). *The Ideas and Methods of William Farr*. Baltimore: Johns Hopkins University Press.

Gail, M.H., Rosenberg, P., and Goedert, J. (1990). Therapy may explain recent deficits in AIDS incidence. *Journal of Acquired Immune Deficiency Syndromes* **3**, 833–835.

Huillard d'Aignaux, J.N., Simon, N., Cousens, S.N., and Smith, P.G. (2001). Predictability of the UK variant Creutzfeldt-Jakob disease epidemic. *Science* **294**, 1729–1731.

Janssen, R.S., Satten, G.A., Stramer, S.L., Rawal, B.D., O'Brien, T.R., Weiblen, B.J., Hecht, F.M., Jack, N., Cleghorn, F.R., Kahn, J.O., Chesney, M.A., and Busch, M.P. (1998). New testing strategy to detect early HIV-1 infection for use in incidence estimates and for clinical and prevention purposes. *Journal of the American Medical Association* **280**, 42–48.

Kaplan, E.H. and Brookmeyer, R. (1999). Snapshot estimators of recent HIV incidence rates. *Operations Research* **47**, 29–37.

Medley, G.F. (2001). Predicting the unpredictable. *Science* **294**, 1663–1664.

Medley, G.F., Anderson, R.M., Cox, D.R., and Billard, L. (1987). Incubation period of AIDS in patients infected via blood transfusion. *Nature* **328**, 719–721.

Rosenberg, P. (1995). The scope of the AIDS epidemic in the United States. *Science* **270**, 1372–1375.

Sartwell, P.E. (1950). The distribution of incubation periods of infectious diseases. *American Journal of Hygiene* **51**, 310–318.

Zeger, S.L., See, L.-C., and Diggle, P.J. (1989). Statistical methods for monitoring the AIDS epidemic. *Statistics in Medicine* **8**, 3–21.

6

Using Public Health Data to Evaluate Screening Programs: Application to Prostate Cancer

RUTH ETZIONI, LARRY KESSLER,
DANTE DI TOMMASO

Cancer surveillance, or the monitoring of population cancer trends, is vital to cancer control research. Changes in cancer incidence or mortality can provide information relevant to treatment advances, new screening or diagnostic technologies, and changes in risk factors in the population. Monitoring cancer trends also allows geographic, demographic, and social subgroups to be compared and provides information on changes over time in the extent of disease at diagnosis, patterns of care, and patient survival.

The importance of population cancer trends is evident in the ongoing debate about prostate-specific antigen (PSA) screening for prostate cancer. Screening tests for PSA, introduced in the United States in 1988, were rapidly adopted (Legler et al., 1998). By 1998, 35% to 40% of men over the age of 65 years without a prior diagnosis of prostate cancer were being tested each year (Etzioni et al., 2002a). Figure 6–1 shows that the adoption of PSA screening was accompanied by great changes in prostate cancer incidence and mortality (National Cancer Institute SEER Program Data 1973–1999, 2002). From 1986 to 1992, the overall age-adjusted incidence nearly doubled, but it has since returned to pre-PSA-screening levels. Mortality rates followed a similar pattern, increasing in the late 1980s before falling by 21% from 1991 to 1999. The incidence of distant stage prostate cancer has also declined sharply since 1990. The absence of re-

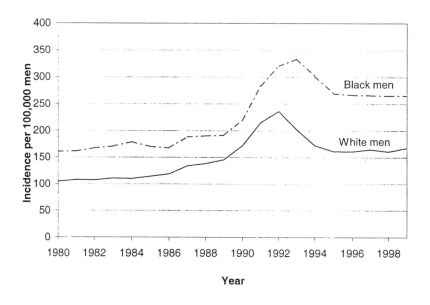

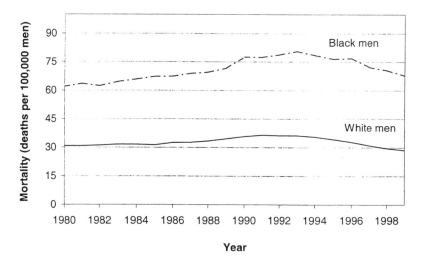

Figure 6–1 Age-adjusted prostate cancer incidence (top) and mortality (bottom) in black and white men in the United States from 1980 to 1999. *Source:* National Cancer Institute SEER Program Data 1973–1999. http://seer.cancer.gov (accessed July 12, 2002), used with permission.

sults from clinical trials about PSA screening has made these changes a focus of attention among researchers and the general public.

What do the observed trends in prostate cancer incidence and mortality say about PSA screening? Declines in disease mortality rates suggest that screening may be effective and have been cited as evidence that screening saves lives (see, for example, Magee and Thompson, 2001). Changes in incidence can also be informative. The introduction of a screening test into a population is followed by a predictable pattern of disease incidence (Feuer and Wun, 1992). First, the incidence increases because the screen identifies cases in which disease was present but not yet clinically apparent. As screening use stabilizes, incidence falls because individuals who would have been diagnosed in later years have been removed from the prevalent pool. After screening has been introduced, the magnitude and duration of the expected incidence peak vary according to the *lead time*, or the time by which the test advances diagnosis, and the extent of overdiagnosis, or overdetection, of latent cancer attributable to the test (Fig. 6–2) (Feuer and Wun, 1992; Etzioni et al., 2002b). Thus, mortality trends provide information on screening efficacy, and incidence trends can provide insight into properties of the screening test. This information is particularly relevant when results from controlled clinical trials are unavailable, as is the case with prostate cancer screening. Two large trials—the European Randomized Screening for Prostate Cancer Trial (Beemsterboer et al., 2000), and the Prostate Lung, Colon and Ovarian Cancer trial (Gohagan et al., 1994)—are ongoing, and results are expected in 2008. In contrast to these controlled studies, the population represents the ultimate, uncontrolled study setting.

Population cancer trends are a complex product of biological, epidemiologic, clinical, and behavioral factors. Thus, any observed patterns in cancer incidence or mortality typically have multiple interpretations. Indeed, declining prostate cancer mortality, rather than being universally interpreted as evidence that PSA screening reduces death from the disease, has been the subject of much debate. Recent ecological analyses of international prostate cancer trends have only added fuel to the fire. For example, one recent study noted that prostate cancer mortality rates were declining in the United States but not in Australia, although PSA screening had been widely used in both places (Oliver et al., 2001). A second study that focused only on the United States and the United Kingdom found that, although PSA screening rates (as measured by prostate cancer incidence) differed greatly between the two countries, prostate cancer mortality rates for 1993 through 1995 were similar (Lu-Yao et al., 2002). Alternative explanations for the declining mortality rates include improved treatment, earlier detection and treatment of recurrent disease, and reduced

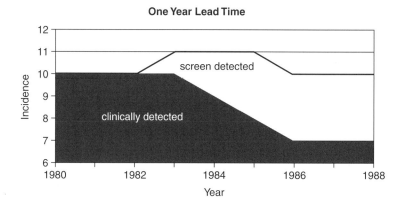

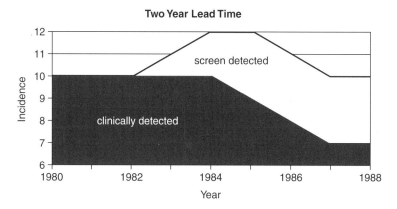

Figure 6–2 Dependence of cancer incidence on the lead time after the introduction of screening. In a hypothetical example, screening is introduced in 1983 against a backdrop of constant disease incidence in the population. Cancer incidence is decomposed into clinically detected cases and screen-detected cases. *A*: (constant, 1-year lead time) and *B*: (constant, 2-year lead time) assume the same dissemination of screening, described in terms of total number of cancer cases screen-detected each year. The number of screen-detected cancer cases from 1980 through 1988 is as follows: 0, 0, 0, 1, 2, 3, 3, 3, 3. *Source*: Feuer, E.J. and Wun, L.M. (1992). How much of the recent rise in breast cancer incidence can be explained by increases in mammography utilization: A dynamic population approach. *American Journal of Epidemiology* **136,** 1423–1436, used with permission.

misattribution of cause of death to prostate cancer in recently diagnosed cases (Feuer et al., 1999; Hankey et al., 1999). Separating the effects of each of these factors requires careful, and often extensive, analysis.

In separating the effects of PSA screening from the effects of other factors on prostate cancer trends, computer modeling is an indispensable tool.

Computer modeling is a powerful technique for projecting the outcomes of interventions in the absence of data from clinical trials (Ramsey et al., 2000). In prostate cancer research, models have compared initial treatments for localized prostate cancer (Fleming et al., 1993), different intervals for PSA testing (Etzioni et al., 1999a), and delayed versus immediate androgen deprivation therapy for recurrent disease (Bayoumi et al., 2000). Cervical and breast cancer screening models have been used to design, monitor, and evaluate national screening programs in several European countries (van den Akker-van et al., 1999). In the United States, models have been used to clarify marked changes in national cancer statistics, such as increased incidences of breast and prostate cancer (Feuer and Wun, 1992; Etzioni et al., 2002b; Wun et al., 1995), and increased survival rates for Hodgkin's disease and testicular cancer (Feuer et al., 1991; Weller et al., 1999).

A model is a structured representation that links potential actions with their consequences. It is, effectively, a formalization of the steps, or health states, between an intervention and an outcome. In complex disease processes, computer models provide a method for systematically organizing and synthesizing relevant information from many sources. The relevant information for projecting the outcomes of prostate cancer screening in the population includes PSA screening rates, the likelihood of a prostate cancer diagnosis resulting from a PSA screening test, the lead time, and the supposed reduction in the risk of prostate cancer death after screen detection.

Here we describe our use of computer modeling to quantify the link between PSA screening and prostate cancer incidence and mortality. The first step in model development is to identify the key variables that link screening to each outcome. For incidence, the key variables are the lead time and the secular trend in incidence (the incidence anticipated in the absence of screening). For mortality, the key variables are the lead time and screening efficacy, described in terms of the reduced annual risk of prostate cancer death after the date at which disease would have been clinically diagnosed. The models provide a quantitative framework for identifying values of the key variables that are consistent with the surveillance data on prostate cancer.

Data resources for both cancer surveillance and PSA screening are described. Then we present an approach to modeling both prostate cancer mortality and incidence, and show how the models identify plausible values for the key variables. The models can be formalized as a statistical framework for inference by developing a likelihood function for the key variables that link PSA screening and prostate cancer incidence is also shown. Finally, we review alternative modeling approaches and other methods that have been used to address the link between PSA screening and population trends in prostate cancer mortality.

DATA RESOURCES

Cancer Surveillance Data

Our primary resource for prostate cancer surveillance data has been the Surveillance, Epidemiology, and End Results (SEER) program of the National Cancer Institute (National Cancer Institute SEER Program Data 1973–1999, 2002.) The SEER program is a system of population-based central tumor registries, that collect clinical, sociodemographic, and follow-up information on all cancers diagnosed in their defined catchment areas. Case ascertainment for SEER began on January 1, 1973, in Connecticut, Iowa, New Mexico, Utah, and Hawaii and in the metropolitan areas of Detroit and San Francisco-Oakland. In 1974–1975, the metropolitan area of Atlanta and the 13-county Seattle-Puget Sound area were added. In 1992, the SEER program expanded to increase coverage of minority populations, especially Hispanics, by adding Los Angeles County and four counties in the San Jose-Monterey area south of San Francisco.

The SEER program currently collects and publishes cancer incidence and survival data from 11 population-based cancer registries and two supplemental registries, covering approximately 14% of the US population. Information on more than 2.5 million cancer cases is included in the SEER database, and approximately 160,000 new cases are added each year. Reported information includes the cancer site and histologic characteristics, date of diagnosis, and stage of disease. Treatment provided within 4 months of diagnosis is also recorded. A variable defined as "clinical stage of disease" indicates whether the disease was localized at diagnosis or had metastasized to regional or distant sites. Since 1983, the extent of disease at diagnosis has been recorded by SEER with the Tumor, Node, Metastasis (TNM) system published by the American Joint Committee on Cancer.

The SEER registries actively follow cases to obtain vital status and underlying cause of death. These data are important for estimating survival after a cancer diagnosis. The mortality data reported by SEER are provided by the National Center for Health Statistics.

The SEER data are updated annually and are provided as a public service in print and electronic formats. Queries, which can be submitted through the SEER Web site (http://seer.cancer.gov), allow the user to generate summary reports from the SEER data base.

PSA Screening Data

Any model linking PSA screening with prostate cancer trends requires a reliable assessment of the frequency of PSA screening in the population. The PSA test was introduced for early detection purposes in 1988, and over the next few years, the number of men tested increased exponentially. Unfortunately, during the early years of screening, men's PSA testing habits were not tracked. The earliest population surveys of PSA screening began in 1993, when a few states added PSA testing questions to their local CDC-sponsored Behavioral Risk Factor Surveillance surveys (CDC, 1999), but these efforts were limited to a few specific regions of the United States. More recently, national surveys of PSA screening have been conducted, but estimates of use in the critical early years are lacking.

Given the sporadic attempts to survey patterns of PSA screening, and the limitations of survey data concerning PSA screening behavior (Jordan et al., 1999), our primary resource for tracking annual PSA screening frequencies has been medical claims records, accessed through the linked SEER-Medicare database (Applied Research Program, Division of Cancer Control and Population Sciences, National Cancer Institute, 2002).

The SEER-Medicare data base links cases diagnosed in SEER with Medicare claims records, thus allowing medical service use to be analyzed by SEER cases. The most recent SEER-Medicare linkage covers services for 1991 through 1998 on diagnoses through 1996; this is due to be updated through 2001 in early 2003. Previous versions of the SEER-Medicare data covered services for 1984 through 1994.

The SEER-Medicare data base contains data on all Medicare-covered services for eligible persons, namely, persons over 65 years and disabled persons under the age of 65 who are entitled to Medicare benefits. We have restricted attention to men over 65 in the interest of obtaining a representative population. Covered services include hospital stays, skilled nursing facility stays, physician and laboratory services, hospital outpatient claims, and home health and hospice care. Nursing home services and self-administered prescription drugs are not covered. Indicators of Health Maintenance Organization (HMO) enrollment are provided with the SEER-Medicare data. In our analyses, we exclude HMO enrollees for all calendar years during which they were covered by the HMO.

The HCPCS (CPT-4) codes provided with the Medicare claims data can be used to identify PSA tests (CPT codes 86316 and 84153). The SEER-Medicare linkage allows us to distinguish pre- from postdiagnostic PSA tests. Because SEER provides only the month of diagnosis, not an exact date, we exclude all tests conducted after the month of diagnosis.

In addition to the SEER-Medicare linked files, Medicare data are available for a 5% sample of Medicare enrollees without cancer (controls) residing in the SEER geographic areas. We use data from cases and controls to estimate annual testing rates and cancer detection rates, which are then provided as model inputs. In estimating the annual testing and cancer detection rates, we weight controls by a factor of 20 to account for the relative fractions of cases and controls in the data. The denominator for the testing rates consists of all men alive and eligible for screening at the start of the year. The numerator consists of all men undergoing at least one PSA test during the year. The cancer detection rate is usually defined as the proportion of men with a PSA test whose test leads to a diagnosis of cancer. However, test results are not included in the Medicare claims files. Thus, we approximate the cancer detection rate by using the frequency of a cancer diagnosis within 3 months of a PSA test.

The SEER-Medicare data have several limitations, the most notable being the age range of the eligible population. Because we use the data on men over the age of 65, our results pertain to this older population. Reliable population-based data for younger men for the period of interest is difficult to find. A second limitation of the medical claims records is that they typically do not provide the reason for the test, that is, whether it was a bona fide screening test or a diagnostic test used to confirm the already suspected presence of prostate cancer. Because only screening tests are able to advance diagnosis and alter the progress of the disease, they account for all of the effect of PSA screening on disease incidence and mortality. Recognizing that the PSA testing rates derived from SEER-Medicare likely overstate the PSA screening frequency, we later introduce a nuisance parameter, p, to adjust screening rates and the rates of cancer detection after a PSA test.

MODEL DEVELOPMENT

In this section, our models of PSA screening and prostate cancer incidence and mortality, as well as their inputs and outputs are described briefly. Detailed descriptions of the models can be found in Etzioni et al. (1999b, 2002b).

Although the goals of the models are different, their organization and structure are similar. Briefly, the models generate PSA testing histories for a large number of hypothetical men. From cancer detection rates, the models then identify the screen-detected cohort—the cohort of men whose diagnosis is advanced by PSA screening. As noted above, the screen-detected cohort accounts for all future effect on prostate cancer incidence and mortality in the population. Using the screen-detected cohort, the models then project the changes in incidence and mortality trends relative to the trends that would have been expected in the absence of PSA screening. For incidence, the model calculates the number of extra prostate cancer cases diagnosed each year, and for mortality, it calculates the number of prostate cancer deaths prevented each year by PSA screening.

A Model of PSA Screening and Prostate Cancer Mortality

The purpose of our model of PSA screening and prostate cancer mortality was to determine whether PSA screening could explain the declines in prostate cancer mortality observed from 1991 through 1994. The primary output of the model was the number of prostate cancer deaths prevented each year. The model followed a series of steps:

1. Generate PSA testing histories, using SEER-Medicare testing rates (Applied Research Program, Division of Cancer Control and Population Sciences, National Cancer Institute, 2002), and dates of death from causes other than prostate cancer, using U.S. life tables.
2. Generate indicators of prostate cancer diagnosis from PSA screening, using cancer detection rates from SEER-Medicare (Legler et al., 1998; Etzioni et al., 2002a), adjusted downward by a factor p. The factor p is the fraction of cases for which a test was used for screening, as opposed to confirming a diagnosis among all cases detected after a PSA test. We used three values for p to reflect low, moderate, and high frequencies of screening relative to diagnostic applications.
3. For each screen-detected case, generate the date at which diagnosis would have occurred in the absence of screening. This date of clinical diagnosis (t_d) is the date of screen diagnosis plus the lead time. The lead time is calculated from a gamma distribution with a mean of 3, 5, or 7 years and is based on published information about lead time associated with PSA testing (Gann et al., 1995; Pearson et al., 1996).
4. For each screen-detected case, generate the date at which death from prostate cancer would have occurred in the absence of screening ($T_1 = t_d + s_1$), where s_1 is the time from the clinical diagnosis to prostate cancer death in the absence of screening. Relative survival curves from SEER among cases diagnosed before the PSA era are used to approximate s_1.
5. For each screen-detected case, also generate the date at which death from prostate cancer would have occurred given screen detection ($T_2 = t_d + s_2$), where $P(S > s_2) = (P(S > s_1))^r$ and S denotes the time from clinical diagnosis to death from prostate cancer. The factor r is the benefit associated with prostate cancer screening and is equivalent to the reduction in the annual risk of death from prostate cancer, or the relative risk in a discrete proportional hazards model.
6. For each year, compute the number of deaths prevented by PSA screening by subtracting the number of screened men dying of prostate cancer in the given year from the number of unscreened men dying of prostate

cancer in the same year. Convert the deaths prevented to an incidence per 100,000 men by dividing the difference by the SEER denominator (population size) for that year.

7. Add the estimate of prevented prostate cancer deaths to the observed prostate cancer deaths for 1988–1994. The total provides a model projection of what prostate cancer mortality would have been in the absence of PSA screening. A decline in the model-projected mortality after 1991 implies that PSA screening cannot account for all of the mortality declines observed since this time.

Figure 6–3 shows the model results for a relative risk *r* of 0.5 and moderate *p*. All of the projected incidence rates show some decline after 1991. Thus, even if PSA screening substantially reduces the annual risk of prostate cancer death, it is unlikely to account for all of the observed decline in mortality.

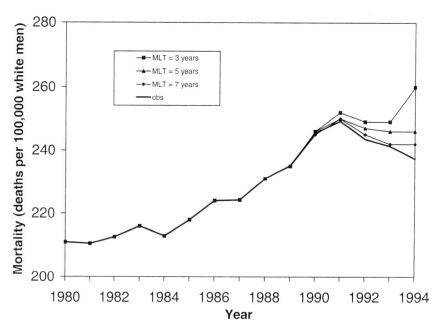

Figure 6–3 Model results for PSA use and prostate cancer mortality. U.S. prostate cancer mortality for white men aged 70 to 84 years; observed (1980–1994) and inflated by deaths prevented by PSA screening (1988–1994). Annual prostate cancer mortality after the date of clinical diagnosis is 50% lower among screen-detected cases than among clinically diagnosed cases (relative risk *r* = 0.5). A moderate value for *p* is assumed. Model results are given for 3 mean lead times (MLT) in years.

A Model of PSA Screening and Prostate Cancer Incidence

The primary goal of our model of PSA screening and prostate cancer incidence was to identify rates of overdiagnosis consistent with PSA screening and observed prostate cancer incidence in the U.S. population from 1988 through 1998. Overdiagnosis was defined as the detection by PSA screening of prostate cancer that, in the absence of the test, would never have become clinically apparent. This modeling effort arose from the fact that overdiagnosis had been, and continues to be, a major concern about PSA screening (Hugosson et al., 2000); because of the high prevalence of the disease, especially in older men, and its indolent course in many cases, the test has a large potential to detect disease that would never have become clinically apparent otherwise.

According to our definition, an overdiagnosed case is a screen-detected case that would never have been diagnosed in the absence of screening. However, this case is simply one in which, without screening, death would have occurred from other causes during the lead time. Thus, overdiagnosis and lead time are closely linked. In fact, knowing the lead time and the expected rates of death from other causes is sufficient to determine the frequency of overdiagnosis. We therefore designed a model to identify plausible lead times, given data on PSA screening rates and the incidence of prostate cancer in the PSA screening era.

As does the mortality model, the incidence model begins by identifying a cohort of screen-detected cases (steps 1 and 2 above). But the primary output of the incidence model is a projection of the excess cases from PSA screening (over and above those that would have been expected without PSA) each year from 1988 through 1998. The steps required to obtain this projection are given below:

1. Generate PSA testing histories, using SEER-Medicare testing rates (Applied Research Program, Division of Cancer Control and Population Sciences, National Cancer Institute, 2002), and the dates of death from causes other than prostate cancer, using US life tables.
2. Generate indicators of prostate cancer diagnosis from PSA screening, using cancer detection rates from SEER-Medicare (Legler et al., 1998; Etzioni et al., 2002a), adjusted downward by the factor p. Once again, we used 3 values for p to reflect low, moderate, and high frequencies of screening relative to diagnostic tests but allowed p to vary with calendar time. Our trajectories for p all reflect increasing use of the test for screening relative to diagnostic purposes.
3. For each screen-detected case, generate a date of clinical diagnosis (t_d). Once again, the lead time is calculated from a gamma distribution with a mean of 3, 5, or 7 years.

4. Compute the number of annual excess cases diagnosed by PSA screening. In a given year t, the number of excess cases, denoted $N(t)$, is equal to the number of cases detected by PSA screening in that year, $R(t)$, less the number of cases previously detected by PSA screening that would have been diagnosed clinically that year, $M(t)$. Thus, the excess cases in a given year may be thought of as a difference between diagnostic gains from screening in that year and diagnostic losses from screening in previous years.

5. Convert the excess cases to an excess incidence per 100,000 men, by dividing the above difference by the SEER denominators (population sizes) for each year.

Whereas the model estimates excess incidence, our observed surveillance data reflect absolute incidence. By definition, the absolute incidence is the sum of the excess incidence (incidence over and above what would have been expected without screening) and the secular trend in incidence (incidence that would have been expected without screening). To project absolute incidence, we add an assumed secular trend to the modeled excess incidence. The secular trend is a projection of what prostate cancer incidence would have been in the absence of PSA screening. The secular trend is effectively an additional nuisance parameter, and inferences are conditional on our assumptions about this parameter.

What would prostate cancer incidence have been without PSA screening? The answer to this question is, of course, not known. However, clues as to the likely incidence in the late 1980s and early 1990s can be gleaned from practice patterns related to prostate care. Before the PSA era, prostate cancer incidence increased steadily. From the late 1970s to the mid-1980s, the principal cause of this increasing trend was the use of transurethral resection of the prostate (TURP) (Potosky et al., 1990; Merrill et al., 1999), a surgical procedure for alleviating symptoms of benign prostatic hyperplasia that frequently resulted in the incidental diagnosis of prostate carcinoma, hence their association with prostate cancer incidence. However, by the early 1990s, medical management of benign disease had led to a marked decline in TURP rates (Merrill et al., 1999; Wasson et al., 2000). These advances would likely have led to smaller increases in incidence, and possibly even declines in incidence, in the absence of PSA screening. Therefore, for our secular trend projections, we consider constant and declining incidence trends, as well as an increasing trend based on historical data, for use in sensitivity analyses.

The results for white men under a constant secular trend and a moderate value for p indicate that, under this assumption, a lead time of 5 years, with an associated overdiagnosis rate of 29% among screen-detected cases, is most consistent with the observed surveillance data (Fig. 6–4).

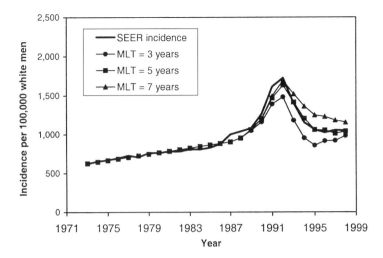

Figure 6–4 Model results for PSA screening and prostate cancer incidence. Observed and model-projected incidence for men aged 70 to 84 years under baseline conditions; constant secular trend and moderate p. The bold curve is the observed, delay-adjusted incidence from SEER (National Cancer Institute SEER Program Data 1973–1999, 2002). The remaining 3 curves represent the model-projected incidence; each corresponds to a specific mean lead time (MLT).

A Maximum Likelihood Framework

In modeling prostate cancer incidence, our goals amount to estimating unknown parameters, principally the mean lead time. The results in Figure 6–4 represent predictions of cancer incidence corresponding to a few isolated points in the space of possible parameter values. To provide a comprehensive and valid approach to estimating parameters, we now describe a maximum likelihood approach. The likelihood function is a function of the parameters of the distribution of the assumed lead time and is conditional on the PSA screening data and assumed secular trend.

Let t denote the year of interest. Denote the observed SEER incidence in year t by $I(t)$, the assumed secular trend in year t by $S(t)$, and the SEER denominator for year t by $D(t)$. Then, the observed number of excess cases in year t (our observed data) is simply $n(t) = D(t)(I(t) - S(t))$. Our model for $n(t)$ is $N(t) = R(t) - M(t)$, where $R(t)$ is the number of cases detected by PSA screening in year t, and $M(t)$ is the number of cases detected previously by screening in which diagnosis would have been made in year t in the absence of PSA screening. Our goal is to derive the likelihood function for $N_1(t), N_2(t), \ldots N_k(t)$, where k is the number of years of follow-up. In our case, k is 11, corresponding to the interval from 1988 through 1998.

$R(t)$ is an observable quantity, given PSA screening and cancer detection rates in year t. Denote the observed value of $R(t)$ by $r(t)$. Now, note that $P(N(t) = n)$ is the same as $P(M(t) = r(t) - n)$. Thus, an equivalent likelihood function for $N(t)$ can be written as a likelihood function for $M(t)$.

Assume that $M(t)$ has a Poisson distribution with a mean of $D(t)\lambda(t)$; $\lambda(t)$ is the proportion of men alive in year t whose prostate cancer was screen-detected before t and who, in the absence of screening, would have been clinically diagnosed at t. We can write $\lambda(t)$ as follows:

$$\lambda(t) = \int_0^t f(s)g(t - s)ds$$

where:

$f(s)$ = the probability density function (pdf) of the interval from time zero (January 1, 1988) to screen detection, and
$g(t - s)$ = the pdf of the lead time.

To derive $f(s)$, note that the risk, or hazard, of screen detection in year s is given by $h(s) = TR(s)CDR(s)p(s)$, where TR is the testing rate, CDR is the cancer detection rate, and p is the adjustment factor for diagnostic versus screening tests. In practice, p is also allowed to be a function of time. Then $f(s)$, the pdf of the interval from time zero to screen detection, may be obtained from $h(s)$ by standard methods for converting a discrete hazard function to a probability density function.

The log-likelihood for $M(t)$ is then given by:

$$l = \sum_t - D(t)\lambda(t) + (r(t) - n(t))\log(D(t)\lambda(t))$$

Given $TR(t)$, $CDR(t)$, $p(t)$, and an assumed secular trend $S(t)$, the log-likelihood is a function of the parameters of the lead time distribution, and, as such, may be maximized using standard techniques. For white men, assuming a constant secular trend and values for p that decrease linearly from 0.5 in 1988 to 0.2 in 1998, we estimated mean lead time to be 6.3 years under an exponential lead-time distribution, and 4.6 years under a gamma lead-time distribution.

CONCLUSION

The models described in this chapter are the latest in a long line of analytic techniques designed to summarize and clarify cancer surveillance data. Statistical methods for summarizing cancer trends include: (*1*) age-period cohort modeling of disease incidence rates (Holford, 1992, Holford et al., 1994) for identifying birth cohort- versus calendar-period influences on cancer incidence trends; (2) join-point regression of disease incidence and mortality (Kim et al., 2000) for identifying the statistical significance of apparent changes in the direction of cancer trends; (3) relative survival modeling (Ederer et al., 1961; Weller et al., 1999) for approximating and modeling "cause-specific survival" after a cancer diagnosis; (4) cancer prevalence statistics (Feldman et al., 1986; Merrill et al., 2000; Merrill, 2001) as a measure of burden of cancer in the population at any given time; and (5) incidence-based mortality methods (Chu et al., 1994) for partitioning cancer mortality according to variables observed at the time of diagnosis, such as disease stage and calendar year of diagnosis. All of these methods have helped us to understand the scope and magnitude of the cancer burden and have helped to define important directions for cancer control research.

Although statistics that summarize cancer surveillance data can provide important insights, quantifying the links between observed trends and specific interventions often requires more in-depth analysis. Information on the use of the interventions of interest is the first requirement. In the past 10 to 15 years, cancer control research has been enhanced greatly by large databases containing records of medical procedure utilization and by the expansion of national survey mechanisms, such as the Behavioral Risk Factor Surveillance System (CDC, 1999) and the National Health Interview Survey (Breen et al., 2001) which track health behaviors in the population. Because data are available on the distribution of cancer control interventions, it is now realistic to consider linking surveillance outcomes to the use of these interventions by the public. Clearly, medical claims data have their limitations; for screening tests, medical procedure codes do not indicate why the test was conducted. Knowing whether the test was used for screening or to confirm a diagnosis is critical and argues for the expansion of surveillance systems to consider including this information with other clinical data collected at the time of diagnosis.

Modeling goes beyond data summaries to quantitatively assess the likelihood that a specific intervention is responsible for trends observed in cancer incidence or mortality. For example, ecologic analyses of the efficacy of PSA screening summarize prostate cancer mortality and PSA screening activities across different geographical areas and attempt to correlate changes in mortality with indicators of PSA screening. Both international (across countries) and national (within countries) ecologic analyses have been conducted, with inconsistent results (Shibata et al., 1998; Bartsch et al., 2001; Crocetti et al., 2001; Oliver et al., 2001; Lu-Yao et al., 2002). In some studies, similar mortality tends have been reported across areas with apparently vastly different PSA testing patterns (see, for example, Lu-Yao et al., 2002). However, these results at best only suggest limited efficacy. Indeed, they may be well in the range of expected results for a beneficial test if the lead time is sufficiently long. Modeling is an ideal tool for projecting expected outcomes under a range of plausible values for lead time, thus allowing us to quantify the evidence in favor of test efficacy.

Other computer models have been used to clarify cancer surveillance data. Feuer et al. (2000) recently used CAN*TROL2 to project the impact of the decline in distant-stage disease on prostate cancer mortality rates. The CAN*TROL2 program is a Windows descendant of the original CAN*TROL program developed to project the effects of cancer control activities for the World Health Organization in the 1980s (Eddy, 1986) CAN*TROL is a macro-level model that uses estimates of standard population-based statistics (birth rates, incidence, stage distributions at diagnosis, mortality) to model the population cancer experience. The effect of cancer control interventions is projected by changing these population statistics. For example, in CAN*TROL, a cancer screening intervention is assumed to affect disease incidence by shifting a user-specified proportion of distant-stage cases to a localized stage at diagnosis. Feuer et al. (2000) used the CAN*TROL2 model to shift each deficit in the number of prostate cancer patients with distant-stage disease to local-regional-stage disease, and they modeled the implications for mortality by modifying disease-specific survival accordingly. Results for their base case assumptions suggested that observed declines in the incidence of distant-stage prostate cancer could have a fairly sizeable and rapid impact on population mortality. The MISCAN microsimulation models, developed in the Netherlands, have also projected the effect of cancer control interventions at the population level (see, for example, van den Akker-van et al., 1999).

This chapter focuses exclusively on screening as a cancer control intervention. Advances in cancer treatment and prevention may contribute to population cancer trends in the same or even more significant ways. A case in point is the recent debate over whether widespread use of mammography or adjuvant therapy for breast cancer is principally responsible for recent declines in breast cancer mortality. Similarly, it is unclear whether declines in mortality from colorectal cancer can be attributed to greater use of screening technologies, changes in diet and other health-related behaviors, or dissemination of more efficacious chemotherapy regimens. We contend that the only way to separate the effects of screening, prevention, and treatment is through computer modeling of the disease process. Efforts to model breast, colorectal, prostate, and lung cancer mortality are under way through the Cancer Intervention and Surveillance Modeling Network of the National Cancer Institute (Cancer Intervention and Surveillance Modeling Network Home Page, 2002). By synthesizing biological and epidemiologic information about the natural history of disease, the prevalence of cancer-control interventions, and the likely clinical effects of these interventions, these models promise to help unravel the complex dynamics of cancer in the population.

REFERENCES

Applied Research Program, Division of Cancer Control and Population Sciences, National Cancer Institute. SEER-Medicare Home Page. http://healthservices. cancer.gov/seermedicare/. (Last accessed May 30, 2002).

Bartsch, G., Horninger, W., Klocker, H., Reissigl, A., Oberaigner, W., Schonitzer, D., Severi, G., Robertson, C., Boyle, P., and the Tyrol Prostate Cancer Screening Group. (2001). Prostate cancer mortality after the introduction of prostate-specific antigen mass screening in the federal state of Tyrol, Austria. *Urology* **58,** 418–424.

Bayoumi, A.M., Brown, A.D., and Garber, A.M. (2000). Cost-effectiveness of androgen suppression therapies in advanced prostate cancer. *Journal of the National Cancer Institute*. **92,** 1731–1739.

Beemsterboer, P.M., de Koning, H.J., Kranse, R., Trienekens, P.H., van der MAAS, P.J., and Schroder, F.H. (2000) Prostate specific antigen testing and digital rectal examination before and during a randomized trial of screening for prostate cancer: European randomized study of screening for prostate cancer, Rotterdam. *Journal of Urolology* **164,** 1216–1220.

Breen, N., Wagener, D.K., Brown, M.L., Davis, W.W., and Ballard-Barbash, R. (2001). Progress in cancer screening over a decade: results of cancer screening from the 1987, 1992, and 1998 National Health Interview Surveys. *Journal of the National Cancer Institute* **93,** 1704–1713.

Cancer Intervention and Surveillance Modeling Network Home Page. http://srab. cancer.gov/cisnet.html. (Accessed July 31, 2002).

Centers for Disease Control and Prevention. (1999). National Center for Chronic Disease Prevention and Health Promotion. Behavioral Risk Factor Surveillance System Home Page. http://www.cdc.gov/nccdphp/brfss/index.htm.

Chu, K.C., Miller, B.A., Feuer, E.J., and Hankey, B.F. (1994). A method for partitioning cancer mortality trends by factors associated with diagnosis: an application to cancer. *Journal of Clinical Epidemiology* **47,** 1451–1461.

Crocetti, E., Ciatto, S., and Zappa, M. (2001). Prostate cancer: Different incidence but not mortality trends within two areas of Tuscany, Italy. *Journal of the National Cancer Institute* **93,** 876–877.

Eddy, D.M. (1986) A computer-based model for designing cancer control strategies. *National Cancer Institute Monograph* **2,** 75–82.

Ederer, F., Axtell, L.M., and Cutler, S.J. (1961). The relative survival rate: a statistical methodology. *National Cancer Institute Monograph* **6,** 101–121.

Etzioni, R., Berry, K.M., Legler, J.M., and Shaw, P. (2002a). Prostate-specific antigen testing in black and white men: an analysis of medicare claims from 1991–1998. *Urology* **59,** 251–255.

Etzioni, R., Cha, R., and Cowen, M.E. (1999a). Serial prostate specific antigen screening for prostate cancer: a computer model evaluates competing strategies. *Journal of Urology* **162**, 741–748.

Etzioni, R., Legler, J.M., Feuer, E.J., Merrill, R.M., Cronin, K.A., and Hankey, B.F. (1999b). Cancer surveillance series: interpreting trends in prostate cancer-Part III: quantifying the link between population prostate-specific antigen testing and recent declines in prostate cancer mortality. *Journal of the National Cancer Institute* **91**, 1033–1039.

Etzioni, R., Penson, D., Legler, J.M., di Tommaso, D., Boer, R., Gann, P.H., and Feuer, E.J. (2002b). Overdiagnosis in prostate-specific antigen screening: lessons from US prostate cancer incidence trends. *Journal of the National Cancer Institute* **94**, 981–989.

Feldman, A.R., Kessler, L.G., Myers, M.H., and Naughton, M.D. (1986). The prevalence of cancer: estimates based on the Connecticut Tumor Registry. *New England Journal of Medicine* **315**, 1394–1397.

Feuer, E.J., Kessler, L.G., Triolo, H.E., Baker, S.G., and Green, D.T. (1991). The impact of breakthrough clinical trials on survival in population based tumor registries. *Journal of Clinical Epidemiology* **44**, 141–153.

Feuer, E., Marriotto, A., and Merrill, R. (2000). Modeling the impact of the decline in distant stage disease on prostate cancer mortality rates. *Cancer* **95**, 870–880.

Feuer, E.J., Merrill, R.M., and Hankey, B.F. (1999). Cancer surveillance series: interpreting trends in prostate cancer—part II: cause of death misclassification and the recent rise and fall in prostate cancer mortality. *Journal of the National Cancer Institute* **91**, 1025–1032.

Feuer, E.J. and Wun, L.M. (1992). How much of the recent rise in breast cancer incidence can be explained by increases in mammography utilization: a dynamic population approach. *American Journal of Epidemiology* **136**, 1423–1436.

Fleming, C., Wasson, J.H., Albertsen, P.C., Barry, M.J., and Wennberg, J.E. (1993). A decision analysis of alternative treatment strategies for clinically localized prostate cancer. Prostate Patient Outcomes Research Team. *Journal of the American Medical Association* **269**, 2650–2658.

Gann, P.H., Hennekens, C.H., and Stampfer, M.J. (1995). A prospective evaluation of plasma Prostate-Specific Antigen for detection of prostate cancer. *Journal of the American Medical Association* **273**, 289–294.

Gohagan, J.K., Prorok, P.C., Kramer, B.S., and Connett, J.E. (1994). Prostate cancer screening in the prostate, lung, colorectal and ovarian screening trial of the National Cancer Institute. *Journal of Urology* **152**, 1905–1909.

Hankey, B.F., Feuer, E.J., Clegg, L.X., Hayes, R.B., Legler, J.M., Prorok, P.C., Ries, L.A., Merrill, R.M., and Kaplan, R.S. (1999). Cancer surveillance series: interpreting trends in prostate cancer—Part I: evidence of the effects of screening in recent prostate cancer incidence, mortality, and survival rates. *Journal of the National Cancer Institute* **91**, 1017–1024.

Holford, T.R. (1992). Analysing the temporal effects of age, period and cohort. *Statistical Methods in Medical Research* **1**, 317–337.

Holford, T.R., Zhang, Z., and McKay, L.A. (1994). Estimating age, period and cohort effects using the multistage model for cancer. *Statistics in Medicine* **13**, 23–41.

Hugosson, J., Aus, G., Becker, C., Carlsson, S., Eriksson, H., Lilja, H., Lodding, P., and Tobblin, G. (2000). Would prostate cancer detected by screening with prostate-specific antigen develop into clinical cancer if left undiagnosed? *British Journal of Urology International* **85**, 1078–1084.

Jordan, T.R., Price, J.H., King, K.A., Masyk, T., and Bedell, A.W. (1999). The validity of male patients' self-reports regarding prostate cancer screening. *Preventative Medicine* **28**, 297–303.

Kim, H.J., Fay, M.P., Feuer, E.J., and Midthune, D.N. (2000). Permutation tests for joinpoint regression with applications to cancer rates. *Statistics in Medicine* **19**, 335–351.

Legler, J., Feuer, E., Potosky, A., Merrill, R., and Kramer, B. (1998). The role of Prostate-Specific Antigen (PSA) testing patterns in the recent prostate cancer incidence decline in the USA. *Cancer Causes and Control* **9**, 519–557.

Levin, D.L., Gail, M.H., Kessler, L.G., and Eddy, D.M. (1986). A model for projecting cancer incidence and mortality in the presence of prevention, screening and treatment programs. Cancer Control Objectives for the Nation: 1985–2000, NCI Monographs, 83–93.

Lu-Yao, G. Albertsen, P.C., Stanford, J.L., Stukel, T.A., Walker-Corkery, E.S., and Barry, M.J. (2002). Natural experiment examining impact of aggressive screening and treatment on prostate cancer mortality in two fixed cohorts from Seattle area and Connecticut. *British Medical Journal* **325**, 725–726.

Magee, C., and Thompson, I.M. (2001). Evidence of the effectiveness of prostate cancer screening. In Thompson, I.M., Resnick, M.I., and Klein, E.A., eds. *Current Clinical Urology: Prostate Cancer Screening.* Totowa, New Jersey: Humana Press, pp. 157–174.

Merrill, R.M. (2001). Partitioned prostate cancer prevalence estimates: an informative measure of the disease burden. *Journal of Epidemiology and Community Health* **55**, 191–197.

Merrill, R.M., Capocaccia, R., Feuer, E.J., and Mariotto, A. (2000). Cancer prevalence estimates based on tumour registry data in the Surveillance, Epidemiology, and End Results (SEER) Program. *International Journal of Epidemiology* **29**, 197–207.

Merrill, R.M., Feuer, E.J., Warren, J.L., Schussler, N., and Stephenson, R.A. (1999). The role of transuretheral resection of the prostate in population-based prostate cancer incidence rates. *American Journal of Epidemiology 150*, 848–860.

National Cancer Institute SEER Program Data 1973–1999. http://seer.cancer.gov/ (Accessed July 12, 2002).

Oliver, S.E., May, M.T., and Gunnell, D. (2001). International trends in prostate-cancer mortality in the "PSA Era." *International Journal of Cancer* **92**, 893–898.

Pearson, J.D., Luderer, A.A., Metter, E.J., Partin, A.W., Chao, D.W., Fozard, J.L., and Carter, H.B. (1996). Longitudinal analysis of serial measurements of free and total PSA among men with and without prostatic cancer. *Urology* **48**, 4–9.

Potosky, A.L., Kessler, L., Gridley, G., Brown, C.C., and Horm, J.W. (1990). Rise in prostatic cancer incidence associated with increased use of trans-urethral resection. *Journal of the National Cancer Institute* **82**, 1624–1628.

Ramsey, S.D., McIntosh, M., Etzioni, R., and Urban, N. (2000). Simulation modeling of outcomes and cost effectiveness. *Hematology/Oncology Clinics of North America* **14,** 925–938.

Shibata, A., Ma, J., and Whittemore, A.S. (1998). Prostate cancer incidence and mortality in the United States and the United Kingdom. *Journal of the National Cancer Institute* **90,** 1230–1231.

Urban, N., Drescher, C., Etzioni, R., and Colby, C. (1997). Use of a stochastic simulation model to identify an efficient protocol for ovarian cancer screening. *Controlled Clinical Trials 18,* 251–270.

van den Akker-van Marle, E., de Koning, H., Boer, R., and van der Maas, P. (1999). Reduction in breast cancer mortality due to the introduction of mass screening in the Netherlands: comparison with the United Kingdom. *Journal of Medical Screening* **6,** 30–34.

Wasson, J.H., Bubolz, T.A., Lu-Yao, G.L., Walker-Corkery, E., Hammond, C.S., and Barry, M.J. (2000). Transurethral resection of the prostate among Medicare beneficiaries: 1984–1997. *Journal of Urology* **164,** 1212–1215.

Weller, E.A., Feuer, E.J., Frey, C.M., and Wesley, M.N. (1999). Parametric relative survival modeling using generalized linear models with application to Hodgkin's Lymphoma. *Applied Statistics* **48,** 79–89.

Wun, L.M., Feuer, E.J., and Miller, B.A. (1995) Are increases in mammographic screening still a valid explanation for trends in breast cancer incidence in the United States? *Cancer Causes and Control* **6,** 135–144.

7

Detecting Disease Clustering in Time or Space

LANCE A. WALLER

One goal of public health surveillance is to detect emerging trends in the incidence or prevalence of a health outcome. These trends occur in time, space, or space–time. The primary focus of this chapter is the detection of clusters of incidence or prevalence of some health event in time or space. The term *disease cluster* means a local anomaly in the data where the observed incidence or prevalence rate for a particular location in space, a particular time interval, or a particular location at a particular time appears to be different from that expected, based on an assumption of a uniform distribution of disease cases among persons at risk, irrespective of time or location. I use the term *disease* in general to refer to the health event of interest.

THE DATA

Public health surveillance data include reported incident or prevalent cases of particular diseases. The goal in making statistical assessments of particular clusters or overall clustering within surveillance data is to quantify the temporal or spatial patterns in these data. Patterns may involve overall trends, cyclical patterns, or localized anomalies (e.g., hot spots of increased incidence or prevalence). The data may include addresses of residences or dates of diagnoses, but confidentiality issues often restrict data to counts of events for specified time periods (e.g., weeks, months, or years), geographic districts (e.g., census tracts, counties, or states), or both. As a result, many assessments of disease clustering based on count data are ecological and require care in interpretation (see Richardson and Monfort, 2000 for an overview of ecological analysis).

Surveillance data by their nature are most often observational and are reported by a variety of persons to a central data repository (often a regulatory agency). Sullivan et al. (1994) review surveillance data collection and quality control issues. One issue of particular importance in interpretating statistical cluster tests is distinguishing between passive and active surveillance systems. Passive surveillance systems receive reports of cases from physicians or others as mandated by law, whereas active surveillance systems involve a data collection agency contacting physicians and others to identify any reported cases (or absence of reported cases). Active surveillance systems provide better reporting and higher quality data at the cost of increased effort (Sullivan et al., 1994).

Patterns in surveillance data (e.g., anomalies, trends, and cycles) result from a combination of two and perhaps more separate processes: the true pattern of disease incidence in time, space, or both; and the pattern of diagnosis and reporting of events, which may exhibit its own temporal or spatial variation. For example, Kitron and Kazmierczak (1997) discuss the impact of passive reporting combined with the lack of accurate diagnosis and imprecise serological results on assessing spatial patterns of Lyme disease incidence. Time periods or areas exhibiting marked local elevations in rates for surveillance data may indicate true raised local risks, increased local awareness, increased local diagnostic efforts, better local reporting, or some combination of these factors. The statistical methods outlined below will not differentiate among these possible sources of variation.

THE PROBABILISTIC AND STATISTICAL TOOLS

To determine when an observed collection of cases represents an anomaly unlikely to have arisen by chance, we must define a chance allocation of disease cases. Most, if not all, statistical models of disease incidence involve an unknown risk (the probability of disease occurrence in a defined time interval) assigned to each individual under surveillance. This individual risk can vary among individuals based on risk factors ranging from fairly straightforward (e.g., the individual's age and gender) to complex (e.g., genetic profiles or cumulative exposures to toxic substances). Models of chronic disease incidence or prevalence typically assume statistical independence between individuals (perhaps adjusted for familial effects), whereas models of infectious disease typically involve an additional component that address the probability of contact between infective and susceptible individuals (which evolves in space and time over the course of an outbreak). Irrespective of the type of disease, statistical models typically assume a random determination of disease for individuals after accounting for known or suspected risk factors in the model.

Clusters are collections of cases in which the temporal or spatial distributions appear to be inconsistent with uniform or equal risk of at-risk individuals, regardless of time or location. This uniform risk is often the null hypothesis in statistical hypothesis tests of disease clustering. All statistical models of disease incidence and prevalence assume a random component that reflects the probability of a particular individual contracting the disease. Thus, in a sense, all models, even clustered ones, involve some sort of random allocation. However, in this chapter the phrase "random allocation" is used to mean a uniform distribution of cases among those at risk, where each individual is subject to the same probability (possibly adjusted for known risk factors) of becoming a case during the study period.

Two primary building blocks for statistically assessing disease clustering in time or space are the Poisson process and general principles of hypothesis testing. The Poisson process represents a basic model of randomness in time or space and underlies many of the null hypotheses used in such tests.

The Poisson process in time has three components: a time interval over which data are collected (say, $(0, t^*)$), a collection of random variables representing the number of events observed up to time t^* (say, $N(t^*)$), and an intensity function, λ. The first two components define a stochastic process. The third defines the number of events expected to occur in a unit of time. A Poisson process in time with intensity λ also meets the following criteria:

   (i) $N(0) = 0$.
   (ii) The numbers of events occurring in nonoverlapping time intervals are independent.
   (iii) The number of events occurring in a time interval of length t^* follows a Poisson distribution with expected value λt^* (Ross, 1996).

Criteria (ii) as written indicates that the Poisson process in time may be less appropriate for infectious than for chronic disease surveillance, because the numbers infected in any time period may depend on the numbers of infectives and susceptibles in the immediately preceding time period.

As a result of these criteria, data generated by an underlying Poisson process in time with intensity λ will have the following properties:

(a) The number of events observed in any finite interval of time, say (t_1, t_2), follows a Poisson distribution with expected value $\lambda(t_2 - t_1)$.

(b) Given the number of events observed within a particular time interval, these events will be uniformly distributed within this time interval.

(c) The inter-event times (times between events) follow an exponential distribution with parameter $1/\lambda$.

Property (b) provides the basis for the use of a Poisson process as a model of randomness or lack of clustering. Property (a) forms the probabilistic structure for many of the hypothesis tests of clustering proposed in the literature (e.g., comparing annual numbers of observed cases to those expected under a Poisson distribution, as detailed below).

The Poisson process in space is an extension of the Poisson process in time and is equivalent to the notion of *complete spatial randomness*, as defined by Diggle (1983) and Cressie (1993). In particular, the Poisson process in space is a stochastic process of event locations in space that meets the following criteria (where the subscript s distinguishes the criteria for a spatial Poisson process with intensity λ from those of the temporal Poisson process):

(i$_s$) The numbers of events occurring in disjoint areas are independent.

(ii$_s$) For $\lambda > 0$, the number of events occurring in a finite planar region R follows a Poisson distribution with mean $\lambda|R|$, where $|R|$ denotes the area of region R.

A point process is said to be stationary if the intensity λ (expected number of events per unit area) is constant across the study area.

Similar to properties (a) to (c) for the Poisson process in time, a Poisson process in space results in the following:

(a$_s$) The number of events observed in two nonoverlapping regions with areas $|R_1|$ and $|R_2|$ are independent Poisson random variables with means $\lambda|R_1|$ and $\lambda|R_2|$, respectively.

(b$_s$) Given the overall number of events observed in a region, these events will be uniformly distributed throughout this region.

Property (c) for the Poisson process in time has no spatial counterpart because interevent times require an ordering of events in time, and no corresponding ordering exists for events in space.

Properties (b) and (b$_s$) describing the uniform distribution of events in time intervals and regions, respectively, form the basis of what is meant by random or nonclustered occurrence of events for many of the tests outlined below. Properties (a) and (a$_s$) represent the probabilistic motivation for the null hypothesis in many statistical tests of clustering where one considers interval or regional counts as random variables following a Poisson distribution with mean (and variance) determined by the number at risk within the interval or region, possibly stratified by common risk factors, such as age. In some cases, a binomial distribution may be preferred, with parameters defined by the population size at risk in each interval or region and a common (perhaps stratum-specific) disease risk as the null hypothesis. For rare diseases, the Poisson and binomial distributions are very close, but for more common outcomes, a Poisson assumption may be less appealing because of the small but positive probability of observing more cases than persons at risk.

To illustrate these concepts, Figure 7–1 shows 3 independent realizations of a uniform distribution of 20 events in time and in space. Even in uniform random patterns, we tend to perceive clusters or collections of nearby events; thus visually assessing the randomness of an observed pattern is very difficult.

Statistical hypothesis testing theory frames the development of several tests described below. For comparing a simple null hypothesis (e.g., the Poisson mean is proportional to λ_0 representing no clustering) to a simple

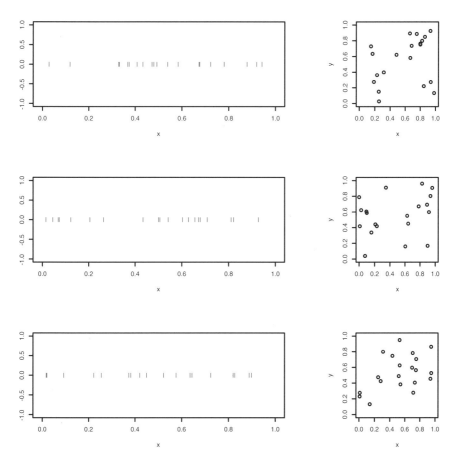

Figure 7–1 Three independent realizations, each of a Poisson process in time (left column) and a Poisson process in space (right column). All realizations contain 20 observations. Even random patterns contain apparent patterns.

alternative hypothesis (e.g., the Poisson mean is proportional to $\lambda_R(t) > \lambda_0$, where $\lambda_R(t)$ represents a higher intensity of cases occurring within region R), the ratio of the likelihood under the alternative hypothesis to the likelihood under the null hypothesis provides the test statistic for a likelihood ratio test (cf. Cox and Hinkley, 1974 for details). If the data appear more likely under the alternative hypothesis than under the null hypothesis, the likelihood ratio tends to be high and leads to extreme values of the statistic and rejection of the null hypothesis in favor of the alternative. Such tests offer the highest statistical power (probability of rejecting the null hypothesis given that the alternative is true) for any test of size α comparing the null hypothesis to this particular alternative hypothesis (Cox and Hinkley, 1974).

Unfortunately, most tests of clustering are not tests of simple alternatives. Rather, there is a wide range of alternative hypotheses consisting of different types of clustering. In many cases, the alternatives are too numerous to allow separate likelihood ratio tests for each, even if the resulting multiple comparisons issues are ignored. Mathematical statistics offers other approaches for testing families of multiple alternatives based on asymptotic theory. A score test has optimal local power properties, where local means small perturbations from the null hypothesis toward specific families of alternative hypotheses. A score test is based on the efficient score, i.e., the partial derivative of the log likelihood with respect to the parameter(s) of interest, evaluated under the null hypothesis, and on the Fisher information, i.e., the second derivative of the log likelihood with respect to the parameter(s) of interest, also evaluated under the null hypothesis (Cox and Hinkley, 1974).

Asymptotic results must be applied cautiously to tests of clustering in time or space. The quantity assumed to approach infinity in the definition of the asymptotic distribution must be considered carefully. In the case of time interval or regional counts, the asymptotics are often expressed in terms of the number of intervals and regions, and not necessarily the number of individual cases (see Tango, 1990a for a specific example). Considering the addition of time intervals that extend observation time may be reasonable, but for spatial clustering, in the context of a particular application, considering the addition of extra regions external to the original study area may not make sense. Subdividing existing regions provides a different sort of asymptotics, termed *infill asymptotics*, where any gains in sample size (number of subregions) can be offset in the loss of statistical precision from decreasing numbers of cases observed in each subregion.

If asymptotic results are in question for a particular application, the general frequentist notion of comparing the observed value of a test statistic to its distribution under the null hypothesis, combined with the availability of modern computers, suggests the use of Monte Carlo (simulation-based) methods of inference. In Monte Carlo testing, one first calculates the test statistic value based on the observed data, and then calculates the same quantity on a large number (say, n_{sim}) of data sets simulated independently under the null hypothesis of interest (e.g., no clustering based on a Poisson process). A histogram of the values associated with the simulated data sets provides an estimate of the distribution of the test statistic under the null hypothesis. The proportion of test statistic values based on simulated data that exceeds the value of the test statistic observed for the actual data set provides a Monte Carlo estimate of the upper tail p-value for a one-sided hypothesis test. Specifically, suppose T_{obs} denotes the test statistic for the observed data and $T_{(1)} \geq T_{(2)} \geq \ldots \geq T_{(n_{sim})}$ denotes the test statistics (ordered from largest to smallest) based on the simulated data sets. If $T_{(1)} \geq \ldots \geq T_{(\ell)} \geq T_{obs} > T_{(\ell+1)}$ (i.e., only the ℓ largest test statistic values based on simulated data exceed T_{obs}) then the estimated p value is

$$\widehat{Prob}[T \geq T_{obs} | H_0 \text{ is true}] = \frac{\ell}{n_{sim} + 1}$$

where we add 1 to the denominator, because our estimate is based on the n_{sim} values from the simulated data plus the value based on the observed data. Diggle (1983) and Cressie (1993) provide further details regarding the application of Monte Carlo tests to spatial point patterns in particular.

CLUSTERING IN TIME

Types of Clusters and Clustering

Before discussing specific testing procedures, we must specify what sort of clustering we seek to detect; i.e., the alternative hypotheses of interest. We follow Besag and Newell (1991) and distinguish between tests to detect clusters and tests of clustering. Tests to detect clusters seek to identify and evaluate particular aggregations of cases as the most likely clusters, whereas tests of clustering seek to assess the overall propensity of events to occur in clusters rather than uniformly in time. The distinction between tests for detecting clusters and tests of clustering is important for appropriately interpreting results. A conclusion of "no significant clustering" does not necessarily preclude the existence of an isolated cluster within a large number of otherwise uniformly distributed cases. Also, detecting a significant cluster need not imply a tendency for the disease in question always to occur in clustered patterns.

In the following sections, tests of seasonality (a particular type of broad temporal clustering where events occur in regularly spaced clusters), tests to detect particular temporal clusters, and tests of temporal clustering are considered. Tango (1984) briefly reviews the literature addressing both areas, and additional detail on some of the more widely used approaches are presented below.

Tests of Seasonality

Edwards (1961) provides one of the most commonly applied statistical tests of seasonality. Suppose the data include counts of the number of events (cases of a disease) for each month, perhaps over a period of years. If seasonality is our primary interest, we ignore long-term temporal trends and combine counts within each month across years, yielding counts y_t, where $t = 1, \ldots, 12$. (Throughout this chapter t denotes index time intervals, and y_t denotes interval counts.) One option is to consider Pearson's chi-square statistic (denoted X^2), where the observed monthly counts are compared with those expected under uniformity (or some other null hypothesis). Edwards (1961) and others note that Pearson's X^2 is an "extremely bad" test of cyclical pattern, because the test statistic provides a summary of how close individual monthly counts are to their null expectations but does not take into account the position of each month within a year. For example, Pearson's X^2 will not distinguish between data that suggest a higher incidence in January and July from data that suggest a higher incidence in January and February, although the latter would seem to offer more evidence for an annual cycle than the former. Pearson's X^2 is a test of the fit of a uniform null hypothesis against all possible deviations from uniformity, and has poor power to detect the specific family of cyclical alternatives.

Edwards (1961) based a statistical test on the following idea: suppose one arranges the months as 12 equally spaced locations on a circle centered at the origin, places a weight at each month corresponding to the square root of the observed monthly count of events, and finds the center of gravity of these points. Under a null hypothesis of a uniform distribution of events throughout the year, the expected location of the center of gravity is at the origin. The direction of deviation from the origin indicates the time of year associated with the maximum number of events, and the distance from the origin indicates the strength of the observed deviation from temporal uniformity. Edwards (1961) proposes the use of the square root transformation as a guard against spurious conclusions of seasonality caused by an outlying value in a single month (i.e., to improve the specificity toward seasonality by limiting the impact of single clusters). Figure 7–2

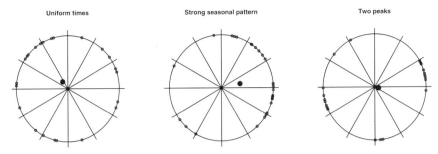

Figure 7–2 Examples of the location of Edwards's (1961) seasonal center of gravity (see text) for a uniform pattern of events, a seasonal pattern of events, and a pattern with 2 peaks per year. The large filled circle represents the center of gravity based on monthly counts, and the small filled circles represent event times. The calculation of the center of gravity assumes that the year is divided into 12 months of equal length (see text).

illustrates the center-of-gravity concept for a pattern of uniformly distributed events, a pattern with a strong seasonal pattern, and a pattern with identical increases in the likelihood of disease at 6-month intervals. In the third example, the pattern will not impact the expected location of the center of gravity and would not be detected by such an approach.

Edwards (1961) proposes $S = 8c^2 y_+$ as a test statistic, where $y_+ = \sum_{t=1}^{12} y_t$ denotes the total number of observed cases and c denotes the distance of the center of gravity from the origin. If $\theta_t = 30(t - 1)$ degrees is defined as the midpoint of month t, $t = 1, \ldots, 12$, then

$$\left(\frac{\sum_t \sqrt{y_t}(\cos \theta_t)}{\sum_t \sqrt{y_t}}, \frac{\sum_t \sqrt{y_t}(\sin \theta_t)}{\sum_t \sqrt{y_t}} \right)$$

provides the coordinates of the center of gravity. Under the null hypothesis of uniformity, S follows a χ^2 distribution with 2 degrees of freedom, and departures cause S to follow a noncentral χ^2 distribution (Edwards, 1961; Walter, 1994).

Edwards's (1961) test is popular for its relative ease of use and calculation but does suffer some shortcomings. Edwards's derivations assume equal at-risk population sizes for each month, months of equal length, and independence between monthly counts (after adjusting for any overall temporal trend). Walter and Elwood (1975) provide a generalization of Edwards's (1961) test to adjust for variation in the numbers at risk each month, thereby avoiding conclusions of seasonal variation in outcome caused only by seasonal variations in the at-risk population. The assumption of equal-length months provides some mathematical simplifications and may appear inconsequential; however, Walter (1994) quantifies the effect of unequal months on the power of Edwards's (1961) statistic. For example, studies with 100,000 individuals (e.g., surveillance of birth trends over several years) can result in a type I error (rejecting the null hypothesis when you should not) rate of almost 55%, caused only by calendar effects. Conceptually, as the sample size increases, so does the pull on the center of gravity toward July and August and away from February. Finally, independence between monthly counts is an assumption in most generalizations and competitors to Edwards's (1961) test, but it is perhaps a questionable assumption for data regarding outbreaks of infectious diseases.

In addition to calendar-effect power problems resulting from large sample sizes mentioned above (Walter, 1994), St. Leger (1976) reports that the asymptotic χ_2^2 distribution for Edwards's (1961) test is inadequate for sample sizes smaller than 100 events. Roger (1977) derives a score test that is asymptotically equivalent to Edwards's (1961) test but that more closely follows a χ_2^2 distribution under the null hypothesis for small sample sizes. Roger's (1977) statistic is

$$R = 2\left[\left\{\sum_t y_t \sin(\theta_t)\right\}^2 + \left\{\sum_t y_t \cos(\theta_t)\right\}^2\right]/y_+$$

and agrees well with a χ_2^2 distribution under the null hypothesis, even for sample sizes as small as 20 events (i.e., fewer than 2 events per month). Roger (1977) assigns weights based on the monthly counts rather than on Edwards's (1961) proposed square root transformation. Roger (1977) also reports adjustments for varying at-risk population sizes.

Other approaches for testing seasonality include Nam's (1995) score tests (uniformly most powerful unbiased) based on prior knowledge of peak and trough seasons. Lee (1996) points out that center-of-gravity approaches such as those described above, can detect only seasonal patterns with a single trough and peak in the year, whereas other patterns (e.g., 2 peaks offset by 6 months, as in Figure 7–2) have little impact on the center of gravity. This feature motivates Lee's (1996) proposal to use the Lorenz curve as a graphical assessment of seasonality. Briefly, Lee (1996) first orders months by increasing incidence rates, then plots the cumulative percentage of cases on the y axis and the cumulative percentage of days on the x axis, providing a plot similar to the PP (probability–probability) plots used to compare distribution functions between two populations (du Toit et al. 1986). Under the null hypothesis of a uniform distribution of events in the study period, the points should lie along the line joining (0,0) and (1,1). Departures from this line suggest some nonuniformity in the temporal distribution of events. Lee (1996) also explores the use of the Gini index (twice the area under the Lorenz curve) both as a test statistic that summarizes the temporal nonuniformity in the data and as a component of an estimated probability that a randomly selected case arrives from a month with elevated incidence. Although presented in the context of a test of seasonality, Lee's approach is described more accurately as a goodness-of-fit test of the null hypothesis of uniform incidence throughout the year (i.e., a test of clustering) than as a test of seasonality, per se.

In addition to the hypothesis testing approaches above, analysts can consider methods based on time series (Diggle, 1990a). However, the focus of time series analyses is often to determine temporal correlations, period length of regular fluctuation, and overall mean trends, rather than to identify particular clusters or directly assess seasonality. Finally, interested readers may consult Fellman and Eriksson's (2000) recent review of statistical approaches for assessing seasonality.

Tests for Detecting Temporal Clusters

In contrast to statistical tests of seasonal patterns in disease data, tests to detect temporal clusters seek to identify anomalies in time series of data and their temporal locations. In particular, a disease cluster typically involves cases occurring in a relatively short period (compared with the length of the entire series of observations) that appear in some sense unusual or inconsistent with the general pattern of events in the rest of the data.

Identifying particular temporal clusters almost always involves retrospectively analyzing surveillance data; that is, we wish to identify past periods with incidence rates that are in some sense statistically different from the rest of the data. Contrast this goal with that of identifying the start of an epidemic in a prospective collection of cases. In retrospective analyses, we survey a history of event times or time interval counts, seeking any indications of aberrations inconsistent with our null model of disease occurrence (perhaps adjusted for seasonality or a temporally varying population at risk). In prospective studies, the goal is to identify a significant increase as close as possible to the actual time of occurrence (e.g., identify an outbreak early in its time course) rather than to scan for anomalies from the large-scale temporal pattern or trend (cf. Farrington et al., 1996).

The scan statistic is a popular tool for detecting temporal clusters retrospectively. First investigated rigorously by Naus (1965) and evaluated in detail in an epidemiologic setting by Wallenstein (1980), Wallenstein and Neff (1987), and Wallenstein et al. (1993), the statistic is simply the maximum number of events observed in a window of predefined fixed length, say w, occurring anywhere in the study period. Using the maximum count, the scan statistic provides a test to detect the most likely cluster rather than to assess overall clustering tendencies or to detect several clusters. Statistical inference follows by determining the distribution of the maximum number of events in an interval of width w under the null hypothesis of a uniform rate of occurrence throughout the entire study period. The literature contains applications to temporal series of poisonings (Hryhorczuk et al., 1992), suicide and attempted suicide (Gould et al., 1994; Hourani et al., 1999), and drug-resistant disease incidence (Singer et al., 1998), among others. Most applications involve data that include time values for each event rather than counts from time intervals (e.g., monthly counts as above), because interval counts can obscure clusters that occur in the specified interval w but across portions of adjacent intervals. Directly calculating the null distribution and associated p-values is complicated because w defines a sliding window of time that occurs anywhere in the study period. Wallenstein (1980) provides some tables for determining p values, and other approximation methods appear in the literature (Wallenstein and Neff, 1987; Glaz, 1993). In addition, Wallenstein et al. (1993) and Sahu et al. (1993) provide power calculations for the scan statistic to detect temporal clusters that correspond to various types of anomalies (e.g., local, constant increases in relative risk, and pulses of increasing and subsequent decreasing relative risk).

Naus (1966) notes that the scan statistic is a generalized likelihood ratio test that compares the null hypothesis of a uniform distribution of events in the study period with alternatives defined by an unknown, but constant, increase in relative risk in a time interval of length w. Nagarwalla (1996) uses the likelihood ratio format to generalize the scan statistic for variable-length time intervals; that is, Nagarwalla's (1996) approach determines the most likely cluster in the study period for a range of interval widths, and provides both the collection of cases and the width of the time interval defining the cluster.

Other approaches in a spirit similar to that of the scan statistic involve monitoring the value of summary statistics (other than the maximum in an interval) over the study period. Proposed approaches include monitoring ratios of the number of cases observed to that expected under the null hypothesis (Stroup et al., 1989), monitoring the time interval between observed cases (Chen et al., 1993; Chen and Goldbourt, 1998), or using cumulative sum (*cusum*) indices popular in industrial quality control applications (Levin and Kline, 1985). Applying such methods involves calculating threshold values, or the value at which the monitored statistic suggests clustering inconsistent with the null hypothesis. Just as comparing the number of cases observed in overlapping windows complicates calculating the tail probability (p-value) of the scan statistic, the repeated nature of monitoring other statistics over subintervals complicates calculating the associated critical values. Although the cited authors each present threshold values based on various distributional assumptions, in many cases Monte Carlo testing is more straightforward (e.g., repeatedly generate data under the null hypothesis, calculate the statistics of interest for each simulated data set, and generate a threshold value based on the simulated statistics).

Tests of Temporal Clustering

Tango (1984) proposed a global index of disease *clustering* using interval count data similar to the seasonality tests described in the section Tests of Seasonality except that Tango considers T equal length intervals that subdivide the entire study period with observed event counts $y_1, y_2, \ldots, y_T$. This approach contrasts with aggregating all disease counts (perhaps over several years) into 12 monthly intervals in seasonality tests. Tango's approach provides a flexible, straightforward index that is applicable to a wide variety of types of clustering, and we present it in some detail.

The null hypothesis of interest for Tango's test is that of a uniform distribution of events to intervals, or more specifically, that the events are equally likely to fall into any interval. Recalling the multinomial conditional distribution of a collection of independent Poisson counts given a fixed total value, conditioning on the total number of observed events, $y_+ = \sum_t y_t$, yields a multinomial distribution of interval counts for the null hypothesis of uniformity with the probability of an event occurring in the tth interval equal to $1/T$ for $t = 1, 2, \ldots, T$. Tango defines

$$r = \left(\frac{y_1}{y_+}, \frac{y_2}{y_+}, \ldots, \frac{y_t}{y_+} \right)^{\tau}$$

as a column vector (letting τ denote transpose) of the relative proportion of cases in each interval, and considers the index

$$C = r^{\tau} Ar = \sum_{t=1}^{T} \sum_{t'=1}^{T} \alpha_{t,t'} r_t r_{t'} \qquad (7\text{--}1)$$

where $A = \{\alpha_{t,t'}\}_{t,t'=1,\ldots,T}$ is a predefined matrix and $\alpha_{t,t'}$ provides a measurement of closeness as defined by some monotonically decreasing function of the temporal distance $d_{t,t'}$ between time periods t and t'. We consider various options for $\alpha_{t,t'}$ and $d_{t,t'}$ below. Note that the index C achieves its maximum value of 1.0 if, and only if, $y_t/y_+ = 1$ for some t and $y_{t'}/y_+ = 0$ for $t' \neq t$, i.e., all observed cases occur in a single time interval.

Tango (1990a) generalizes the index in Eq. 7–1 for applications involving unequal time intervals, interval-specific covariates, or both. The generalized index includes a vector of expected proportions under the null hypothesis of interest. Let

$$\boldsymbol{p} = (p_1, p_2, \ldots, p_t)^\tau$$

where p_t denotes the proportions of cases expected under the null hypothesis in time interval $t, t = 1, 2, \ldots, T$. For example, $p_t = n_t/n_+$, where n_t denotes the number at risk in the tth time interval corresponding to a null hypothesis in which each individual is equally likely to experience the disease. One could also adjust $\boldsymbol{p}$ based on covariates such as age. Tango's (1990a) generalized index is

$$C_G = (\boldsymbol{r} - \boldsymbol{p})^\tau \boldsymbol{A}(\boldsymbol{r} - \boldsymbol{p}) = \sum_{t=1}^{T}\sum_{t'=1}^{T} \alpha_{t,t'}(r_t - p_t)(r_{t'} - p_{t'}) \qquad (7\text{–}2)$$

The index C_G is similar to a weighted version of the familiar chi-square goodness-of-fit test (e.g., Pearson's X^2), in the sense that C_G is a sum of weighted "observed-minus-expected" elements. Instead of squares of each element, as in Pearson's statistic, each summand consists of the product of a pair of elements from two time intervals weighted by the closeness of the intervals ($a_{t,t'}$). The statistic is also similar to indices of spatial correlation (e.g., Moran's I or Geary's c; see Walter, 1992a,b).

The choices of $d_{t,t'}$ and $a_{t,t'}$ define the clustering alternatives of interest. For detecting temporal clusters, $d_{t,t'} = |t - t'|$ provides a natural temporal distance, whereas for detecting seasonality with cycle length ℓ, one could consider $d_{t,t'} = \min\{|t - t'|, \ell - |t - t'|\}$. As a starting point, Tango (1995) suggests

$$a_{t,t'} = \exp(-d_{t,t'}/\delta)$$

where δ represents a tuning parameter that increases sensitivity of the test to large or small clusters using large or small values of δ, respectively.

Whittemore and Keller (1986), Whittemore et al. (1987), and Rayens and Kryscio (1993) show that Tango's index is a member of the class of U statistics, a family of nonparametric tests that includes the familiar Wilcoxon rank-sum test (Cox and Hinkley, 1974). The above authors derive an asymptotic normal distribution for Tango's index. However, Tango (1990b) and Rayens and Kryscio (1993) note that, although the asymptotic derivation is correct, it applies most directly to increasing values of T (the number of time intervals subdividing the study period). They also note that the convergence with respect to increasing values of y_+ (the total number of observed cases) is too slow to be useful for most disease-clustering investigations. Instead, Tango (1990b) derives a chi-square approximation based on the substantial amount of skewness remaining in the distribution of C_G, even for large numbers of cases. Specifically, consider the standardized statistic

$$C_G^* = \frac{C_G - E(C_G)}{\sqrt{\mathrm{Var}(C_G)}}$$

with expectation and variance given by

$$E(C_G) = \frac{1}{y_+}\, tr(AV_p)$$

and

$$\mathrm{Var}(C_G) = \frac{2}{y_+}\, tr[(AV_p)^2]$$

where

$$V_p = \mathrm{diag}(p) - pp^\tau$$

is the asymptotic variance of r (Agresti, 1990), $\mathrm{diag}(p)$ denotes a matrix with the elements of p along the diagonal and zeros elsewhere, and $tr(\cdot)$ denotes the trace function (the sum of the diagonal elements of a matrix). Tango's (1990b, 1995) chi-square approximation requires calculating the skewness, $\gamma(C_G)$, of C_G via

$$\gamma(C_G) = 2\sqrt{2}\, \frac{tr[(AV_p)^3]}{(tr[(AV_p)^2])^{1.5}}$$

By transforming the standardized statistic C_G^* by the degrees of freedom adjusted for skewness, Tango (1995) derives the asymptotic chi-square distribution

$$\nu + C_G^* \sqrt{2\nu} \overset{a}{\sim} \chi_\nu^2 \tag{7-3}$$

where $\nu = 8/[\gamma(C_G)]^2$. Tango (1990b) shows this chi-square approximation to be adequate for sample sizes with as few as one case expected per time interval.

Rayens and Kryscio (1993) also note that Tango's chi-square approximation holds under particular clustering alternative hypotheses defined by p_A, with increased incidence defined for intervals in the clusters of interest, assuming that the incidence counts in different intervals remain independent. This assumption allows ready calculation of the statistical power of Tango's index for a particular clustering alternative. In addition, Cline and Kryscio (1999) provide Markov chain Monte Carlo algorithms for determining the distributions of Tango's index, Pearson's X^2, and other similar statistics under alternative hypotheses generated under a family of contagion models, where interval counts are no longer assumed to be independent.

As an alternative to Tango's approach, Best and Rayner (1991) propose using collections of the orthogonal components of Pearson's X^2 statistic to test for temporal clustering, arguing that these components offer score tests with optimal power properties for particular clustering alternatives. However, as illustrated in Tango (1992) and Best and Rayner (1992), the components of Pearson's X^2 must be used carefully because some types of clustering can be significant in some components of Pearson's X^2 but not in others.

Tango's approach offers a fairly straightforward general-purpose index for detecting a variety of clustering patterns in temporal data recorded as interval counts from equal- or unequal-length intervals. The test may be tuned to particular clustering patterns of interest (single clusters at pre-specified times, seasonality, etc.) through the user's choice of the distance measure $d_{t,t'}$ and the closeness function $\alpha_{t,t'}$. Although at first glance the notation may appear somewhat dense, any statistical package allowing basic matrix operations (e.g., transpose and trace) will perform the calculations (see the Appendix for an S-plus implementation), and the chi-square approximation works well in practice for various sample size configurations with respect to number of cases and number of intervals (Rayens and Kryscio, 1993).

CLUSTERING IN SPACE

Types of Clusters and Clustering

Next, I consider statistical tests of clustering in space. The approaches described below have similarities to those for detecting temporal clusters and clustering. In particular, Besag and Newell's (1991) contrast between tests of clustering and tests to detect clusters remains important. As with temporal tests, some tests involve data with specific locations for each individual (but in space rather than time) and other tests involve counts of cases within regions that partition the study area. Tests for specific locations usually evaluate the nearest neighbor structure or estimates of local intensities of events, and tests based on regional counts compare observed counts to those expected under the null hypothesis.

Besag and Newell (1991) also distinguish between general and focused tests (either of clustering or to detect clusters). General tests seek to detect clusters and clustering anywhere in the study area, whereas focused tests seek to detect clusters and clustering around predefined foci of putative excess risk. Examples of foci include hazardous waste sites, high-voltage power lines, or fields treated with pesticides. The same distinction (general versus focused) could be made for temporal tests, but examples of temporally local foci are less common in the literature than their spatial counterparts.

The distinction between point location and regional count data naturally categorizes analytical methods. In the following sections, I further subdivide tests into general and focused tests within these categories.

Point Location Data

People tend to aggregate into towns and cities, and population density generally varies over space. As a result, investigations of clusters and clustering in spatial health surveillance data rarely involve homogeneously distributed populations at risk. Thus, to assess whether the observed pattern of cases differs from the expected pattern, the pattern expected under a null hypothesis of no clustering must first be determined. The spatial Poisson process with a constant intensity function (complete spatial randomness, as defined in Types of Clusters and Clustering, above) is not quite appropriate when the population at risk itself exhibits a nonuniform spatial distribution. Rather, a null hypothesis equating the spatially varying intensities (numbers of expected events per unit area) of cases with those of the population at risk (number at risk per unit area) seems more appropriate. The intensity of the cases is denoted as $\lambda_0(s)$, where s represents a location in the study area, indicating that the intensity depends on location. We also define $\lambda_1(s)$ to be the intensity function of the population at risk. The null hypothesis becomes "no clustering of case locations above that observed in the population at risk"; i.e., a hypothesis of proportional intensity functions, $H_0:\lambda_0(s) = \rho\lambda_1(s)$, where ρ = (number of cases/number at risk).

Assessing clustering and clusters based on such a null hypothesis requires some information regarding the spatial distribution of individuals at risk. Several methods consider drawing a sample of controls from the at-risk population and comparing the spatial distributions of the case and control locations. In epidemiology, the term controls often reflects nondiseased individuals. In practice, many assessments of clusters and clustering define controls as either a random sample from the population at risk (for a rare disease), or, often more conveniently, as cases of some other disease, unrelated to the disease of interest and suspected to be distributed among the population at risk according to the null hypothesis (Diggle, 1990b; Lawson, 2001). In perhaps a slight abuse of notation, $\lambda_1(s)$ denotes the intensity function of both the population at risk and that of the controls (assumed to be a simple random sample of the population at risk). If the controls are identified via some mechanism other than simple random sampling (e.g., members of a particular health care system where the probability of membership varies over the study area), one would need to account for sampling when assessing their spatial properties (see Kelsall and Diggle, 1995a for related discussion).

Directly testing a null hypothesis of equal intensities involves estimating the two intensity functions, as illustrated below. However, with chronic diseases, an equivalent null hypothesis is often considered, in which cases are assumed to be drawn independently from the at-risk population in which each individual experiences an equal probability of contracting the disease. Here, the cases represent a simple random sample of the at-risk population under the null hypothesis. In theory, such random thinning of the set of all locations for at-risk individuals does not alter the properties of the spatial process. In particular, the underlying intensity functions are the same under such thinning and satisfy the null hypothesis. This formulation of the null hypothesis is referred to as random labeling and provides a mechanism for Monte Carlo testing of the null hypothesis, even for approaches that do not directly estimate the 2 spatial intensities.

Cuzick and Edwards (1990) consider a random labeling approach based on the nearest neighbor properties observed in point data, including y_+ case locations and, say, z_+ control locations (giving $m = y_+ + z_+$ locations in all), where the test statistic represents the number of the q nearest neighbors of cases that are also cases. The analyst defines q and then determines the nearest neighbor adjacency matrix $B = \{b_{j,j'}\}$ where

$$b_{j,j'} = \begin{cases} 1 \text{ if location } j, \text{ is among } q \text{ nearest neighbors of location } j, \\ 0 \text{ otherwise.} \end{cases} \tag{7-4}$$

Cuzick and Edwards's (1990) q nearest neighbor test statistic is

$$T_q = \sum_{j=1}^{m} \sum_{j'=1}^{m} b_{j,j'} \delta_j \delta_{j'}$$
$$= \delta^\tau B \delta, \tag{7-5}$$

where $\delta_j = 1$ if location j represents a case, $\delta_j = 0$ if location j represents a control location, and $\delta = (\delta_1, \delta_2, \ldots, \delta_m)^\tau$ is the vector of case indicators for all (case and control) locations. Eq. 7–5 simply accumulates the number of times $\delta_j = \delta_{j'} = 1$ (both locations are cases), and location j' is in the q nearest neighbors of location j.

For inference, Cuzick and Edwards (1990) provide an asymptotic normal distribution; however, Monte Carlo tests under the random labeling hypothesis can be applied to any sample size. To implement them, one conditions on the observed set of m locations and repeatedly randomly assigns y_+ of the locations to be cases. Locations do not need to be reassigned; rather, they are randomly relabeled as cases or controls. For each randomly generated set of y_+ cases, the test statistic is calculated from Eq. 7–5, and the result is stored. As described at the end of the section Types of Clusters and Clustering, above, the ranks of the test statistic based on the observed data among these based on the randomly labeled data allow the p-value associated with the test to be calculated.

As described above, the Cuzick and Edwards (1990) approach is a general test of clustering. Cuzick and Edwards also describe its use as a focused test of clustering by considering the q nearest neighbors to a fixed set of foci locations and by defining the test statistic as the total number cases among the q nearest neighbors of the foci.

Kelsall and Diggle (1995a,b) present a related approach that directly assesses the equality of the case and control intensity functions. The approach considers a surface defined by the natural logarithm of the ratio of the estimated intensity functions for cases ($\widehat{\lambda}_0(s)$) and that for controls ($\widehat{\lambda}_1(s)$), i.e.,

$$\log\left[\frac{\widehat{\lambda}_0(s)}{\rho\widehat{\lambda}_1(s)}\right]$$

where s denotes any location in the study area (not necessarily the location of a particular case or control). The approach involves so-called "kernel estimation" of the intensity functions wherein a small kernel function is placed at each case location and the value of all kernel functions at a location s^* are summed to estimate the intensity function of cases at location s^*. Estimating the intensity function for controls is similar. To illustrate the concept, imagine marking case locations on a tabletop and placing identically shaped mounds of soft modeling clay over each event. Mounds of clay overlap for close events, and clay accumulates in such areas. When viewed across the tabletop, the surface of the clay reflects the kernel estimate of the intensity function of cases.

Typically, kernel functions are symmetric functions with a peak at the event location and decreasing value as one moves away from the event location; e.g., a bivariate Gaussian density (see Wand and Jones, 1995 for an overview). The bandwidth of the kernel (how far away from an event location the kernel assigns appreciable weight) affects the estimate more than the particular shape of the estimate, where wider bandwidths (e.g., a wider variance in a bivariate Gaussian kernel) result in smoother estimated surfaces. The bandwidth is similar in spirit to the window width of the scan statistic. However, instead of counting each event where it occurs, decreasing fractions of each event are counted as one moves further away from its kernel center (the location of that particular observed case or control). Algorithms for selecting bandwidth are beyond the scope of this chapter. See Wand and Jones (1995) for a general description and Kelsall and Diggle (1995a,b) for a description relating to this application.

Kelsall and Diggle's (1995a,b) approach provides a log-relative risk surface with peaks that indicate areas of elevated case intensity over the control intensity. These peaks suggest the locations of clusters; thus, the approach provides a means to detect individual clusters. Under the null hypothesis, the log-relative risk surface is identically equal to zero at all locations, regardless of any spatial nonuniformity of the density of the at-risk population.

To identify whether the observed peaks differ significantly from the null value of zero, Kelsall and Diggle (1995b) propose a Monte Carlo approach based on the random labeling hypothesis. One conditions on the observed set of case and control locations and generates a large number of data sets by repeatedly assigning at random a sample of y_+ of the m observed (case and control) locations as cases and calculating the log-relative risk surface for each simulated data set. The value of each simulation-based log-relative risk surface is calculated at the same grid of points over the study area, and a distribution of the log-relative risk at those points under the null hypothesis is obtained. Effectively, this approach conducts a Monte Carlo test at each grid point. Contour lines that show where the observed log-relative risk surface exceeds, say, the 95th percentile of the simulated values indicate areas that suggest increased relative risk above that arising from random variation under the null hypothesis. Such tolerance contours are generated in a pointwise manner; thus, an overall significance level for clustering is best handled through some summary statistic (Kelsall and Diggle 1995a).

Kelsall and Diggle (1995b) consider a focused version of the approach in which the estimated log-relative risk is plotted as a function of decreasing exposure to the foci, rather than as a map over the study area. Again, random relabeling generates pointwise tolerance bands around the log-relative risk under the null hypothesis and indicates any exposures that exhibit suspicious increases in relative risk.

The intensity function relates to the expected (or mean) number of events in a unit area and is only one property of a spatial point pattern.

Other researchers (notably Diggle and Chetwynd [1991] and Chetwynd and Diggle [1998]) consider approaches based on observed properties that relate to the covariance and interaction between events. Such approaches relate more to tests of clustering than to tests to detect clusters, and they require definition of additional properties of point processes. Interested readers are referred to the cited references for more details.

Regional Count Data

Several features of regional count data merit special mention. First, confidentiality restrictions often limit access to, and availability of, individual location data. Data aggregated to regional counts are more widely available, and the literature contains a variety of proposed tests of clustering and tests to detect clusters for such data. As mentioned above for point data, the tendency for people to reside in cities and towns results in a nonuniform density of the population at risk across the study area. Unlike point data, regional counts often allow inclusion of population counts (even stratified by disease risk correlates such as age and income) for the same set of regions based on census values. As a result, most methods for regional count data ignore the use of controls and assume that census data provide sufficient information on the spatial distribution of the at-risk population.

Second, although census districts are often designed to contain approximately the same number of people, the observed population counts may vary considerably, particularly in urban areas in which the districts are geographically small and the population mobile. For instance, rezoning a former residential area for industrial use can reduce the number of residents from 1000s to fewer than 100 between census periods.

Another result of the spatial nonuniformity of the population at risk is a spatially varying local sample size for inference. Although the properties of spatial Poisson processes suggest independent regional counts (for chronic diseases), these counts will not be identically distributed because their associated expected (mean) values and variances depend on the at-risk population size in that region. This variability is more pronounced in spatial analysis than in temporal analysis because time intervals are often similar in size (e.g., years or months) whereas spatial regions may vary widely geographically and in population size.

Third, the ecologic (aggregate) nature of regional count data raises the possibility of the so-called ecologic fallacy of attributing associations observed in groups of people to individuals. Epidemiologists are familiar with concerns regarding the ecologic fallacy, but they may not have considered the related spatial issue, termed the modifiable areal unit problem (MAUP) by geographers, wherein results based on aggregated data depend on the set of regions in which aggregation occurs; that is, different results may be obtained from data aggregated to different sets of regions (e.g., results based on census tract data may differ from those based on ZIP code data). Monmonier (1996) provides a convincing visual example based on Dr. John Snow's famous map of London cholera cases from 1854. If correlations or statistical (e.g., regression) models are fit to aggregated data, the MAUP effect directly corresponds to an ecologic fallacy, in that the observed association between variables depends on how individuals are grouped.

In summary, the nonuniform and ecologic nature of regional counts provides a necessary context for interpretating statistical tests of clustering and clusters. Various approaches may be more or less sensitive to these data features, but few, if any, will be immune to their effects.

Regarding particular methods, we first consider Kulldorff's (1997) spatial scan statistic, a spatial analog to the temporal scan statistic described in Tests for Detecting Temporal Clusters, above. As in the temporal case, the primary goal of a scan statistic is to find the collection of cases least consistent with the null hypothesis (i.e., the most likely cluster) and to provide a significance value representing the detected cluster's unusualness. Kulldorff (1997) considers circular windows with variable radii (similar to Nagarwalla's [1996] variable width temporal scan statistic), ranging from the smallest observed distance between a pair of cases to a user-defined upper bound (e.g., one-half the width of the study area). Loader (1991) and Nagarwalla (1996) note that variable-width, one-dimensional scan statistics represent collections of local likelihood ratio tests of a null hypothesis of a spatially invariant disease rate compared with alternatives wherein the disease rate in the window is greater than that outside the window. Kulldorff (1997) uses this structure to evaluate each potential cluster. The maximum observed likelihood ratio statistic provides a test of overall general clustering, and significance is determined by Monte Carlo testing. Notationally, let y_{IN} and n_{IN} denote the number of cases and persons at risk inside a particular window, respectively, and similarly define y_{OUT} and n_{OUT} for outside the window. The overall test statistic is

$$T = \max_{\text{all windows}} \left(\frac{y_{IN}}{n_{IN}}\right)^{y_{IN}} \left(\frac{y_{OUT}}{n_{OUT}}\right)^{y_{OUT}} I\left(\frac{y_{IN}}{n_{IN}} > \frac{y_{OUT}}{n_{OUT}}\right)$$

where $I(\cdot)$ denotes the indicator function (i.e., we only maximize over windows where the observed rate inside the window exceeds that outside the window). Kulldorff's (1997) approach has seen considerable application and is available using SaTScan, a free software package developed and distributed by the U.S. National Cancer Institute (United States National Cancer Institute, 1998).

Turnbull et al. (1990) and Besag and Newell (1991) present two methods similar to the scan statistic but based on windows defined by quantities other than geographic distance. Turnbull et al. (1990) consider windows containing the same number of persons at risk and centered at each region by aggregating neighboring regions until the accumulated population of each region reaches a user-defined population radius. Because all windows contain the same number of persons at risk, the same number of cases is expected in each under the null hypothesis of equal risk. However, because the windows overlap, the counts are not statistically independent. As with the temporal scan statistic, the maximum number of cases observed in any window forms the test statistic. Inference follows via Monte Carlo testing.

Whereas Turnbull et al. (1990) create comparable disease rates by stabilizing the denominator (the population size in each window), Besag and Newell (1991) consider stabilizing the numerator (the number of cases defining potential clusters). Turnbull et al.'s (1990) approach seeks to detect the largest number of observed cases in aggregations of the same number of individuals at risk. Besag and Newell (1991) propose a method to detect the collection of a fixed number of cases that appears least consistent with the null hypothesis (i.e., the most likely cluster). To implement their test, the cluster size of interest is defined as, say, k cases, collections of k cases centered at each census region are considered, and the most unusual collections of k cases are identified as possible clusters. For each potential cluster (collection of k cases centered at a particular region), the number of neighboring regions that contain the k nearest cases is determined, and significance is assessed on the basis of the probability of observing k cases in fewer regions (the probability of observing a more tightly clustered collection of k cases). For each region, the other regions are ordered by increasing distance to the region under consideration (denoted region 0). Let n_{j+} denote the cumulative population size associated with regions containing the closest k cases to region j, L a random variable representing the number of regions containing a collection of k cases, l as the observed value of L for this particular collection of k cases, and λ as the overall disease rate for the study area. The underlying regional Poisson probabilities define the statistical significance for a particular collection of k cases as

$$P[L \leq l] = 1 - \sum_{s=0}^{k-1} \frac{\exp(-n_{j+}\lambda)(n_{j+}\lambda)^s}{s!}$$

The process is repeated for each collection of k cases. This approach assigns a separate p value to each collection of k cases.

Although both the spatial scan statistic and Turnbull et al.'s (1990) approach assess clustering by a test to detect the most likely cluster, Besag and Newell's test specifically detects clusters or anomalies in the data set. Besag and Newell (1991) propose a map of the study area showing all potential clusters that attained a given significance level (say 5%). If pressed for an overall test of clustering, Besag and Newell (1991) suggest using the number of potential clusters that attained the predefined significance level and determining significance by Monte Carlo testing.

Also, although scan statistic approaches are usually applied as general tests of clustering and clusters, they can also be applied in a focused situation by considering potential clusters around each focus, rather than at each region.

In addition to scan-type tests of clustering, Tango's index defined in Eq. 7–2 can easily be applied to spatial as well as temporal data, by defining the elements of the matrix A in terms of geographic instead of temporal distance. Tango (1995) presents the index as a spatial test in some detail, and describes different possible choices for the elements $a_{j,j'}$ of matrix A, where j, j' denote two regions in the study area. Again, Tango (1995) suggests $a_{j,j'} = \exp(-d_{j,j'}/\delta)$ for a starting point that provides a test of general clustering, where δ (as in Tests for Detecting Temporal Clusters, above) increases sensitivity to large or small clusters. Inference follows via the chi-square approximation.

Tango's index is structurally similar to Pearson's X^2 statistic and to Moran's I, a widely applied index of spatial autocorrelation. Rogerson (1999) contrasts the methods by pointing out that Pearson's X^2 compares observed-to-expected regional counts without regard to any spatial patterns in lack of fit and Moran's I examines spatial patterns without stressing differences between observed and expected counts, whereas Tango's index provides a test that addresses both aspects. To more closely mirror the structure of Moran's I statistic, Rogerson (1999) proposes replacing A with W, where $w_{j,j'} = a_{j,j'}/\sqrt{p_j p_{j'}}$, and p_j is the jth element of p, the vector of proportions of the expected number of cases in each region. Inference follows using Tango's (1995) chi-square approximation with W in the place of A. Other definitions of the matrix A yield tests sensitive to other types of clustering. Tukiendorf (2001) describes a recent application of Tango's index in assessing patterns of leukemia in Poland.

For focused testing in regional count data, Lawson (1993) and Waller et al. (1992, 1994) propose a test based on a weighted sum of deviations of observed case counts from those expected under the null hypothesis. This approach is, again, similar to the notion of a weighted version of a chi-square goodness-of-fit statistic similar to Pearson's X^2. However, in the focused setting, the weights are functions of the putative exposure experienced by individuals residing in each region; whereas in the general setting they are functions of the proximity of regions to one another. Specifically, Waller et al. (1992) propose the test statistic

$$U = \sum_{j=1}^{J} x_j (y_j - E_j)$$

where x_j denotes the exposure experienced by individuals in the jth region, J denotes the number of regions, and y_j and E_j denote the observed and expected number of cases, respectively, in the jth region. The statistic U is a score test with optimal local power in comparing a null hypothesis of a constant disease rate, i.e.

$$H_0 : E_j = n_j \lambda \text{ for all } j$$

to the alternative hypothesis,

$$H_A : E_j = n_j \lambda (1 + x_j \varepsilon)$$

where λ is the overall (null) disease rate, n_j is the population at risk in region j, and ε is a small positive number related to the increase in relative risk (under H_0, $\varepsilon = 0$). For both H_0 and H_A, the observed disease counts are assumed to be independent Poisson random variables. As a score test, U has an asymptotic normal distribution with mean zero and variance $\sum_{j=1}^{J} x_j^2 E_j$, assuming λ is known.

Implementing the score tests requires a measure of exposure x_j for each region. Relevant, monitored exposure data may be interpolated to each region. In practice, some sort of surrogate for exposure is used, perhaps based on geographic distance of regions to the foci. Waller et al. (1992, 1994) use the inverse distance of a region from the nearest foci as a surrogate for exposure, and Tango (1995) suggests other distance-decay surrogates. Waller and Poquette (1999) use both inverse distance and Tango's functional forms of exposure to illustrate the effect of using a misspecified exposure function on the statistical power of the score test.

Not surprisingly, the score test is equivalent to a score test for trend in Poisson random variables (Rothman 1986) because the test of focused clustering does, in effect, test for a trend in independent Poisson random variables (increasing expected rates with increasing exposure). Finally, Tango (1995) illustrates that the score test outlined above reflects a focused version of Tango's index using shared levels of exposure rather than simple geographic proximity between regions.

AN EXAMPLE OF SPATIAL CLUSTERING METHODS: LEUKEMIA IN UPSTATE NEW YORK

To illustrate some of the spatial clustering methods, I describe leukemia data reported and analyzed by Waller et al. (1992, 1994). The data are available in Lange et al. (1994) and on the StatLib website (StatLib, 1994). The data include incident leukemia cases from 1978 to 1982 in an eight-county region of upstate New York, divided into 790 census regions (tracts in Broome County, block groups in the other seven counties). In total, the data include 592 cases among 1,057,673 people at risk. Waller et al. (1994) consider foci defined by inactive hazardous waste sites documented as containing trichloroethylene (TCE) by the New York State Department of Environmental Conservation (1987). Other analyses of these data appear in the literature (e.g., Rogerson [1999], Ghosh et al. [1999], Gangnon and Clayton [2000, 2001], and Ahrens et al. [2001]) and the interested reader is referred to these studies for further details.

Waller et al. (1994) apply the approaches of Besag and Newell (1991) and of Turnbull et al. (1990) to the New York leukemia data described above for $k = 8$ and 10 cases, and for population radii = 2500, 5000, 10,000, and 20,000 people, respectively. Both methods suggest that the most likely clusters occur in Cortland County (the center of the study region), but in both cases, the observed test statistic values are not unusual when compared with the distribution of values obtained by repeatedly assigning the 592 cases at random to the 1,057,673 people at risk (a Monte Carlo test of significance). These methods indicate little evidence of general clusters in the data set for specified population radii and values of k. In contrast to the results of the spatial scan statistic (Fig. 7–3, in which the dots represent census region centroids and not individual cases), the collection of cases in Cortland county now appears to be statistically significant, along with a second collection in the southern portion of the study region. This southern collection of cases occurs near and in the city of Binghamton, an area in which the data are aggregated to regions containing more individuals. As a result, the cluster identified by the spatial scan statistic contains many more cases and people than any of the clusters considered by the other two tests for the values of k and the population radii considered. In short, the different results are based on different suspected clusters.

Waller et al. (1994) also applied focused tests to the leukemia data. Table 7–1 illustrates results for each of eleven TCE sites. As above, the observed differences in Table 7–1 do not necessarily indicate inconsistency between methods, but rather indicate different results for different types of clusters (different alternative hypotheses). Consider, for example, site 1, where the collection of the nearest 8 cases is not significant at the 0.05

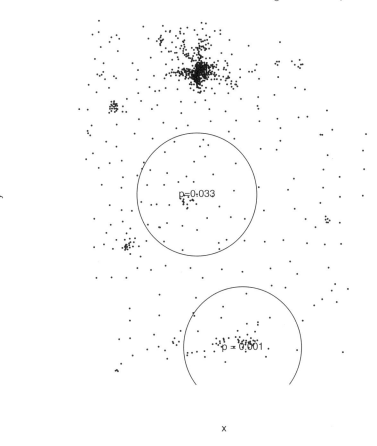

Figure 7–3 Example of the output of the spatial scan statistics applied to leukemia (all types) incidence in an 8-county region of upstate New York from 1978 to 1982. The points represent centroids of 790 census tracts, and the circles represent the 2 most likely clusters reported by the spatial scan statistic.

level, but the collection of the nearest 10 cases is. Such a situation would arise when the 9th and 10th nearest cases have distances to the focus similar to that of the 8th nearest case. The rate based on 8 cases is not particularly unusual, but one based on 10 cases appears to be high. In contrast, the score test reports statistically significant deviations from expectation for all sites except 6, 10, and 11. These data indicate patterns of excess cases (above expectations) in census regions nearest the waste sites and continuing as one moves farther away. In this case, evidence is stronger for a gradual increase in risk as one nears a TCE site than for abrupt increases around each site (conclusions are based on the score and the Besag and Newell, 1991 results, respectively).

Table 7–1 Results of focused clustering tests for leukemia around inactive hazardous waste sites containing trichloroethylene in an eight-county region of upstate New York

Focus	Besag and Newell p value*		Score test p value*
	$k = 8$	$k = 10$	
Nearest focus	0.602	0.334	<0.001
1	0.07	0.01	<0.01
2	0.06	0.07	<0.01
3	0.73	0.47	0.01
4	0.73	0.47	0.01
5	0.13	0.14	0.02
6	0.25	0.17	0.39
7	0.26	0.12	0.01
8	0.49	0.24	0.02
9	0.49	0.28	0.03
10	0.73	0.88	0.78
11	0.88	0.72	0.21
Nearest focus	0.60	0.33	<0.01

*We report no adjustment to p-values for multiple testing.

Sources: Adapted from Waller, L.A., Turnbull, B.W., Clark, L., and Nasca, P. (1994). Spatial pattern analysis to detect rare disease clusters. In Lange, N., Ryan, L., Billard, L., Brillinger, D., Conquest, L., and Greenhouse, J., eds. *Case Studies in Biometry*, New York: John Wiley and Sons, pp. 3–23. © 1994. Reprinted by permission of John Wiley & Sons, Inc.

The results in Table 7–1, even with small p values, do not provide conclusive evidence of focused clustering in the data. Waller et al. (1994) calculate expected rates based on the overall 5-year rate of leukemia in the study area, without adjusting for common risk factors, such as age or occupation. Waller and McMaster (1997) consider age adjustments for one county in the study area (Broome County, containing the city of Binghamton) and find small differences from the results reported here. Ahrens et al. (2001) consider additional adjustments based on more detailed, individual-level data. Applying the score test based on more realistic exposure surrogates may provide different results from those presented above.

CONCLUSION

As outlined above, each statistical test of clustering originates from some mathematical model that provides the type of spatial pattern expected in the absence of clustering. Tests rely on data summaries (statistics) to reveal particular deviations from the null hypothesis (i.e., the model of non-clustering). Different tests are sensitive to different types of clusters (Waller and Jacquez, 1995). The distinction between tests of clustering and tests to detect clusters, and the distinction between general and focused tests, offer broad classes of differing sets of alternative hypotheses. The issue of varying sensitivity between methods to particular types of clusters is particularly important in interpreting the results of different tests applied to the same data. Tests designed to detect different types of clusters may support different conclusions for the same data.

The first step in choosing a statistic is to consider of the sorts of alternatives to non-clustering that are of interest. Is the intent to determine a general pattern of clustering or to detect the most likely clusters? Are there putative foci of increased risk? The answers to these questions narrow the list of appropriate approaches considerably.

The data structure further refines the set of appropriate methods. Do the data include point locations or interval and regional counts? What data are available to describe the temporal or spatial pattern of the at-risk population (e.g., census counts, or a set of control locations)? Are the data sufficient to reveal the types of clusters of interest?

After narrowing the options appropriate for the questions of interest and the data at hand, the statistical power of the tests can be compared. Several such comparisons appear in the literature (Waller and Lawson, 1995; Tango, 1995, 1999; Waller, 1996; Hill et al., 2000) and at times provide sobering results regarding the power to detect local increases in the relative risk of disease in the range reasonably expected from environmental exposures (e.g., local relative risks of 2 or 3 compared with the background rate of disease). Also, the temporal and spatial structure of the population at risk affects power, in the sense that tests more easily detect clusters in areas with more persons at risk than in areas with fewer persons at risk (Rudd, 2001).

For tests of clustering in time or space, Tango's (1995) index provides a straightforward approach that can be applied flexibly to counts from time intervals or regions. The index requires the case counts, the size of the population at risk and a location in time or space for each interval or region, respectively. As noted by Rogerson (1999), Tango's (1995) method provides a compromise between an assessment of goodness-of-fit (how close are the observed counts to the expected counts?) and an assessment of spatial autocorrelation (are high rates near other high rates?). The method is flexible in that users can define different measures of proximity to detect different types of clusters.

Tango's (1995) test is a test of clustering and, as such, provides a global significance value to assess the overall tendency of cases to cluster within the population, although it does not indicate where any potential clusters might occur. Rogerson (1999) decomposes Tango's index into a sum of local statistics, providing one method for identifying particular clusters but Kulldorff's (1997) spatial scan statistic provides a somewhat more straightforward approach for identifying the most likely cluster within a spatial data set.

The score test (Lawson, 1993; Waller et al., 1992, 1994) provides a basic method of assessing focused clustering in regional count data, and requires the same input as Tango's index as well as an exposure surrogate for each region. As mentioned above, the score test can be seen as a focused version of Tango's index.

Methods for point data typically involve additional implementational considerations (e.g., selection of controls and more involved calculations) but offer potentially more detailed results. In addition, analyses of point data are less subject to the ecological fallacy and the related modifiable areal unit problem.

In summary, this review provides an overview of common data issues and inferential considerations in statistical approaches for assessing temporal or spatial clustering. The review is by no means complete and readers interested in more detailed development and data analysis examples are referred to special issues of the *American Journal of Epidemiology* (1990), *Statistics in Medicine* (1993, 1995, 1996, 2000), the *Journal of the Royal Statistical Society Series A* (2001), and texts by Elliott et al. (1992, 2000), Lawson (2001), and Lawson et al. (1999).

REFERENCES

Agresti, A. (1990). *Categorical Data Analysis*. New York: Wiley.

Ahrens, C., Altman, N., Casella, G., Eaton, M., Hwang, J.T.G., Staudenmayer, J., and Stefanescu, C. (2001). Leukemia clusters in upstate New York: How adding covariates changes the story. *Environmetrics* **12**, 659–672.

American Journal of Epidemiology (1990). **132**, Supplement, S1–S202.

Besag, J. and Newell, J. (1991). The detection of clusters in rare diseases. *Journal of the Royal Statistical Society Series A* **154**, 143–155.

Best, D.J. and Rayner, J.C.W. (1991). Disease clustering in time. *Biometrics* **47**, 589–593.

Best, D.J. and Rayner, J.C.W. (1992). Response to Tango's comments. *Biometrics* **48**, 327.

Chen, R. and Goldbourt, U. (1998). Analysis of data associated with seemingly temporal clustering of a rare disease. *Methods of Information in Medicine* **37**, 26–31.

Chen, R., Connelly, R.R., and Mantel, N. (1993). Analysing post-alarm data in a monitoring system in order to accept or reject the alarm. *Statistics in Medicine* **12**, 1807–1812.

Chetwynd, A.G. and Diggle, P.J. (1998). On estimating the reduced second moment measure of a stationary spatial point process. *Australian and New Zealand Journal of Statistics* **40**, 11–15.

Cline, G.A. and Kryscio, R.J. (1999). Contagion distributions for defining disease clustering in time. *Journal of Statistical Planning and Inference* **78**, 325–347.

Cox, D.R. and Hinkley, D.V. (1974). *Theoretical Statistics*. London: Chapman and Hall.

Cressie, N.A.C. (1993). *Statistics for Spatial Data, Revised Edition*. New York: Wiley.

Cuzick, J. and Edwards, R. (1990). "Spatial clustering for inhomogeneous populations" (with discussion). *Journal of the Royal Statistical Society Series B* **52**, 73–104.

Diggle, P.J. (1983). *Statistical Analysis of Spatial Point Patterns*. London: Academic Press.

Diggle, P.J. (1990a). *Time Series: A Biostatistical Introduction*. Oxford: Clarendon Press.

Diggle, P.J. (1990b). A point process modelling approach to raised incidence of a rare phenomenon in the vicinity of a prespecified point. *Journal of the Royal Statistical Society Series A* **153**, 349–362.

Diggle, P.J. and Chetwynd, A.G. (1991). Second-order analysis of spatial clustering for inhomogeneous populations. *Biometrics* **47**, 1155–1163.

du Toit, S.H.C., Steyn, A.G.W., and Stumpf, R.H. (1986). *Graphical Exploratory Data Analysis*. New York: Springer.

Edwards, J.H. (1961). The recognition and estimation of cyclic trends. *Annals of Human Genetics* **25**, 83–86.

Elliott, P., Cuzick, J., English, D., and Stern, R., eds. (1992). *Geographical and Environmental Epidemiology: Methods for Small-Area Studies*. Oxford: Oxford University Press.

Elliott, P., Wakefield, J.C., Best, N.G., and Briggs, D.J., eds. (2000). *Spatial Epidemiology: Methods and Applications*. Oxford: Oxford University Press.

Farrington, C.P., Andrews, N.J., Beale, A.D., and Catchpole, M.A. (1996). A statistical algorithm for the early detection of outbreaks of infectious disease. *Journal of the Royal Statistical Society, Series A* **159**, 547–563.

Fellman, J. and Eriksson, A.W. (2000). Statistical analysis of the seasonal variation in demographic data. *Human Biology* **72**, 851–876.

Gangnon, R.E. and Clayton, M.K. (2000). Bayesian detection and modeling of spatial disease clustering. *Biometrics* **56**, 922–935.

Gangnon, R.E. and Clayton, M.K. (2001). A weighted average likelihood ratio test for spatial clustering of disease. *Statistics in Medicine* **20**, 2977–2987.

Ghosh, M., Natarajan, K., Waller, L.A., and Kim, D. (1999). Hierarchical Bayes GLM's for the analysis of spatial data: an application to disease mapping. *Journal of Statistical Planning and Inference* **75**, 305–318.

Glaz, J. (1993). Approximations for the tail probabilities and moments of the scan statistic. *Statistics in Medicine* **12**, 1845–1852.

Gould, M.S., Petrie, K., Kleinman, M.H., and Wallenstein, S. (1994). Clustering of attempted suicide—New Zealand national data. *International Journal of Epidemiology* **23**, 1185–1189.

Hill, E.G., Ding. L., and Waller, L.A. (2000). A comparison of three tests to detect general clustering of a rare disease in Santa Clara County, California. *Statistics in Medicine* **19**, 1363–1378.

Hourani, L.L., Warrack, A.G., and Coben, P.A. (1999). Suicide in the U.S. Marine Corps, 1990 to 1996. *Military Medicine* **164**, 551–555.

Hryhorczuk, D.O., Frateschi, L.J., Lipscomb, J.W., and Zhang, R. (1992). Use of the scan statistic to detect temporal clustering of poisonings. *Journal of Toxicology—Clinical Toxicology* **30**, 459–465.

Journal of the Royal Statistical Society Series A (2001). **164**, 1–207.

Kelsall, J.E. and Diggle, P.J. (1995a). Non-parametric estimation of spatial variation in relative risk. *Statistics in Medicine* **14**, 2335–2342.

Kelsall, J.E. and Diggle, P.J. (1995b). Kernel estimation of relative risk. *Bernoulli* **1**, 3–16.

Kitron, U. and Kazmierczak, J.J. (1997). Spatial analysis of the distribution of Lyme disease in Wisconsin. *American Journal of Epidemiology* **145**, 558–566.

Kulldorff, M. (1997). A spatial scan statistic. *Communications in Statistics-Theory and Methods* **26**, 1481–1496.

Lange, N., Ryan, L., Billard, L., Brillinger, D., Conquest, L., and Greenhouse, J., eds. (1994). Case Studies in Biometry. New York: Wiley.

Lawson, A.B. (1993). On the analysis of mortality events associated with a pre-specified fixed point. *Journal of the Royal Statistical Society, Series A* **156**, 363–377.

Lawson, A.B., Böhning, D., Lesaffre, E., Biggeri, A., Viel, J.-F., and Bertollini, R. eds. (1999). *Disease Mapping and Risk Assessment for Public Health.* Chichester: Wiley.

Lawson, A.B. (2001). *Statistical Methods in Spatial Epidemiology.* Chichester: Wiley.

Lee, W.C. (1996). Analysis of seasonal data using the Lorenz curve and the associated Gini index. *International Journal of Epidemiology* **25**, 426–434.

Levin, B. and Kline, J. (1985). The cusum test of homogeneity with an application in spontaneous abortion epidemiology. *Statistics in Medicine* **4**, 469–488.

Loader, C.R. (1991). Large-deviation approximations to the distribution of scan statistics. *Advances in Applied Probability* **23**, 751–771.

Monmonier, M. (1996). *How to Lie with Maps*, 2nd ed. Chicago: University of Chicago Press.

Nagarwalla, N. (1996). A scan statistic with a variable window. *Statistics in Medicine* **15**, 845–850.

Nam, J. (1995). Interval estimation and significance testing for cyclic trends in seasonality studies. *Biometrics* **51**, 1411–1417.

Naus, J. (1965). The distribution of the size of the maximum cluster of points on a line. *Journal of the American Statistical Association* **60**, 532–538.

Naus, J.I. (1966). A power comparison of two sets of non-random clustering. *Technometrics* **8**, 493–517.

Rayens, M.K. and Kryscio, R.J. (1993). Properties of Tango's index for detecting clustering in time. *Statistics in Medicine* **12**, 1813–1827.

Richardson, S. and Monfort, C. (2000). Ecological correlation studies. In Elliott, P., Wakefield, J.C., Best, N.G., and Briggs, D.J., eds. *Spatial Epidemiology: Methods and Application.* Oxford: Oxford University Press, pp. 203–220.

Roger, J.H. (1977). A significance test for cyclic trends in incidence data. *Biometrika* **64**, 152–155.

Rogerson, P.A. (1999). The detection of clusters using a spatial version of the chi-square goodness-of-fit statistic. *Geographical Analysis* **31**, 130–147.

Ross, S. (1996). *Stochastic Processes*, 2nd ed. New York: Wiley.

Rothman, K.J. (1986). *Modern Epidemiology.* Boston: Little, Brown and Company.

Rudd, R.A. (2001). *The Geography of Power: a Cautionary Example for Tests of Spatial Patterns of Disease.* Master of Science in Public Health Thesis. Department of Biostatistics, Rollins School of Public Health, Emory University.

Sahu, S.K., Bendel, R.B., and Sison, C.P. (1993). Effect of relative risk and cluster configuration on the power of the one-dimensional scan statistic. *Statistics in Medicine* **12,** 1853–1865.

Singer, R.S., Case, J.T., Carpenter, T.E., Walker, R.L., and Hirsh, D.C. (1998). Assessment of spatial and temporal clustering of ampicillin- and tetracycline-resistant strains of Pasteurella multocida and P-haemolytica isolated from cattle in California. *Journal of the American Veterinary Medical Association* **212,** 1001–1005.

St. Leger, A.S. (1976). Comparison of two tests for seasonality in epidemiologic data. *Applied Statistics* **25,** 280–286.

Statistics in Medicine (1993). **12,** 1751–1968.

Statistics in Medicine (1995). **14,** 2289–2501.

Statistics in Medicine (1996). **15,** 681–952.

Statistics in Medicine (2000). **19,** 2201–2593.

StatLib (1994). *Case Studies in Biometry* datasets available from http://lib.stat.cmu.edu/datasets/csb.

Stroup, D.F., Williamson, G.D., and Herndon, J.L. (1989). Detection of aberrations in the occurrence of notifiable disease surveillance data. *Statistics in Medicine* **8,** 323–329.

Sullivan, K.M., Gibbs, N.P., and Knowles, C.M. (1994). Management of the surveillance system and quality control of data. In Teutsch, S. M. and Churchill, R.E., eds. *Principles and Practice of Public Health Surveillance.* New York: Oxford University Press, pp. 86–95.

Tango, T. (1984). The detection of disease clustering in time. *Biometrics* **40,** 15–26.

Tango, T. (1990a). An index for cancer clustering. *Environmental Health Perspectives* **87,** 157–162.

Tango, T. (1990b). Asymptotic distribution of an index for disease clustering. *Biometrics* **46,** 351–357.

Tango, T. (1992). Letter regarding Best and Rayner's (1991) "Disease clustering in time." *Biometrics* **48,** 326–327.

Tango, T. (1995). A class of tests for detecting 'general' and 'focused' clustering of rare diseases. *Statistics in Medicine* **14,** 2323–2334.

Tango, T. (1999). Comparison of general tests for spatial clustering. In Lawson, A., Böhning, D., Lesaffre, E., Biggeri, A., Viel, J.-F., and Bertollini, R., eds. *Disease Mapping and Risk Assessment for Public Health.* Chichester: Wiley, pp. 111–117.

Tukiendorf, A. (2001). An ecological analysis of leukemia incidence around the highest Cs-137 concentration in Poland. *Cancer Causes and Control* **12,** 653–659.

Turnbull, B.W., Iwano, E.J., Burnett, W.S., Howe, H.L., and Clark, L.C. (1990). Monitoring for clusters of disease: application to leukemia incidence in upstate New York. *American Journal of Epidemiology* **132,** Supplement. S136–S143.

United States National Cancer Institute (1998). *SaTScan Version 2.1* available from http://www.nci.nih.gov/prevention/bb/satscan.html.

Wallenstein, S. (1980). A test for detection of clustering over time. *American Journal of Epidemiology* **111,** 367–372.

Wallenstein, S. and Neff, N. (1987). An approximation for the distribution of the scan statistic. *Statistics in Medicine* **6,** 197–207.

Wallenstein, S., Naus, J., and Glaz, J. (1993). Power of the scan statistic for detection of clustering. *Statistics in Medicine* **12,** 1829–1843.

Waller, L.A. (1996). Statistical power and design of focused clustering studies. *Statistics in Medicine* **15,** 765–782.

Waller, L.A. and Jacquez, G.M. (1995). Disease models implicit in statistical tests of disease clustering. *Epidemiology* **6,** 584–590.

Waller, L.A. and Lawson, A.B. (1995). The power of focused tests to detect disease clustering. *Statistics in Medicine* **14,** 2291–2308.

Waller, L.A. and McMaster, R.B. (1997). Incorporating indirect standardization in tests for disease clustering in a GIS environment. *Geographical Systems* **4,** 327–342.

Waller, L.A. and Poquette, C. (1999). The power of focused score tests under misspecified cluster models. In Lawson, A, Böhning, D., Lesaffre, E., Biggeri, A., Viel, J.-F., and Bertollini, R., eds. *Disease Mapping and Risk Assessment for Public Health.* Chichester: Wiley, pp. 257–269.

Waller, L.A., Turnbull, B.W., Clark, L.C., and Nasca, P. (1992). Chronic disease surveillance and testing of clustering of disease and exposure: application to leukemia incidence and TCE-contaminated dumpsites in upstate New York. *Environmetrics* **3,** 281–300.

Waller, L.A., Turnbull, B.W., Clark, L.C., and Nasca, P. (1994). Spatial pattern analyses to detect rare disease clusters. In Lange, N., Ryan, L., Billard, L., Brillinger, D., Conquest, L., and Greenhouse, J., eds, *Case Studies in Biometry.* New York: Wiley, pp. 3–23.

Walter, S.D. (1992a). The analysis of regional patterns in health data I: distributional considerations. *American Journal of Epidemiology* **136,** 730–741.

Walter, S.D. (1992b). The analysis of regional patterns in health data II: the power to detect environmental effects. *American Journal of Epidemiology* **136,** 742–759.

Walter, S.D. (1994). Calendar effects in the analysis of seasonal data. *American Journal of Epidemiology* **140,** 649–657.

Walter, S.D. and Elwood, J.M. (1975). A tests for seasonality of events with a variable population at risk. *British Journal of Preventive and Social Medicine* **29,** 18–21.

Wand, M.P. and Jones, M.C. (1995). *Kernel Smoothing.* Boca Raton: Chapman & Hall/CRC.

Whittemore, A. and Keller, J.B. (1986). On Tango's index for disease clustering in time. *Biometrics* **42,** 218.

Whittemore, A.S., Friend, N., Brown, B.W., and Holly, E.A. (1987). A test to detect clusters of disease. *Biometrika* **74,** 631–635.

APPENDIX

```
#############################################
# Splus code for Tango (1995)
#############################################
# Input:
# cases = vector of interval or region counts
# pop   = vector of interval or region population size
# x     = vector of x-coordinates of interval
#         or region centers.
# y     = vector of y-coordinates of interval
#         or region centers.
#############################################
# Set up case and population proportions

r <- cases/sum(cases)
p <- pop/sum(pop)
# assuming constant background rate
#############################################
# Find distance matrix
dist <- matrix(0,length(cases),length(cases))
for (i in 1:length(cases)) {dist[i,] ,- sqrt( (x[i]-x) ^2 + (y[i]-y) ^2 )}
#############################################
# Set A matrix and tau constant
tau <-1
A <- matrix(0,length(cases),length(cases))
A <- exp(-dist/tau)
#############################################
# Calculate exp'd value and variance under null
Vp <- diag(p) - p%*%t(p)
EC <- (1/sum(leuk$cases))*sum(diag(A %*% Vp))
VarC <- (2/(sum(leuk$cases)*sum(leuk$cases)) )*
          sum(diag(A %*% Vp %*% A %*% Vp))
gamma <- sqrt(2*sqrt(2)* (sum(diag(A %*% Vp %*% A %*% Vp %*% A %*% Vp))/
          (sum(diag(A%*% Vp %*% A %*% Vp))) ^(1.5)))nu <- 8/(gamma ^2)
#############################################
# Calculate observed value of test statistic
C <- t(r-p) %*% A %*% (r-p)
# Standardized version
Tstat <- (C - EC)/sqrt(VarC)
Tstat.chisq <- nu + Tstat*sqrt(2*nu)
# Find chi-square approximation p-value
pval.chisq <- 1-pchisq(Tstat.chisq,df=nu)
# Print out results
print( paste("Tango's index = ",round(Tstat.chisq,5),
   " p = ",round(pval.chisq,5)) )
```

8

Outbreak Detection: Application to Infectious Disease Surveillance

PADDY FARRINGTON, NICK ANDREWS

An important function of public health surveillance is to detect unusual clusters or outbreaks of disease and initiate timely interventions. With the surveillance of infectious disease, interventions may include removing contaminated foodstuffs, vaccinating or prophylactically treating individuals at risk, or changing production or industrial procedures. Whatever the context, the intervention must be undertaken as soon as possible after the outbreak starts, on a timescale often measured in days rather than weeks or months.

To ensure timely public health intervention, a system for detecting outbreaks must meet several requirements. First, it must detect outbreaks before they have fully developed, while the number of cases is still low. Second, it must detect outbreaks early, often before reports are complete or the data have been fully validated. Third, it must be capable of monitoring large numbers of data series. Finally, it must form an integral part of the surveillance and intervention process so that detection can be followed by action.

Some outbreak detection systems focus on a single health event (e.g., influenza, a type of cancer, or spontaneous abortion) and thus can incorporate detailed epidemiologic information. In contrast, others deal with a wide range of events (e.g., salmonella infections, which account for several thousand serotypes and phage types) and must be able to scan large databases.

This chapter describes the methodological issues involved in outbreak detection and give examples from a range of statistical techniques. Its focus is infectious disease detection because most outbreak detection systems have been applied to infectious disease. However, the methods we describe apply more generally, and we have drawn examples from related areas, such as monitoring birth defects.

Formal statistical methods have traditionally played only a minor part in outbreak detection, in contrast with other areas of epidemiology (e.g., clinical trials or epidemiologic study design) where statistical methodology has been central. The statistical literature on retrospective detection of temporal and spatial clusters of disease is extensive, but the statistical problem of prospective outbreak detection has received less attention. Recently, surveillance systems have been computerized, large amounts of data have been generated, and substantial computing power has become available. These three factors have provided an impetus for developing computer-assisted outbreak detection systems. Some systems now in routine use are reviewed in subsequent sections.

Devising a definition of an outbreak that can be used in a computer-assisted detection system requires statistical thinking. In most systems, a threshold is established above which observations are deemed aberrant. Specifying the threshold is a statistical problem requiring some allowance for random fluctuations in the data. A statistical perspective is required at other levels as well, e.g., for reporting delays, treating outliers, accounting for trends or seasonality in the data series, applying multiple sequential testing, and dealing with overdispersion.

Beyond the issues of statistical methods and computing wizardry, the primary issue in developing an effective computer-assisted outbreak detection system is that it must win the trust of the epidemiologists who undertake the interventions. The most technically advanced system will be worthless if it does not carry the conviction of those who use it. Developing a useful detection system therefore requires the collaborative efforts of epidemiologists, statisticians, and computer programmers.

METHODOLOGICAL ISSUES

Definition of an Outbreak

An often overlooked requirement for detecting outbreaks is to agree on a definition of outbreak. An outbreak has been defined by the Centers for Disease Control and Prevention (CDC) as two or more cases of infection by a common agent that are epidemiologically linked in some way, e.g., by exposure to the same contaminated foodstuff (CDC, 2000). Although useful in detecting outbreaks retrospectively, this definition is of little use in identifying outbreaks prospectively because it presupposes that detailed epidemiological information is available on the cases, when this information is usually obtained only after the outbreak investigation has begun.

To be useful for prospective detection, suitable proxy events must be defined, typically unusual temporal or spatial/temporal clusters of cases. The aim of a prospective outbreak detection system is to detect these events as they occur and target them for more detailed investigation. Thus, in practice, an outbreak is first identified when the number of reported cases exceeds expected levels. This triggering event is referred to as an aberration. An aberration signals only a potential outbreak because it may identify only chance clusters or artefacts of the reporting system.

Once an aberration is detected, further investigations are needed to establish whether it indicates a genuine outbreak. An outbreak detection system combines the statistical detection of aberrations and the epidemiological protocols and resources for classifying aberrations as worthy or not of detailed epidemiological investigation. In this chapter, we deal primarily with the statistical issue of detecting aberrations, although we touch on other issues.

The above definition of an outbreak requires the specification of a baseline count and a decision mechanism to judge whether current counts significantly exceed this baseline. Accordingly, most outbreak detection systems involve calculating threshold values that depend on baselines derived from historical data. A reported organism count that exceeds the threshold may trigger further epidemiological investigations. These investigations determine common epidemiological factors and, if an outbreak is confirmed, may lead to control measures. Methods for calculating baselines and thresholds are discussed in subsequent sections.

Ideally, the threshold value θ would be chosen to satisfy some criterion of the form

$$P(X > \theta \,|\, \text{no outbreak}) = \alpha$$

where X is the disease count in some predetermined time period and α is the nominal false detection rate, that is, the probability of triggering an investigation when no outbreak is occurring. In fact, the best we can do is to aim to satisfy the weaker criterion

$$P(X > \theta \,|\, \text{no aberration}) = \alpha$$

Here α is the probability of triggering an investigation when no genuine aberration exists, i.e. the probability that the threshold is exceeded by chance.

The timescale on which outbreaks are to be defined must be carefully considered. For example, if a detection system is based on weekly reports, should an aberration be declared only if the current weekly count is in excess of the weekly threshold? The issue arises because the relationship between the timescale and the threshold is non-linear when the false detection rate is kept constant. For example, if X_k denotes the number of cases aggregated over k successive reporting periods, and θ_k is the corresponding threshold chosen so that

$$P(X_k > \theta_k \mid \text{no aberration}) = \alpha$$

then generally $\theta_k < k\theta_1$. Thus, it is quite possible for, say, consecutive weekly reports to lie below the weekly threshold but the monthly total to lie above the monthly threshold. In this case, a detection system based on weekly counts would then miss more diffuse outbreaks occurring over longer periods. No simple statistical solution to this problem exists because no single system can detect every outbreak. A useful definition of a threshold requires careful discussion with the epidemiologists involved.

The threshold θ is most commonly defined as the upper endpoint of a prediction interval for the current observation, calculated from past observations. The calculation does not use the current observation. A prediction interval is similar conceptually to a confidence interval, except that it applies to a random quantity (in our case, the current count) rather than a parameter (such as the average baseline value). A prediction interval for the count will be wider than a confidence interval for the baseline because it allows for the uncertainty in the calculation of the baseline and the variability of the current count around this baseline.

Suppose, for example, that the baseline is to be calculated from the average of the observed counts over the past 8 weeks: 92, 131, 88, 93, 102, 116, 100, 120. (The current count of, say, 162 is excluded.) The baseline for the current count is the average of the previous eight values: 105.2. The prediction interval is calculated around this baseline value, and again the current value is excluded. Details of the calculation are given in Example 1: The Centers for Disease Control System, below; a 95% prediction interval for the current count is 66.6 to 143.8, calculated on the assumption that the counts are normally distributed. An appropriate threshold with $\alpha = 0.025$ is 143.8. The current observed count of 162 lies above the threshold and would therefore be declared aberrant.

Reporting Delays

Perhaps the most important difference between retrospective and prospective outbreak detection is that prospective studies must account for reporting delays, although this issue is rarely discussed. Retrospective outbreak detection is usually undertaken with complete data, for which reporting delays can be ignored. For infectious diseases, the data are typically assembled and analyzed by date of event, ideally date of infection, or date of onset or specimen collection if infection date is not available. As is standard practice in most statistical analyses, the data are validated, errors are corrected, missing fields are entered, and so on.

In contrast, for prospective detection, the data must be analyzed as it accumulates. Because the purpose of this system is to initiate timely interventions, little if any time is available for data validation. However, the data are often subject to reporting delays whereby the most recent infections are the least likely to have been reported. Thus current and recent counts are underestimated when data are ordered by date of infection or specimen. Such underestimation is a serious problem because the most recent data are precisely those on which outbreak detection is based. A clear understanding of the reporting system and the delays inherent in it is essential in designing an effective prospective outbreak detection system. Two approaches can be taken toward this problem. The first is to apply to recent data a correction factor based on an estimate of the delay distribution. This method is routinely used to correct for reporting delays in AIDS cases (Brookmeyer and Gail, 1994). However, this method poses several difficulties. First, it requires that all dates of onset or specimen collection be available. It also necessitates organism-specific calculations, because delays result from identification procedures that may vary between organisms. A more fundamental objection is that the data are imputed rather than observed. Imputing data is reasonable when a description of current trends, assumed to vary continuously, is required. However, imputing outbreaks, which involve discontinuities in the time series, is perhaps more questionable.

The second approach is to analyze the data by dates of receipt of the case reports, which are always available. In this case the historical series should also be ordered by date of report for comparability. The main advantage of this method is that it is based on actual rather than imputed data, although reporting delays inevitably affect detection sensitivity and specificity. An indirect benefit is that attention shifts to improving the surveillance and reporting system rather than tinkering with putative adjustments of dubious trustworthiness.

The mean of the reporting delay distribution affects the timeliness of outbreak detection. The longer the delay, the later the outbreak is deu ˙ ˙d. The variance of the reporting delay distribution affects the sensitivity of the detection system. The greater the variance in reporting delays, the more spread out the reports will be, and the less peaked will be the distribution.

This variability reduces the sensitivity of the system by reducing the chance that the fixed threshold will be exceeded. In a surveillance system involving many reporting centers, all centers should work to the same protocol, with the same procedures and deadlines, to minimize the variability of reporting delays. Also, all centers should concurrently attempt to reduce the average reporting delay. Settling for a slightly higher mean delay may be preferable if doing so substantially reduces the variance. The mean reporting delay should ideally be small in relation to the time scale over which an outbreak might develop. For national outbreaks of food-borne infection, for example, an outbreak might span several weeks; thus, delays between infection date and reporting of data should be kept to 1 or 2 weeks.

Systematic Variation

Typically, infectious diseases undergo large-scale systematic variations in incidence that are not outbreaks. These variations may follow seasonal cycles, epidemic cycles, or secular trends. For instance, in temperate climates, respiratory syncytial virus infections peak in early winter, rotavirus infections peak in late winter or early spring, and most salmonella infections peak in summer. Some infections, such as parvovirus B19, undergo regular epidemic cycles with a period of several years, whereas others, such as the influenza B virus, have an irregular epidemic cycle. Some infections emerging as major health problems, such as verocytotoxin-producing *Escherichia coli* O157 in the United Kingdom display an increasing secular trend. Others, such as measles or other infections controlled by mass vaccination, are declining in importance.

Although the primary aim of an outbreak detection system is to detect sudden departures from regular patterns, regular features may sometimes be of interest. For example, tracking the once-yearly rise in influenza cases to identify the start of the epidemic season can help in heightening public awareness and reinforcing control measures.

Regular fluctuations in incidence of infection can easily be incorporated into statistical models, but the complex patterns displayed by some infections cannot. For example, the wide variation in *Salmonella typhimurium* DT104 reports in the United Kingdom (Fig. 8–1) makes modeling the entire historical series a complex task that is unlikely to produce reliable baselines for the current period. More generally, past data values not occurring at similar points in previous years or epidemic cycles may have little relevance when establishing baselines for the period of interest. Thus, modeling the data series as a whole may serve little purpose. However, if the data series displays no seasonal or epidemic cycles, one can borrow strength between periods to provide a better baseline for the current period.

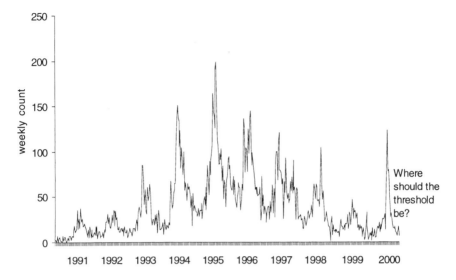

Figure 8–1 Weekly counts of *Salmonella typhimurium* DT104 in England and Wales from 1991 to 2000, illustrating the difficulty of setting an appropriate decision threshold.

Outbreak detection based on spatial temporal data is a possible exception to the notion of using only directly comparable time periods in calculating baselines. In this case, information on all time periods might provide useful information on the spatial correlation structure.

Influence of Past Aberrations

The baseline level of infection in the absence of outbreaks must be calculated so as to eliminate the impact of past outbreaks or other aberrations. Failing to adjust for past aberrations can result in unrepresentative baselines and thresholds that are too high. An example is the impact of the aberrant central peak in the time series for *Salmonella Gold Coast* (Fig. 8–2). Unless the threshold is adjusted, it will be biased upwardly, and future outbreaks will be more difficult to detect.

In statistical terms, past aberrations correspond to outliers in the data series. The easiest way to correct for such outliers is simply to omit the corresponding data points from baseline calculations. Alternatively, the outliers can be down-weighted (Farrington et al., 1996). Past aberrations can usually be identified easily by inspection. However, no satisfactory algorithm for recognizing them has been devised. In outbreak detection, the approach to treating outliers among the baseline values should be driven by the need to avoid bias, even at the expense of obtaining more conser-

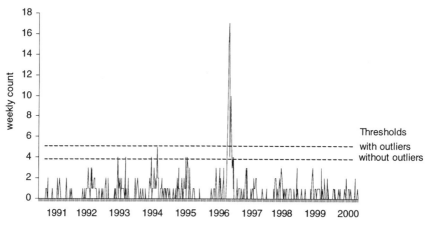

Figure 8–2 Weekly counts Reports of *Salmonella Gold Coast* in England and Wales from 1991 to 2000, illustrating the effect of not adjusting the decision threshold for past outbreaks.

vative (i.e., lower) thresholds. This treatment differs from that in other settings, where outliers require careful consideration because they may indicate a failure of the model or inaccuracies in the data (Altman, 1999).

For systems in long-term operation, the impact of past aberrations might be controlled by incorporating prospectively acquired information into a dynamic memory for later reference, although such a system has yet to be implemented. For example, an infection count that exceeds its threshold in a given reporting period could be flagged as a possible outbreak and this information stored. When that data point is later used as a baseline, it may be excluded or down-weighted, or it might simply result in a warning.

Complexity and Robustness of Outbreak Detection Systems

An important question in devising outbreak detection systems is how complex the models should be. The answer differs for organism-specific detection systems and generic systems. An organism-specific detection system is geared to detecting outbreaks of a single infective organism or a group of infections with similar epidemiologic features, such as influenza infections or water-borne infections. Organism-specific systems can incorporate much knowledge of the epidemiologic features of the infection. For example, the influenza season in the United Kingdom begins in September each year and past epidemics are well known, and thus this information can be used to calculate suitable baselines. More generally, relatively complex modeling tools involving user intervention can be used. Time-series methods based on autoregressive integrated moving average (ARIMA) models are possible contenders for such systems.

In contrast, generic detection systems are designed to scan large databases of hundreds or thousands of organisms with differing epidemiologies and frequencies. These systems require computer-aided outbreak detection because such a task cannot be performed manually. For example, surveillance of a nonspecific disease, such as gastroenteritis, requires monitoring large numbers of infective organisms that may be associated with clinical illness. Subtypes may also be distinguished for epidemiologic purposes. Thus, large amounts of data relating to different organisms must be processed within a short time. For example, in 2000, the central database of the U.K. Communicable Disease Surveillance Centre tracked the weekly reports of 4200 distinct organism types. Processing this volume of data within hours each week requires relatively simple methods (e.g., simple regression models) that do not rely on frequent resetting of organism-specific parameters.

For practical purposes, a single robust algorithm is required to handle the wide variety of organisms reported in generic detection systems. The algorithm must be robust in several ways. First, it must handle both common and rare organisms because the frequency of outbreaks among organisms is vastly different. For example, many rare salmonella infections have expected weekly frequencies of less than 0.1, whereas other infections, such as *Samonella enteritidis* PT4, generate hundreds of reports each week. Second, the algorithm must cope with different seasonalities and trends. Third, it must have a mechanism to handle past outbreaks. Fourth, it should not require the resetting of infection-specific parameters; rather, it should ideally be a wholly automated procedure that can run week after week with minimal user intervention.

A consequence of the need for robustness is that detailed modeling of the transmission dynamics of the infection usually cannot be incorporated, because such modeling is incompatible with the need for rapid, routine data processing. More generally, complex or computer-intensive statistical procedures are inappropriate in this context. The system should be built on simple yet robust statistical models.

REVIEW OF STATISTICAL METHODS

Many statistical studies have been published on the detection of temporal and spatio-temporal cluster (see, for example, the review of temporal and cyclical clustering by Tango, 1984). Most have focused on detecting retrospective clusters, i.e., clusters that may have occurred in a specific time interval in the past. This setting contrasts with that of detecting outbreaks prospectively, i.e., as they arise. Prospective detection differs from retrospective detection not only in the methodological problems it poses (see Methodological Issues, above) but also in the types of hypotheses to be tested. In prospective detection, interest focuses on the null distribution of disease counts at the current time t, given the history of the process prior to time t. This requires that an appropriate outbreak-free distribution be specified and that a decision rule be formulated under which the current observed value is classified as aberrant or not. In contrast, most statistical procedures for retrospective cluster detection are designed to identify clusters in a time interval (t_1,t_2) with $t_1 < t_2 < t$, where t is the current time and t_1, t_2 are often left unspecified. Many of these methods can be adapted for use in prospective detection.

In this section we review some statistical methods developed for detecting aberrations prospectively or used in retrospective detection but likely to be useful prospectively. Our aim is not to review cluster detection and its applications exhaustively, but to illustrate the diversity of techniques. Most examples are of detecting infectious disease outbreaks, but a few are of prospective detection of clusters of congenital abnormalities.

Regression Methods

A conceptually simple, hence appealing, approach to detecting aberrations prospectively is to estimate the distribution of counts at time t, $f(y|t)$ by regressing the observed counts y_i, $i = 1, 2, \ldots, n$ at previous times t_i. For large counts, $f(y|t)$ might be assumed $N(\mu, \sigma^2)$; for low counts, a Poisson distribution may be appropriate. The expected count μ is estimated from the predicted value at time t, and an upper threshold is derived from prediction limits. An advantage of this method is that the regression equation can readily incorporate terms for trend and seasonality. A shortcoming is that it ignores any serial correlation between counts. For rare organisms, serial correlation is not an issue because most cases are sporadic, at least in nonoutbreak conditions.

Example 1: The Centers for Disease Control system
The simplest version of a regression method is used in the aberrant report detection system described by Stroup et al. (1989), which is a routine monitoring system applied to monthly counts of notifiable diseases in the United States. The output, which appears each month in the *Morbidity and Mortality Weekly Report* of the CDC, displays a barchart of the observed-over-expected ratios (Fig. 8–3). The system does not incorporate time trends, and it handles seasonality by comparing the counts for the current month with those for the comparable month, the previous month and the subse-

quent month in the 5 previous years. For example, the March 2002 count is compared with counts in February, March, and April of the years 1997 to 2001. The predicted value is the mean of the 15 baseline values. A 95% confidence or prediction interval for the current value may be calculated from the sample mean and variance of the baseline observations, and the current observed-over-expected ratio is declared aberrant if it lies outside the corresponding prediction interval. Figure 8–3 displays 95% confidence intervals; we illustrate here the alternative approach based on prediction intervals.

Let $\bar{x}$ denote the sample mean of the k baseline values and s the sample standard deviation. Then a $100\ (1 - \alpha)\%$ prediction interval for the current value is

$$\left(\bar{x} - z_{\alpha/2} \times s \times \sqrt{1 + \frac{1}{k}}, \bar{x} + z_{\alpha/2} \times s \times \sqrt{1 + \frac{1}{k}}\right) \qquad (8\text{–}1)$$

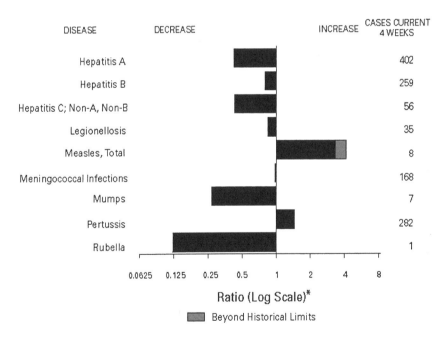

Figure 8–3 Sample selected notifiable disease reports United States, comparison of provisional 4-week totals ending February 24, 2001, with historical data. *Source:* Centers for Disease Control and Prevention. (2001). *Morbidity and Mortality Weekly Report* **50,** 151. *Ratio of current 4-week total to mean of 15 4-week totals (from previous, comparable, and subsequent 4-week periods for the past 5 years). The point where the hatched area begins is based on the mean and 2 standard deviations of these 4-week totals.

The constant $z_{\alpha/2}$ in this expression is the $(1 - \alpha/2)$ quantile of the normal distribution. For example, for a 2.5% nominal false detection rate α we would use a 95% prediction interval, for which $z_{\alpha/2} = 1.96$. (In the numerical illustration in Definition of an Outbreak, above we used the 0.975 quantile of the t distribution on $8 - 1 - 7$ degrees of freedom, 2.365.) The threshold value is the upper endpoint of this interval. For example, if $\bar{x} = 246.2$, $s = 38.7$, and $k = 15$, the threshold value is 324.5; thus a report in excess of 324 would be classified as aberrant.

The considerable advantages of this system are its simplicity and the ease with which the output can be conveyed to the epidemiological community by a simple graphic. This approach, or a simple variation of it, is widely used in detecting nosocomial outbreaks (see, for instance, Birnbaum, 1984). A main shortcoming is that it does not correct for past outbreaks. These can seriously distort the baselines, inflating the mean and hence producing an artificially low observed-over-expected ratio. Another shortcoming is that the normality assumption, although valid for the substantial counts of some notifiable diseases, is unlikely to hold for less common infections. Kafadar and Stroup (1992) discussed the impact of serial correlation on their method, and concluded that the simple estimation method described above is preferable to more complex resampling schemes, unless detailed information is available on the underlying correlation structure. An evaluation of the system is described in Stroup et al. (1993).

Example 2: Explicit modeling of trend and seasonality

In a pioneering application, Serfling (1963) used regression techniques to quantify the mortality attributable to influenza in cities in the United States. Although the focus of his application differs from that of outbreak detection, many ideas are directly transferable (see, for instance, Costagliola et al., 1991; Costagliola, 1994; Flahault et al., 1995 for applications to detection of outbreaks of influenza and gastro-enteritis).

Essentially, the model fitted is a normal errors regression, with a linear secular time trend and sinusoidal seasonal components. Thus the expected value at time t is given by the regression equation

$$E(Y|t) = \alpha + \beta t + \gamma \cos(\omega t + \varphi) \tag{8-2}$$

Serfling (1963) fitted his model in three stages. First, he estimated the secular trend from selected periods of low incidence, mid-May to mid-September. He then estimated the seasonal parameters from the detrended data for nonepidemic years after identifying the epidemic years by inspection. Finally he estimated the (null) residual variance from the sum of squared residuals corresponding to nonepidemic years.

This procedure may be adapted easily to the construction of suitable thresholds for future periods based on prediction intervals and, hence, applied to the prospective detection of temporal clusters. The expected value obtained is adjusted for past epidemics and incorporates adjustments for trend and seasonality. However, the method involves considerable empirical judgment, particularly in identifying past epidemic years, and is thus not well suited for automation. Furthermore, an explicit functional specification of the seasonal component is unlikely to work when applied to a broad spectrum of organisms with different, or occasionally nonexistent, seasonalities.

Example 3: Poisson regression

Examples 1 and 2 use normal errors regression, which is suitable when the number of events is large, but inappropriate when events are infrequent. Parker (1989) described a cluster detection system that used Poisson regression to detect changes in an uncommon event—abortion-related mortality in the United States. The model is a log-linear model of the form

$$Y_t \sim P(\mu_t), \log(\mu_t) = \alpha + \beta_t \tag{8--3}$$

where Y_t is the observed incidence rate of abortion-related deaths at time t. When calculating a prediction interval, some allowance should be made for the asymmetry of the Poisson distribution, so that the false-positive probability (i.e., the probability of the current count exceeding the threshold when there is no outbreak) remains constant over a broad range of expected values. Thresholds derived from symmetric prediction intervals are unsuitable.

A solution is to use a transformation to produce an approximately symmetric distribution, calculate a symmetric interval on this scale, and transform the results back to the original scale. When the counts are Poisson, a 2/3-power transformation induces approximate symmetry (Farrington et al., 1996). When this transformation is used the endpoints of an approximate $100(1 - \alpha)\%$ prediction interval for the count at time t are

$$\hat{\mu}_t \times \left\{ 1 \pm \frac{2}{3} z_{a/2} \times \sqrt{\frac{1}{\hat{\mu}_t} + V_t} \right\}^{3/2}$$

where $\hat{\mu}_t = \exp(\hat{\alpha} + \hat{\beta}t)$ is the estimated baseline value and

$$V_t = \text{var}(\hat{\alpha}) + t^2 \, \text{var}(\hat{\beta}) + 2t \, \text{cov}(\hat{\alpha}, \hat{\beta})$$

All components of the calculation may be obtained from the output of standard regression software. For example, suppose that the prediction interval for the current count is to be obtained from the previous 8 weeks' counts: 3, 2, 5, 8, 6, 7, 5, and 9 at weeks 0–7 (the current week is 8). A Poisson model fitted to these data yields $\hat{\alpha} = 1.222$, $\hat{\beta} = 0.1315$, $\text{var}(\hat{\alpha}) = 0.100094$, $\text{var}(\hat{\beta}) = 0.004467$, and $\text{cov}(\hat{\alpha}, \hat{\beta}) = -0.018654$. It follows that $\hat{\mu}_8 = \exp(\hat{\alpha} + 8\hat{\beta}) = 9.718$ and $V(\hat{\mu}_8) = 0.0875$. Hence the upper 95% prediction limit is

$$9.718 \times \left(1 + \frac{2}{3} \times 1.96 \times \sqrt{\frac{1}{9.718} + 0.088}\right)^{3/2} = 19.1$$

Counts higher than 19 would be regarded as aberrant, with a nominal false detection rate of 2.5%.

Unlike normal errors regression, this approach is applicable to rare events (e.g., those in a hospital setting). However, the Poisson assumption is unlikely to hold in many circumstances, and some method of handling extra-Poisson variation is required.

Example 4: The Communicable Disease Surveillance Centre system

The detection system in use at the Communicable Disease Surveillance Centre (CDSC) in the United Kingdom, described by Farrington et al. (1996), is specifically designed to handle a wide variety of organism frequencies and temporal patterns. The basic model is a quasilikelihood loglinear regression model:

$$\log(\mu_i) = \alpha + \beta_{t_i}, \quad E(Y_i) = \mu_i, \quad V(Y_i) = \varphi\mu_i \qquad (8\text{--}3)$$

Seasonality is handled as in the CDC system (Example 1). To try to reduce the influence of past outbreaks, baseline values with high residuals are given lower weights in the regression. For a baseline count with standardized residual s_i, the weight is γs_i^{-2} if $s_i > 1$ and γ otherwise, for some appropriately chosen constant γ. Anscombe residuals are used (Davison and Snell, 1991). The model is reestimated three times: first, to adjust for past outbreaks; again, to estimate the dispersion parameter φ; and a third time with the parameter β set to zero if the trend is not significant.

To ensure a broadly constant false positive rate over the wide range of organism frequencies, the threshold is calculated after applying a 2/3 power transformation, as in the Poisson model (Example 3). The threshold value at time t is the upper $100(1 - \alpha)\%$ prediction limit:

$$\mu_U = \hat{\mu}_t \left\{ 1 + \frac{2}{3} z_{\alpha/2} \left(\frac{\hat{\varphi}\hat{\mu}_t + \text{var}(\hat{\mu}_t)}{\hat{\mu}_t^2} \right)^{1/2} \right\}^{3/2}$$

The power 2/3 was chosen because it is the transformation to approximate symmetry for the Poisson distribution. The rationale for this model is that the distribution for rare organisms is approximately Poisson and hence $\varphi \approx 1$, whereas for more frequent organisms normal approximations are valid. When $\varphi = 1$, the expression for the upper prediction limit is the same as that for the Poisson model in Example 3: Poisson Regression, above.

At the CDSC, the model is run automatically every week on all 250 to 350 different organism types reported. For each organism, 99.5% prediction limits are calculated, and a list is produced of all organisms exceeding their threshold. Farrington et al. (1996) discussed the assumptions underlying the model and evaluated its performance. Figure 8–4 shows a sample output screen from the system, displaying the geographical distribution, age distribution, and time series of cases, along with summary statistics.

Example 5: Smoothing the baselines

An attractive method of obtaining the baselines is the compound smoothing procedure proposed by Stern and Lightfoot (1999) who used it for routine detection of Salmonella outbreaks in Australia. A baseline time period is defined, and the past counts within this period are smoothed. A first set

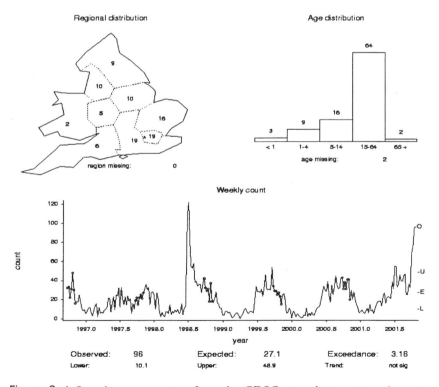

Figure 8–4 Sample output screen from the CDSC exceedance system (see text for explanation).

of residuals is calculated (raw data minus the smoothed data). These residuals are smoothed using the same smoother as was applied to the raw data. The smoothed residuals are added to the smoothed data to provide a set of "polished" baselines $\hat{\mu}_t$. A second set of residuals is calculated from the raw data, minus the polished baselines, and an estimate $\hat{\sigma}$ of the standard deviation σ is obtained from these.

The baseline value for the current time point is then calculated from the polished baselines that correspond to the same time points in previous years. Finally, the threshold is calculated as $\hat{\mu}_t + z_{\alpha/2}\hat{\sigma}$ where $z_{\alpha/2}$ is the $(1 - \alpha/2)$ quantile of the standard normal distribution.

A great advantage of the method is that it is easily programmed and is therefore suitable for large databases. Also, it can be used with data subject to seasonal variation. Choosing a smoother bandwidth (or window) requires some care to achieve the right balance between sensitivity and false positive rate. Stern and Lightfoot (1999) used monthly data from a 5-year period, and a compound smoother made up of a sequence of five moving averages applied in successive passes.

Time Series Methods

Time series methodology is an obvious candidate for detection systems. After all, the surveillance data upon which the detection system is based are time series data. Furthermore, time series methods, unlike regression methods, exploit the correlation structure of the data. However, two main problems are associated with the more complex time series methods used in the present context. First, these methods generally require an initial transformation of the time series to achieve stationarity. Second, the model-fitting techniques required, at least for the more complex Box-Jenkins models, are difficult to automate, in that they generally require careful interpretation of a panoply of autocorrelation functions.

Example 6: Exponential smoothing

Applying exponential smoothing to monitoring surveillance data was first suggested by Healy (1983). The method was used by Ngo et al. (1996) to detect nosocomial outbreaks. Exponential smoothing is essentially a weighted procedure for predicting the current count in a stationary series by giving greater weight to more recent observations and less weight to observations from the more distant past. Thus, the prediction at time $t + 1$, $\hat{y}_{t+1}$, is related to the observed values $y_t, y_{t-1}, \ldots$ by:

$$\hat{y}_{t+1} = \alpha y_t + \alpha(1 - \alpha)y_{t-1} + \alpha(1 - \alpha)^2 y_{t-2} + \ldots$$

$$= \alpha y_t + (1 - \alpha)\hat{y}_t$$

The forecast error e_t is defined as

$$e_t = y_t - \hat{y}_t$$

and the estimated forecast error variance at time point t, s_t^2, based on the last k values, is

$$s_t^2 = \frac{1}{k} \sum_{i=t-k+1}^{t} e_i^2$$

The forecast error variance may be used to define the threshold as the upper limit of the prediction interval:

$$\hat{y}_t \pm z_{\alpha/2} \times s_t$$

It may also be used to adjust the choice of the constant α. Once several predictions have been obtained using a starting value of α, the forecast error variance is calculated. A slightly different value of α is then chosen and the predictions are recalculated, along with the forecast error variance. The optimal value of α is that which minimizes the forecast error variance.

   To illustrate the method, suppose that we choose $\alpha = 0.1$ and $y_1 = \hat{y}_1 = 84$. The first forecast is for $t = 2$, giving $\hat{y}_2 = \alpha y_1 + (1 - \alpha)\hat{y}_1 = 0.1 \times 84 + 0.9 \times 84 = 84$. Suppose that we observe $y_2 = 96$. Thus, the forecast error at $t = 2$ is $e_2 = 96 - 84 = 12$. The forecast for $t = 3$ is $\hat{y}_3 = 0.1 \times 96 + 0.9 \times 84 = 85.2$. Suppose that the observed value turns out to be 80; thus, the forecast error at $t = 3$ is $e_3 = 80 - 85.2 = -5.2$. An initial estimate of the forecast error variance is $(12^2 + 5.2^2)/2 = 85.52$. The forecast for $t = 4$ is $\hat{y}_4 = 0.1 \times 80 + 0.9 \times 85.2 = 84.68$. The 95% prediction limits are $84.68 \pm 1.96 \times \sqrt{85.52}$, namely 66.6 to 102.81. After more values are obtained, and the estimate of the forecast error variance is reasonably stable, the procedure can be rerun using, say, $\alpha = 0.2, 0.3, \ldots$ and an optimal value of α selected.

   In the nosocomial application envisaged by Ngo et al. (1996) the forecast error was found not to be sensitive to the choice of the smoothing constant α. However, the method as described is only applicable to stationary series. In particular, recent outbreaks would seriously affect the accuracy of the forecasts.

Example 7: Box-Jenkins models
Watier et al. (1991) described the construction of a warning system for outbreaks of salmonella infection using Box-Jenkins time series models.

They fitted a seasonal autoregressive integrated moving average (SARIMA) model to data on *Salmonella bovismorbificans*. The model may be written

$$(y_t - y_{t-12}) = \alpha(y_{t-1} - y_{t-13}) + \varepsilon_t + \beta\varepsilon_{t-12} \qquad (8\text{--}4)$$

where y_t is the count in period t. Before fitting the model, Watier et al. identified past outbreaks and replaced these counts with those that would have been expected if there had been no outbreak. They calculated an alert threshold from the upper limit of a suitably chosen prediction interval on the one-step forecast, adjusting for small fluctuations in seasonal effects.

Watier et al. (1991) carefully considered the methodologic problems inherent in devising outbreak detection systems, and their approach adjust for many of these difficulties. The authors noted that their approach is applicable to other salmonella serotypes. However, automating the system in a way that guarantees robustness for a wide variety of organisms would be difficult.

Choi and Thacker (1981) also described a time series approach for detecting outbreaks of influenza. They compared the performance of this method to that of Serfling (1963) (see Example 2), and concluded that the time series method is superior. However they also noted that the two methods yield comparable results if, in the regression method, counts in epidemic years are replaced by expected values rather than excluded.

Statistical Process Control Methods

The problem of detecting outbreaks of infectious diseases prospectively is similar to that of detecting aberrances in industrial production processes. Several proposed approaches are directly inspired by, or related to, methods of statistical process control. For instance, many of the methods used for nosocomial surveillance are similar to Shewart charts (Birnbaum, 1984; Parkhurst et al., 1985). Shewart charts are typically used to track the characteristics of a production process (for example, a quality index, or the proportion of defective items) over time. Upper and lower control boundaries are defined, and the process is said to go out of control if a boundary is crossed. In outbreak detection, the process that is being tracked is the count of events over time, the prediction limits playing the role of control boundaries. In this section we consider three further methods which share a flavor of statistical process control methodology. Other such methods have been proposed (e.g., the short memory scheme of Shore and Quade (1989) based on the distribution of cases in the current and previous periods) but will not be considered further here.

Example 8: Cumulative sum techniques

Cumulative sums (cusums) were introduced by Page (1954) and have been used in outbreak detection in recent decades (e.g., the onset of influenza epidemics in the United Kingdom (Tillett and Spencer, 1982) and salmonella outbreaks in the United States (Hutwagner et al., 1997)).

One definition of the cusum is as follows. Given counts y_i normally distributed $N(\mu_t, \sigma^2)$ in the absence of an outbreak, the (one-sided) cusum at time t is defined iteratively by

$$C_0 = 0, \; C_t = \max\{0, C_{t-1} + (y_t - \mu_t - k\sigma)\} \tag{8-5}$$

where k is a constant depending on the size of the effect of interest; for example, if changes in the mean of the order of σ are of interest, then $k = 0.5$.

In the absence of any systematic departure from the expected values μ_i, the cusum remains at or close to zero. However, if an outbreak occurs, the cusum registers a change in level. The values μ_i in Figure 8–5, for example, are baseline counts, most easily derived from corresponding periods in the past in which no outbreaks occurred. This definition can be extended to Poisson data (see for example Lucas, 1985).

If the cusum exceeds a specified threshold value $h\sigma$, the process is said to be "out of control" and an alert is declared. The cusum is then reset to zero and the process starts again. The parameters h and k together define

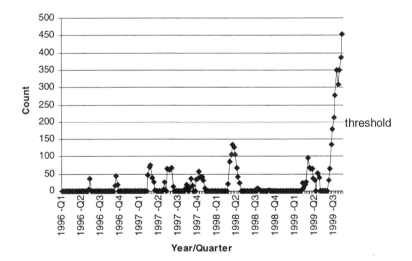

Figure 8–5 Cusum of crytosporidium weekly counts 1996 to 1999 (baseline = 80, standard deviation = 25, k = 1, h = 8).

the Average Run Length (ARL), i.e., the average time between alerts when the process is in control. The reciprocal of the ARL is thus the false detection rate. Tables of ARLs for a range of values of h and k are available (see for instance Wetherill and Brown, 1991). For outbreak detection, it is probably advisable to set h and k empirically after suitable simulation studies based on real data.

If the counts vary seasonally, the baselines μ_t can be calculated from counts in comparable periods in previous years, as described in Example 1. The standard deviation is likely to vary with time of year, and standardized cusums are best used:

$$C_0 = 0, \; C_t = \max\left\{0, \; C_{t-1} + \left(\frac{y_t - \mu_t}{\sigma_t} - k\right)\right\}$$

For example, baselines might be calculated from counts from the 3 adjacent months (comparable, previous, and subsequent) in the previous 5 years. Suppose that $y_1 = 321$ in March 2002. The baseline μ_1 is estimated by the mean of the 15 counts from February, March and April from 1997 to 2001. These counts are also used to estimate the standard deviation σ_t. Suppose that $\hat{\mu}_1 = 298.2$, $\hat{\sigma}_1 = 23.4$. Using the value $k = 1$, we obtain

$$C_0 = 0$$

$$C_1 = \max\left\{0, \; 0 + \frac{321 - 298.2}{23.4} - 1\right\}$$

$$= 0$$

If now $y_2 = 363$ in April 2002, and the corresponding baseline, calculated from the March to May counts in the previous 5 years, is $\hat{\mu}_2 = 290.8$ with $\hat{\sigma}_2 = 31.7$, then

$$C_2 = \max\left\{0, \; 0 + \frac{363 - 290.8}{31.7} - 1\right\}$$

$$= 1.18,$$

and so on.

Because cusums are sensitive to small changes in the numbers of reports, they are well suited for detecting the timing of onsets of epidemics, such as influenza, or monitoring series of relatively uncommon infections. However, for the same reason, they are sensitive to small changes in reporting efficiency and other artefacts of the reporting process. Thus, they may lack robustness when used with surveillance data unless the baselines are frequently reset.

Example 9: Methods based on time to failure

When events are very rare, methods based on monitoring aggregate total cases in discrete time periods will fail, because even a single report is unusual in a statistical sense. This problem can be circumvented by specifying a minimum outbreak size that must be exceeded for the count to qualify as an outbreak. A contrasting approach is to base detections not on total reports, but on the intervals between them. Such an approach was developed by Chen (1978) for tracking congenital abnormalities.

Assuming that events arise in a stationary Poisson process, inter-event times follow an exponential distribution with mean μ, say. The detection threshold is specified by parameters (n, τ), and an aberrance is declared if the intervals between $n + 1$ consecutive events are all less than τ. The false detection probability is $(1 - e^{-\tau/\mu})^n$ when there is no change in the underlying rate. Similarly, the sensitivity of detection is $(1 - e^{-\gamma\tau/\mu})^n$ when the rate of events increases by a factor γ.

The background rate, and hence μ, may be determined from historical data. Appropriate values of n and τ are selected to yield acceptable sensitivity and false detection probabilities. The analysis is undertaken whenever an event occurs. Chen et al. (1993) proposed supplementing the method with a further confirmatory procedure, to reduce the false detection probability.

Methods based on time to failure overcome some of the shortcomings of other approaches when events are rare (e.g., events connected with very uncommon Salmonella serotypes) and might be useful for detecting low-level point-source outbreaks. Barbujani (1987) reviewed this method and others for monitoring congenital malformations.

Example 10: Derivative-based methods

All methods described previously, other than the last, are based on a threshold value, above which reports are declared aberrant. An intuitively appealing alternative suggested by Nobre and Stroup (1994) is to base monitoring on changes in the first derivative of the data series with respect to time. Two potential advantages of this approach are that departures from the norm might be detected earlier, before reports reach the threshold value, and that long series of historical data are not required.

For simplicity, consider a simple exponentially smoothed model (see Example 6). The forecast error $e_t = y_t - \hat{y}_t$ may be written:

$$e_t = y_t^1 + (1 - \alpha)y_{t-1}^1 + (1 - \alpha)^2 y_{t-2}^1 + \ldots,$$

where $y_t^1 = y_t - y_{t-1}$ is the first numerical derivative. The forecast error is thus a weighted sum of the previous values of the numerical derivative. In the absence of systematic deviations from stationarity, the forecast error will remain close to zero. Nobre and Stroup further smoothed the forecast error and converted it into an index function that varies between -1 and $+1$. Departures of the index function beyond suitable limits then indicate aberrant behavior.

Nobre and Stroup (1994) extended this approach to data series that can be modeled by polynomial functions and discussed an application to data on measles in the United States. The main shortcoming of the approach is its lack of specificity in some circumstances, in that small fluctuations in the data can produce large derivatives. The authors proposed to remedy this problem by introducing further constraints on the detection criterion.

Methods Incorporating Spatial Information

All methods described thus far are based on detecting changes in the temporal pattern of reports and use data aggregated over geographical areas. National detection systems are unlikely to be more effective in detecting local outbreaks than more traditional surveillance methods conducted by epidemiologists and other staff from their experience of local conditions. However, in some circumstances national systems might be enhanced by incorporating information on spatial heterogeneity.

Although much has been published on detecting space–time interactions (see, for instance, Knox [1964] and Mantel [1967] for some early work), little has been written on corresponding methods for outbreak detection. In the following subsections, we describe three methods that, to our knowledge, have not been used to detect infectious disease outbreaks but could potentially be used.

Spatial cusum statistics

Raubertas (1989) described a generalization of the cusum statistic that uses spatial information. Suppose that there are s geographical units, and that S is an $s \times s$ proximity matrix of values s_{kl} representing the closeness of geographical units k and l, with $0 \le s_{kl} \le 1$. For example,

$$s_{kl} = \exp(-d_{kl}/\tau)$$

where d_{kl} is the distance between units k and l and τ is a scale parameter. A contrasting choice is

$$s_{kl} = \begin{cases} 1 & \text{if } d_{ij} \le \tau \\ 0 & \text{otherwise} \end{cases}$$

Now let x_{ki} denote the disease count in geographical unit k at time i, with expectation $n_k\lambda$. Define the pooled count

$$z_{ki} = \sum_{l=1}^{s} s_{kl}\, x_{li}$$

Similar pooling is used to define the reference values θ_{ki}. A cusum for each location is then defined as follows:

$$C_{ki} = \max\{0, C_{k,i-1} + (z_{ki} - \theta_{ki})\}$$

This cusum will go "out of control" if the mean rate in the neighborhood of unit k increases. Raubertas (1989) discussed the ARL for these cusums under a variety of proximity measures.

This spatial cusum method requires monitoring several cusums that each correspond to a spatial unit. Rogerson (1997) proposed another cusum that also uses measures of spatial proximity but that combines information from all geographical units. His method is based on Tango's test of spatial clustering and allows a single cusum to be tracked.

Sequential monitoring of space-time interactions

Rogerson (2001) proposed a method for prospectively detecting emerging clusters based on a local version of Knox's test for space–time interaction (Knox, 1964). As with the Knox test, occurrences of cases within a pre-specified critical distance and time period indicate clustering in space and time. Given n points located in space and time, there are $n(n-1)/2$ distinct pairs of points. These pairs can be classified as close in time, space, both, or neither, giving rise to a 2×2 table. The Knox test statistic is N_{st}, the number of pairs that are close in both space and time.

Rogerson (2001) proposed a local version of this statistic, suitable for prospective monitoring. Suppose that $i-1$ cases are distributed in space and time, and that an i-th case arises. Let $N_{st}(i)$ denote the number of cases that are close to this i-th case in both space and time. Rogerson obtains expressions for the expectation and variance of $N_{st}(i)$ conditional on the observed value of $N_{st}(i-1)$ and relevant marginals. The standardized test statistic Z_i can then be monitored using a cusum chart. This approach is suitable for routine use and provides an attractive method for detecting spatial clusters as they emerge in time.

A prospective spatial scan statistic

The scan statistic has long been used for retrospective detection of temporal and spatial temporal clusters in epidemiology (see Wallenstein [1980] and Wallenstein et al. [1989]). Kulldorff (2001) adapted the method for use in prospective monitoring of emerging clusters.

Consider a given spatial location ω (if the data are grouped in geographical regions, use the centroid of a region), and count the number of cases within a distance δ of this location that occurred in the time interval $(t - \tau, t]$ where t represents the current time point. Here δ and τ are some constants. This region of space-time can be regarded as a cylinder C centered on ω, of radius δ and height τ. Let n be the total number of cases arising at all locations at any time up to t, and n_c the number of cases within the cylinder.

Under a Poisson model, the likelihood ratio conditional on the total number of cases n is

$$\frac{L_1(C)}{L_0(C)} = \left(\frac{n_C}{\mu(C)}\right)^{n_C}\left(\frac{n - n_C}{n - \mu(C)}\right)^{n - n_C}$$

where $\mu(C)$ is the expected count in the cylinder under the null hypothesis of homogeneity. The scan statistic is defined as the maximum ratio over all cylinders C for which the count is greater than expected:

$$S = \max\left\{\frac{L_1(C)}{L_0(C)}\middle| C : n_C \geq \mu(C)\right\}$$

The p-value for an observed value of S is obtained by Monte Carlo methods. The approach is therefore computer-intensive, and as such is better suited to disease-specific surveillance rather than generic detection systems. Kulldorff (2001) discusses various other aspects of this method and its implementation.

VALIDATION AND IMPLEMENTATION

The main challenge in setting up a computer-assisted detection system is to design it in such a way that epidemiologists who undertake the interventions will use it. Our experience suggests that this requirement is by far the most challenging. In the following sections, two key elements of a useful system are discussed: good sensitivity and low false detection rate, and the perception that the system will contribute to detecting outbreaks.

Sensitivity and False Detection Rate

The sensitivity of an outbreak detection system is measured by the proportion of true outbreaks detected by the system. The false detection (or false positive) rate is measured by the proportion of apparently aberrant reports not associated with outbreaks. A low sensitivity or a high false detection rate is likely to jeopardize confidence in the system. Thus, to be of practical use, an outbreak detection system have high sensitivity and a low false detection rate.

Most outbreak detection systems are based on a statistical criterion, such as a prediction interval. A shortcoming of all such statistical mechanisms is their inability to differentiate between statistical significance and practical importance. For example, one or two isolations of a rare organism might constitute an unusual event in statistical terms but would not necessarily warrant further epidemiologic investigations unless the organism was highly pathogenic. In practice, the sensitivity of the system might be controlled primarily by the resources available for further investigations rather than by a requirement that every aberrant count be detected.

Controlling the false detection rate is perhaps more difficult, particularly when large numbers of organisms are processed or large numbers of locations are investigated. Because large-scale multiple testing is involved, the false positive detection rate is likely to be high. Also, because outbreak detection is in effect a sequential procedure, false detection rates are likely to exceed nominal type I error probabilities. Some adjustment to significance levels or prediction intervals is therefore in order, although it is probably best achieved informally. For example the detection system described in Example 4 uses thresholds defined by 99.5% prediction limits. The value of 99.5% was chosen so that a list of weekly potential outbreaks would fit comfortably on a single sheet of paper.

When the data include rare organisms, sporadic occurrences of the organisms are unusual, and will be detected if the system is working correctly. In most cases, sporadic reports or very low counts are of little interest. Thus the detection criterion should be strengthened by specifying that the current count exceed not only the threshold but also some fixed value. Such a criterion is used in the systems described in Examples 4 and 5. Further, the false detection rate should be broadly constant over the range of organism frequencies (see Example 4).

Evaluating an outbreak detection system is in itself a methodological challenge. Estimating the false detection rate is especially difficult because lack of external evidence that an identified excess is attributable to an outbreak does not necessarily establish that it is not an outbreak. Simulation studies can be used to evaluate the system's performance under controlled conditions, but these studies are unlikely to reflect the vagaries of surveillance data. Examples of quantitative investigations of the performance of different systems may be found in Stroup et al. (1993), Farrington et al. (1996), Hutwagner et al. (1997) and Stern and Lightfoot (1999).

Perception and Usage

The ultimate test of an outbreak detection system is whether it is perceived as useful by epidemiologists and other public health professionals. Unfortunately, the track record of computer-based, statistical methods of outbreak detection has been mixed, perhaps partly due to unrealistic expectations. Computer-based systems are widely used in hospitals to track nosocomial infections, but are no substitute for infection control staff who are in the best position to identify outbreaks (Birnbaum, 1987). Similarly, the most effective outbreak detection mechanism for community outbreaks is a network of epidemiologists and microbiologists who, through experience and knowledge of the community they serve, can rapidly recognise unusual increases in infections without resorting to more complex statistical methods. Sometimes the public themselves are involved, as has been reported for water-borne infections:

> It is our experience that the population frequently and rapidly contacts communal authorities for complaints of taste, smell or turbidity of drinking water and requests for quality control. Such enquiries could serve as an early warning system. Repeatedly, outbreaks were first recognised by astute lay persons or medical personnel, before routine run of algorithms through central databases.
>
> Maurer and Sturchler, 2000

In some settings, automated detection systems are unlikely to detect outbreaks more rapidly than workers in the field, but this is not universally the case. For example, Farrington et al. (1996) detailed a case study of an outbreak of *Salmonella agona* in the United Kingdom in 1995 that was repeatedly flagged by the national computer-based detection system several months before the outbreak was noticed by workers in the field. The real difficulty, we believe, lies at the next stage: setting up appropriate protocols for deciding which signals to investigate and which to ignore and for communicating effectively the role and limitations of automated systems. Such protocols are all the more necessary because overburdened epidemiologists may not welcome the suggestion that outbreaks are occurring on their patch when their only evidence is on a printout from a system with which they are only remotely familiar.

The statistician should not merely formulate the statistical models but should participate broadly in implementing of the system, and developing appropriate outputs and procedures for determining whether an apparently aberrant count is genuine and worthy of further investigation. Appropriate tasks might include providing enhanced graphical output, additional analyses, and feedback to reporting sites.

Computer-based outbreak detection systems should complement more traditional methods but not replace them. Such systems can add value to a surveillance program in three areas. First, a computer-assisted detection system can act as a safety net that routinely scans reports and identifies problems that may have been overlooked. This function is particularly important for collecting data on large numbers of infections that cannot be processed manually. Second, the system may detect national outbreaks that escape local detection because they do not give rise to substantial local increases in cases. Third, computer-based procedures can bring about improvements in surveillance data collection.

FUTURE DIRECTIONS

Improvements in computerized data collection, such as availability of accurate spatial information, and efficient computer-intensive statistical techniques, are likely to transform the field of outbreak detection. Data-mining techniques, neural networks (Black, 2002) and Markov Chain Monte Carlo methods are obvious contenders; such methods are discussed further in Chapter 9.

Nevertheless, statisticians will still have to grapple with problems of reporting delays, incomplete data, and high false detection rates. The single greatest challenge and most pressing requirement in automated outbreak detection is to improve the decision tools required to translate signals into actions. Such progress requires a broad conception of the role of the statistician. A possible avenue is to improve interactive data presentation, through, for example, dynamic temporal or spatial temporal presentation of emerging surveillance data, as prefigured by the work of Carrat and Valleron (1992).

Finally, the scope of detection systems is likely to expand beyond single countries to encompass regions and continents. Diseases, after all, do not respect national boundaries. Coordinated multinational surveillance systems are increasing in use, particularly throughout the European Union (Fisher et al., 1994), and are likely to become more important. Extensions of national early warning systems for use in multinational settings are therefore required.

REFERENCES

Altman, D.G. (1999). *Practical Statistics for Medical Research*. London: Chapman & Hall/CRC Press.

Barbujani, G. (1987). A review of statistical methods for continuous monitoring of malformation frequencies. *European Journal of Epidemiology* **3,** 67–77.

Birnbaum, D. (1984). Analysis of hospital surveillance data. *Infection Control* **5,** 332–338.

Birnbaum, D. (1987). Nosocomial infection surveillance programs. *Infection Control* **8,** 474–479.

Black, J. (2002). Applications of artificial neural networks in epidemiology: prediction and classification. PhD Thesis. Monash University, Victoria, Australia.

Brookmeyer, R. and Gail, M.H. (1994). *AIDS Epidemiology: A Quantitative Approach.* New York: Oxford University Press.

Carrat, F. and Valleron, A.-J. (1992). Epidemiologic mapping using the "kriging" method: Application to an influenza-like illness epidemic in France. *American Journal of Epidemiology* **135,** 1293–1300.

Centers for Disease Control and Prevention (2000). Guidelines for confirmation of foodborne disease outbreaks. *Morbidity and Mortality Weekly Report* **49** (SS01), 54–62.

Chen, R. (1978). A surveillance system for congenital malformations. *Journal of the American Statistical Association* **73,** 323–327.

Chen, R., Connelly, R.R., and Mantel, N. (1993). Analysing post-alarm data in a monitoring system in order to accept or reject the alert. *Statistics in Medicine* **12,** 1807–1812.

Choi, K. and Thacker, S.B. (1981). An evaluation of influenza mortality surveillance, 1962–1979. 1: Time series forecasts of expected pneumonia and influenza deaths. *American Journal of Epidemiology* **113,** 215–226.

Costagliola, D., Flahault, A., Galinec, D., Gamerin, P., Menares, J., and Valleron, A.-J. (1991). A routine tool for detection and assessment of epidemics of influenza-like syndromes in France. *American Journal of Public Health* **81,** 97–99.

Costagliola, D. (1994). When is the epidemic warning cut-off point exceeded? *European Journal of Epidemiology* **10,** 475–476.

Davison, A.C. and Snell, E.J. (1991). Residuals and diagnostics. In Hinkley, D.V., Reid, N., and Snell, E.J., eds. *Statistical Theory and Modelling.* London: Chapman and Hall.

Farrington, C.P., Andrews, N.J., Beale, A.D., and Catchpole, M.A. (1996). A statistical algorithm for the early detection of outbreaks of infectious disease. *Journal of the Royal Statistical Society, Series A* **159,** 547–563.

Fisher, I.S.T., Rowe, B., Bartlett, C.L.R., and Gill, O.N. (1994). Salm-net: Laboratory-based surveillance of human salmonella infections in Europe. *PHLS Microbiology Digest* **11,** 181–182.

Flahault, A., Garnerin, P., Chauvin, P., Farran, N., Saidi, Y., Diaz, C., and Toubiana, J. (1995). Sentinelle traces of an epidemic of acute gastroenteritis in France. *Lancet* **346,** 162–163.

Healy, M.J.R. (1983). A simple method for monitoring routine statistics. *The Statistician* **32,** 347–349.

Hutwagner, L.C., Maloney, E.K., Bean, N.H., Slutsker, L., and Martin, S.M. (1997). Using laboratory-based surveillance data for prevention: an algorithm for detecting salmonella outbreaks. *Emerging Infectious Diseases* **3,** 395–400.

Kafadar, K. and Stroup, D.F. (1992). Analysis of aberrations in public health surveillance data: estimating variances on correlated samples. *Statistics in Medicine* **11,** 1551–1568.

Knox, E.G. (1964). The detection of space-time interactions. *Applied Statistics* **13,** 25–29.

Kulldorff, M. (2001). Prospective time periodic geographical disease surveillance using a scan statistic. *Journal of the Royal Statistical Society, Series A* **164**, 61–72.

Lucas, J.M. (1985). Counted data CUSUMs. *Technometrics* **27**, 129–144.

Mantel, N. (1967). The detection of disease clustering and a generalised regression approach. *Cancer Research* **27**, 209–220.

Maurer, A.M. and Sturchler, D. (2000). A waterborne outbreak of small round structured virusw, campylobacter and shigella co-infections in La Neuville, Switzerland, 1998. *Epidemiology and Infection* **125**, 325–332.

Ngo, L., Tager, I.B., and Hadley, D. (1996). Application of exponential smoothing for nosocomial infection surveillance. *American Journal of Epidemiology* **143**, 637–647.

Nobre, F.F. and Stroup, D. (1994). A monitoring system to detect changes in public health surveillance data. *International Journal of Epidemiology* **23**, 408–418.

Page, E.S. (1954). Continuous inspection schemes. *Biometrika* **41**, 100–115.

Parker, R.A. (1989). Analysis of surveillance data with poisson regression: a case study. *Statistics in Medicine* **8**, 285–294.

Parkhurst, S.M., Blaser, M.J., Laxson, L.B., and Wang, W.-L.L. (1985). Surveillance for the detection of nosocomial infections and the potential for nosocomial outbreaks. *American Journal of Infection Control,* **13**, 7–15.

Raubertas, R.F. (1989). An analysis of disease surveillance data that uses the geographic locations of the reporting units. *Statistics in Medicine* **8**, 267–271.

Rogerson, P.A. (1997). Surveillance systems for monitoring the development of spatial patterns. *Statistics in Medicine* **16**, 2081–2093.

Rogerson, P.A. (2001). Monitoring point patterns for the development of space-time clusters. *Journal of the Royal Statistical Society, Series A* **164**, 87–96.

Serfling, R.E. (1963). Methods for current statistical analysis of excess pneumonia-influenza deaths. *Public Health Reports* **78**, 494–506.

Shore, D.L. and Quade, D. (1989). A surveillance system based on a short memory scheme. *Statistics in Medicine* **8**, 311–322.

Stern, L. and Lightfoot, D. (1999). Automated outbreak detection: a quantitative retrospective analysis. *Epidemiology and Infection* **122**, 103–110.

Stroup, D.F., Williamson, G.D., Herndon, J.L., and Karon, J.M. (1989). Detection of aberrations in the occurrence of notifiable diseases surveillance data. *Statistics in Medicine* **8**, 323–329.

Stroup, D.F., Wharton, M., Kafadar, K., and Dean, A.G. (1993). Evaluation of a method for detecting aberrations in public health surveillance data. *American Journal of Epidemiology* **137**, 373–380.

Tango, T. (1984). The detection of disease clustering in time. *Biometrics* **40**, 15–26.

Tillett, H.E. and Spencer, I.-L. (1982). Influenza surveillance in England and Wales using routine statistics. *Journal of Hygiene Cambridge* **88**, 83–94.

Wallenstein, S. (1980). A test for detection of clustering over time. *American Journal of Epidemiology* **111**, 367–372.

Wallenstein, S., Gould, M., and Kleinman, M. (1989). Use of the scan statistic to detect time-space clustering. *American Journal of Epidemiology* **130**, 1057–1064.

Watier, L., Richardson, S., and Hubert, B. (1991). A time series construction of an alert threshold with application to *S. bovismorbificans* in France. *Statistics in Medicine* **10**, 1493–1509.

Wetherill, G.W. and Brown, D.W. (1991). *Statistical Process Control: Theory and Practice*. London: Chapman and Hall.

9

On-line Monitoring of Public Health Surveillance Data

PETER DIGGLE, LEO KNORR-HELD,
BARRY ROWLINGSON, TING-LI SU,
PETER HAWTIN, TREVOR N. BRYANT

The Ascertainment and Enhancement of Gastrointestinal Infection Surveillance and Statistics (AEGISS) project aims to use spatial statistical methods to identify anomalies in the space–time distribution of nonspecific, gastrointestinal infections in the United Kingdom, using the Southampton area in southern England as a test case. Health-care providers are asked to report incident cases daily. Regionwide incident data are then sent electronically to Lancaster, where a statistical analysis of the space–time distribution of incident cases is updated. The results are then posted to a Web site with tabular, graphical and map-based summaries of the analysis.

Here we use the AEGISS project to discuss the methodologic issues in developing a rapid-response, spatial surveillance system. We consider simple, exploratory statistical methods together with more sophisticated methods, based on hierarchical space–time stochastic process models defined either at individual or small-area levels. The chapter is a report of work in progress. Currently, the Web-based AEGISS reporting system uses only simple summaries of the incident data, but its ultimate aim is to display the results of formal predictive inference in a hierarchical model of space–time variation in disease risk.

PROBLEMS OF COLLECTING DATA FOR SURVEILLANCE

Routine surveillance requires a compromise between the sensitivity and specificity of detection and the quality of data derived from daily routine clinical activity. Currently, the poor quality of routinely collected surveillance data on gastroenteric outbreaks severely limits the spatial resolution and speed of detection.

Several factors hinder the routine collection of surveillance data in clinical practice. The focus on treating patients' immediate clinical needs can override efforts to maintain the overall health of the community and to prevent communicable disease. Self-limiting and only occasionally dangerous diseases do not receive priority over diseases with a lower incidence but with greater morbidity and mortality. Providers may find that supplying data for surveillance is a burden, particularly if they do not use the information and reap no immediate benefits from it, such as health gains or financial support.

These problems may be more prevalent in surveillance of food- and waterborne disease than in surveillance of other diseases. A further problem is that, even though a case definition of gastroenteric disease has been adopted ("any disease of an infectious or toxic nature caused by, or thought to be caused by, the consumption of food or water" [Joint FAO/WHO Expert Committee on Food Safety, 1984]), defining cases may be difficult because a wide range of organisms and other agents can cause gastroenteric symptoms. The public is usually only aware of the threat of gastroenteric disease after an outbreak, yet food poisoning is a major health and economic burden and occasionally can cause severe morbidity and some mortality.

Current surveillance of gastroenteric disease in the United Kingdom relies on general practitioners reporting cases of suspected food poisoning through a statutory notification scheme, voluntary laboratory reports of the isolation of gastrointestinal pathogens and standard reports of general outbreaks of infectious intestinal disease by public health and environmental health authorities. However, statutory notification is not widely practiced and surveillance relies heavily on laboratory reports and reports of local outbreaks. Most statutory notifications are made only after a laboratory reports that a gastrointestinal pathogen has been isolated. As a result, detection is delayed and the ability to react to an emerging outbreak is reduced.

Effective intervention for an outbreak of gastroenteric disease depends on collecting accurate and timely information. For example, clinical management of simple diarrhea consists of advice on symptom relief and fluid replacement, and a return visit is recommended if symptoms persist longer than a few days. Considerable time can elapse between onset of symptoms and testing of a fecal sample taken on a return visit to investigate persisting symptoms. Because of this delay, and because samples are tested for only the most common pathogens, tests of most samples reveal no pathogens, and no further epidemiological investigation is conducted. Furthermore, because a pathogen may not be identified until 2 weeks of more after the onset of symptoms the patient may have limited recall of exposure to risk factors, particularly factors related to food. In a reporting pyramid for all infectious intestinal disease, just one in every 136 cases in the community is estimated to reach national surveillance (Food Standards Agency, 2000). Consequently, patients with mild diarrhea who become infected from a common source may be lost to surveillance, hindering early detection of a point source outbreak. In exceptional cases of severe symptoms, such as blood in the stool or severe dehydration, or in explosive outbreaks in a community, a fecal sample is collected promptly. However, the attitude of individual clinicians towards fecal sample collection in routine cases varies widely; a sixfold difference in sampling rates has been observed among general practitioners within a single medical center (Turner, 2000). This variability greatly distorts the already sparse spatial and temporal information reaching public health authorities.

Changes in access to health care have caused even fewer cases of food- and waterborne disease to be ascertained by public health authorities. For example, telephone consultations with a nurse or physical examinations at walk-in medical centers are given with increasing frequency but are not included in any surveillance scheme.

In summary, the present system of food- and waterborne disease surveillance in the United Kingdom is a highly specific, pathogen numerator-based system but is insensitive and overly retrospective. It is effective for detecting cases related to particular pathogens and their individual subtypes (e.g., *salmonella PT4* in eggs), but is limited largely to population-level trend analysis. Thus, either outbreaks must reach high levels or must be sufficiently unusual and persistent to be identified against "background noise."

ASCERTAINMENT AND ENHANCEMENT OF GASTROINTESTINAL INFECTION SURVEILLANCE AND STATISTICS

The aim of the AEGISS project is to improve the quality, spatial resolution, and timeliness of case ascertainment for food- and waterborne disease so that real-time spatial temporal statistical techniques can be applied. These techniques will improve intervention and prevention activities, and will reduce the burden of gastrointestinal disease in local communities. Key issues are whether the analysis of most minor cases can be used to identify point sources or other risk factors before these cases become contaminated with serious pathogens, and whether spatial statistical analysis can identify outbreaks from a point source contaminated with mixed pathogens.

The benefits of applying spatial temporal statistical analysis to all cases of nonspecific gastroenteric symptoms could be substantial. By collecting a minimum data set on every case of acute onset of gastroenteric symptoms, the AEGISS project aims to avoid the variation found in current sampling and reporting. However, this approach lacks diagnostic specificity. Associating microbiologic results from routinely collected fecal samples with the output from spatial temporal statistical analyses would provide specificity. Further diagnostic specificity could be obtained by analyzing a risk factor questionnaire administered during the patient's first visit, to enhance recall. Combining all three approaches would allow high sensitivity to be matched with enhanced specificity. The remainder of the chapter focuses on the first approach—the use of spatial temporal statistical analyses for early detection of unexplained variation in the spatial temporal incidence of nonspecific gastroenteric symptoms.

Recent developments in information technology support the AEGISS project. A private secure network (National Health Service Network) enables primary care physicians within the United Kingdom to receive and transmit health data, whereas commercial clinical systems allow surveillance data to be captured and forwarded. These systems help clinicians to report complete data by prompting for additional information when a notifiable disease code is entered in the patient's electronic health record during a consultation. Much of the patient information is already in digital form, and the clinician records only the date of onset of symptoms and travel history. These data can be transmitted instantaneously to the surveillance database, leading to virtually real-time epidemiology. Data from patient risk factor questionnaires can be entered using scanning technology to allow immediate analysis. Fecal microbiology reports from collaborating laboratories are also received by the health network and are merged to form a common dataset. The data set allows reports of pathogens that have been isolated and identified to be compared among laboratories daily and the spatial and temporal distribution of all gastrointestinal pathogens in a population to be monitored. Finally, linking the three data sources— clinician reports of patient contact, patient risk factor questionnaires and routine fecal microbiology reports—will produce sufficiently timely surveillance to maximize opportunities for intervention, prevention and education in controlling gastrointestinal infection. A key feature of the AEGISS project is the feedback to the primary care system through Web-based reporting, which will provide general practitioners with a contemporary picture of the prevalence and incidence of gastrointestinal disease in their local areas.

STATISTICAL FORMULATION

Problem Definition

For the spatial temporal statistical analysis in the AEGISS project, a *case* is any reported case of acute gastroenteric symptoms, indexed by date of onset and residential location. The primary statistical objectives of the analysis are to estimate the risk, $\rho(x,t)$ say, that at time t an individual living at location x will report symptoms of nonspecific gastrointestinal infection, and to identify quickly any anomalous variations in this space–time risk surface. We estimate risk through a multiplicative decomposition of the space–time intensity of incident cases, with separate terms for the spatial intensity of the population at risk (assumed to be constant over time), known spatially or temporally varying risk factors available as covariate information, and residual space–time variation, which we regard as anomalous. Details of our modelling strategies are given in later sections.

Any anomalies identified by the analysis would become subject to follow-up investigations, including microbiologic analysis. In principle, and as reflected in the notation $\rho(x,t)$ for risk, we would wish to treat the underlying disease process as spatially and temporally continuous. However, in practice the limitations of the available data may force us to work at a spatially aggregated level, a temporally aggregated level, or both. In particular, spatial aggregation could be effected in at least two ways: by recording counts in a set of discrete subareas to partition the study area, or by using a general practice (GP) as the basic unit for data analysis.

Data Sources and Limitations

Incident cases

The primary source of data for the AEGISS project is the daily reporting by GPs of nonspecific incident cases, identified by the unit post code of the patient's residence, the date of symptom onset, and an indication of whether or not the patient has recently traveled outside the area. For the analyses in this chapter, only cases resident in the study area and diagnosed between August 1, 2001 and February 28, 2002 are considered (Fig. 9–1). The study area consists of most of the county of Hampshire, the southern half of Wiltshire and a small part of West Sussex. It contains a mix of urban and rural subareas, with a total population of approximately 1.3 million.

A limitation of the data is that participation in the project is voluntary. At the time of writing, 106 practices are included in the accumulating data base, but only 99 have reported cases during the study period, and not all of these can be guaranteed to have reported all relevant cases.

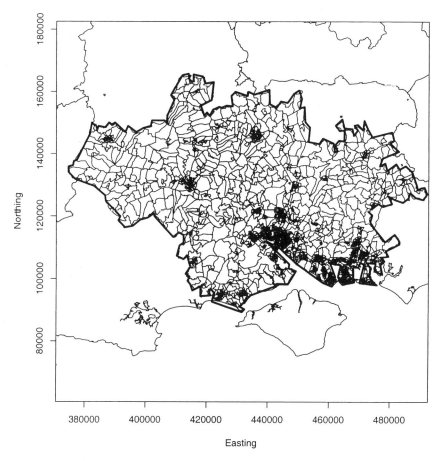

Figure 9–1 The study area for general practice–reported data. Boundaries within the study area identify census enumeration districts (EDs).

Incompleteness of reporting is a major obstacle to effective surveillance, and efforts to engage the remaining practices in the study region are continuing. Inconsistencies in reporting rates between GPs, or by particular GPs at different times, would also lead to spurious patterns of variation. As discussed in Point Process Models and Discrete Spatial Models, below, time-constant variations in reporting rates between GPs can be handled by incorporating GP effects into the statistical model for the risk surface, but time-varying individual reporting rates would inevitably be confounded with the variation in the underlying disease, which is our inferential focus. Consistency of reporting behavior over time is therefore paramount if the full potential of any surveillance system is to be realized.

A further limitation of the data is the delay between onset and reporting of symptoms. We see that approximately 60% of all cases reported between August 1, 2001 and February 28, 2002 are reported within 7 days of onset of symptoms, and approximately 80% within 14 days (Fig. 9–2).

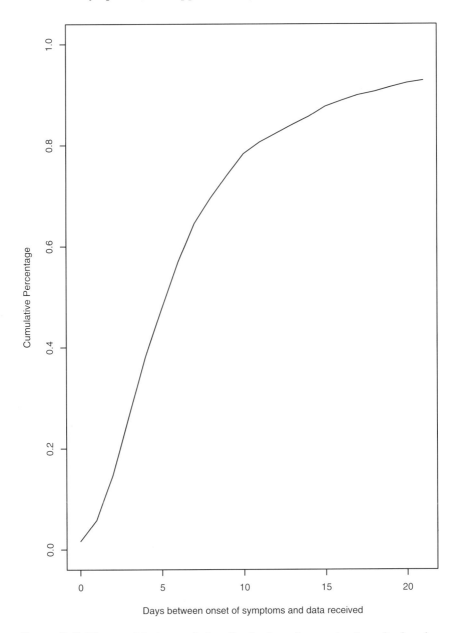

Figure 9–2 The empirical cumulative distribution of reporting lags, in days between onset of symptoms and reporting of the case to the database.

Our current on-line implementation uses date of symptom onset as the relevant date for each case but builds in a 7-day reporting lag to trap most cases for the day in question. More prompt reporting would add value to the surveillance system but is limited by the behavior of individual patients and by delays in their securing GP appointments. Hence, the choice of reporting lag involves an uneasy compromise between the conflicting requirements of timeliness and completeness.

A secondary source of data for the project is NHS Direct, a 24-hour phone-in clinical advice service. A potential advantage of the NHS Direct data over the GP data is that they are less likely to suffer from localized inconsistencies in reporting rates over time. Also, reporting delays are likely to be shorter. On the other hand, the overall pattern of use of this relatively new service may not yet have stabilized.

Integrating the NHS Direct data with the GP-reported data creates difficulties. One problem is that, in many cases, an inquiry to NHS Direct results in the inquirer being advised to see their GP, but the data available do not identify the resulting duplication of cases. A second difficulty is that NHS Direct data are indexed by date of reporting, rather than by date of symptom onset. Also, these data do not include an indicator for recent foreign travel.

The NHS Direct data analyzed in Point Process Models, below cover the entire county of Hampshire and include a total of 3374 cases reported between August 1, 2000 and August 26, 2001 (Fig. 9–3). Each case identifies the date and residential location of any inquiry relating to gastroenteric symptoms.

Population at risk

Estimates of the population at risk, also called denominators, are required for converting incidence data to risk estimates. These estimates can be obtained in different ways, according to the required spatial resolution. We consider three options.

First, for modeling small-area variations in risk, data on the underlying population are available from the national census. These data include population counts in 5-year age-bands at the level of Census Enumeration Districts (EDs), each of which has an average size close to 200 households or 450 people. In the exploratory analysis of the GP data reported in Exploratory Analysis of the General Practice–Reported Data, below we used ED-level data from the 1991 census, because the 2001 census data were not yet available. The study area consists of 2894 EDs with a mean population of 463 (range, 48 to 1145). For analyses at the ED-level, census counts can be used directly to calculate area-level denominators. Enumeration Districts represent the smallest aggregation units widely used in the United

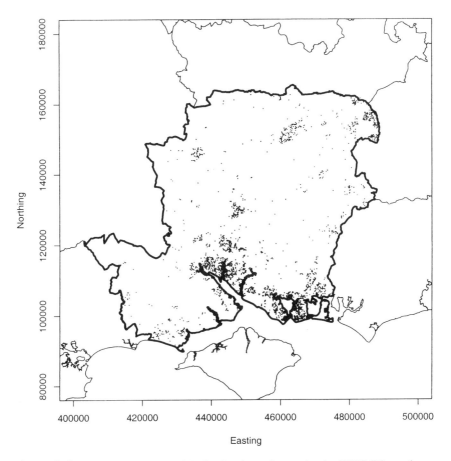

Figure 9–3 Study-area and spatial distribution of cases in the NHS Direct data.

Kingdom. Larger aggregation units include local authority wards or counties (Hampshire, Wiltshire, and West Sussex are separate counties). However, in the current context, in which we aim to detect local variations in disease risk, we would ideally work at the finest spatial resolution consistent with the resolution of the available data. In this connection, Best et al. (2000) describe one way to combine information at disparate spatial scales; for example, individual-level case information together with area-level denominators.

A second option is to use GPs as the basic units for data analysis. In this case, the corresponding population sizes are the known capitation figures for each GP. Finally, for individual-level models, a spatially continuous population density surface, $\lambda_0(x)$, must be specified. Census ED counts and corresponding ED areas could be used to calculate a piecewise constant approximation to $\lambda_0(x)$, possibly in conjunction with some smoothing to alleviate the discontinuities at ED boundaries. Alternatively, denominator information for individual-level analyses may be constructed by using historical incident case data from time periods that are known, with hindsight, to include no recognized major outbreaks. This information could then be used to construct a pseudopopulation distribution at the individual level, by applying a nonparametric smoother to the raw point distribution. The second approach would be the more natural for analyzing the NHS Direct data, because the level of usage of this service may not be uniform across the whole population. Hence, the use of census population counts could be misleading.

Temporal and Spatial Resolution

Each case is indexed by the date of onset of acute gastroenteric symptoms. Hence, time is necessarily treated discretely, although a 1-day resolution is sufficiently fine to be treated as effectively continuous. As described below, the area-level and the GP-based models in effect treat the spatial dimension as a discrete set of locations (EDs or individual general practices, respectively), whereas individual-level models treat space as a continuum. Implementing discrete spatial models, which are known as *Markov random fields*, requires the user to define neighborhood relationships between different spatial units. In a Markov random field model, observed or latent random variables, S_i say, are attached to each spatial unit i. The key assumption is that the conditional distribution of S_i, given all other S_j, depends only on those S_j for which unit j is a neighbor of unit i. Also, the neighborhood relationship must be symmetrical. In area-based models, the conventional approach is to treat as neighbors any two area units that share a common boundary. However, this treatment is questionable when the area units are EDs, which vary enormously in size between urban and rural areas. A possible refinement would be to introduce additional weights for each pair of contiguous spatial units; for example, based on the length of the common boundary or on the inverse distance between the centroids of the units.

In the current application, a GP-based approach is arguably more natural than an area-based approach because the GPs are the reporting units for the incident cases. Also, a GP-based approach may be more practical in the sense that follow-up of identified anomalies in GP reporting rates will be administratively easier than follow-up based on a set of residential locations. On the other hand, the definition of neighborhoods for GPs remains problematic, not least because the effective catchments of different GPs in urban areas overlap spatially.

Individual-level models apparently avoid the arbitrary division of space into discrete units. However, each unit post-code in the United Kingdom is associated with a point location x, which corresponds notionally to the centroid of the area covered by that post code. In urban areas, a unit post code typically covers a single street, or even a single multioccupancy building, and the treatment of post codes as point locations is not an unreasonable approximation. In rural areas, treating post codes as point locations, although standard practice, is more questionable because a unit post code may cover a substantial area.

The implicit assumption in all of the above discussion is that, at least in the short term, the population at risk is stable over time. However, this assumption does not preclude incorporating time variation in the natural incidence pattern through covariate adjustments. In particular, the overall incidence pattern exhibits seasonal variation and day-of-the-week effects, which should be included in any parametric model of spatial temporal variation.

Hierarchical Space–Time Stochastic Models

All of our models for space–time variation in risk can be described as hierarchical, in the sense that they combine a model for a latent stochastic process, representing the unexplained space–time variation in disease risk, with a model for the observed data conditional on this latent process. For Bayesian inference, we would add a third layer to the hierarchy, consisting of a prior distributional specification for the model parameters. In Bayesian terminology, the latent process is sometimes referred to as a parameter, and a model parameter as a hyperparameter. Whether or not we adopt the Bayesian viewpoint, the important difference between the two sets of unknowns is that model (or hyper) parameters are intended to describe global properties of the formulation, whereas the latent stochastic process describes local features.

If large amounts of data are available, specifying the hyperprior for Bayesian inference is not very important in the current application given the correctness of the model. The reason is that our goal is inference for the unobserved risk surface, uncertainty in which reflects the number and pattern of recent incident cases, whereas estimation of global model parameters can be based on abundant historical data over a much longer period. It follows that prediction error will dominate estimation error, and predictive inferences will therefore be relatively insensitive to the choice of a prior.

We consider two qualitatively different classes of hierarchical models, corresponding to the choice between the use of spatially aggregated data and individual-level data. For individual-level data, we formulate our models as Cox (1955) point processes, in which a latent stochastic process $S(x,t)$ defines the intensity of an inhomogeneous Poisson process model for the cases. For area-level data, we use discrete spatial models in which latent variables, S_{it}, are attached either to spatial subareas or to individual GPs as the discrete spatial units, $i = 1, \ldots, I$, for analysis, and unit-level numbers of cases are modeled as binomial or Poisson counts conditional on S_{it}. The point process approach is a natural first choice for the NHS Direct data, whereas Markov random field modeling, using GPs as the spatial units, seems more natural for the GP-reported data. However, spatially discrete GP effects may also be incorporated into area-based or point process models. In Point Process Models and Discrete Spatial Models, below, we consider the two modeling approaches, in each case giving an illustrative analysis of data from the AEGISS project. However, we emphasize that these analyses represent work in progress and are not definitive.

EXPLORATORY ANALYSIS OF THE GENERAL-PRACTICE–REPORTED DATA

In this section, an exploratory analysis of GP-reported incident cases over the period August 1, 2001 to February 28, 2002 is described. The analysis is conducted at the ED level. Let y_{it} denote the number of incident cases on day t resident in the i-th ED and n_i the corresponding number of people resident in the i-th ED, as determined by the 1991 census.

Temporal Trends

The total number of incident cases over the period in question, and resident within the study area is 2624, a mean of 12.4 cases per day. A simple estimate of the whole-area risk per 100,000 people on day t is $R(t) = 100,000 \sum_i y_{it}/\sum_i n_i$. However, at current reporting levels, a time-plot of $R(t)$ is extremely noisy. Smoother estimates are produced by averaging over a k-day time-window; hence,

$$R_k(t) = 100,000 \sum_i \left(\sum_{u=0}^{k-1} y_{i,t-u}/k \right) / \sum_i n_i \qquad (9\text{--}1)$$

The estimate $R_{14}(t)$ shows some (long-term) seasonal variation, a known feature of gastroenteric infections that would have been more evident had a full year's data been available (Fig. 9–4).

The data also show a clear day-of-the-week effect. The raw numbers of cases reporting onset of symptoms on each day of the week (Sunday to Saturday) are: 416, 467, 358, 351, 314, 377, and 341. The highest numbers are on Sunday and Monday (the weekend effect).

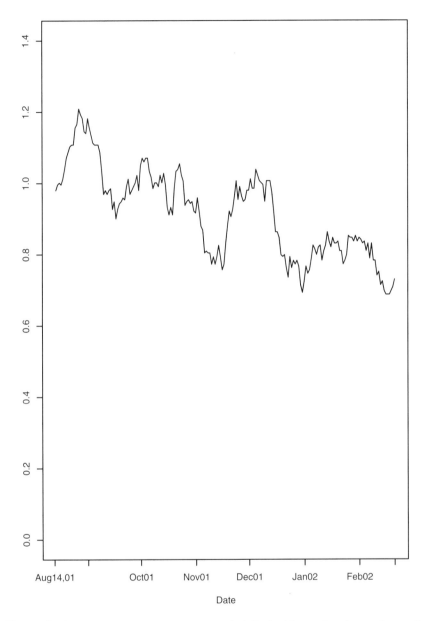

Figure 9–4 Smoothed estimates, $R_{14}(t)$, of daily incidence for the entire study region.

Spatial Variation

To display spatial variation in estimated risk, we apply a similarly ad hoc smoothing method. We define the *m-neighbors* of the *i-th* ED as the set, N_i, consisting of the *m* EDs with centroids closest to the centroid of the *i-th* ED. The smoothed estimate of risk per 100,000 people in the *i-th* ED at time *t* is

$$R_{m,k}\,(i,t) = 100,000 \sum_{u=0}^{k-1} \sum_{N_i} y_{i,t-u} \Big/ \left(k \sum_{N_i} n_i\right) \qquad (9\text{–}2)$$

Estimates $R_{18,14}(i, t)$ for two Saturdays in February 2002, separated by 14 days, are shown in Figure 9–5. The maps are restricted to the north east

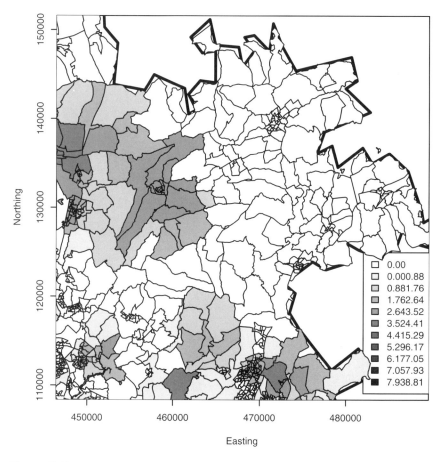

Figure 9–5 Smoothed estimates, $R_{18,14}(i,t)$, of ED-level risk for two Saturdays in February 2002.

portion of the study area, because many of the EDs in the more densely populated parts of the study region are too small to be visible as shaded polygons on the printed page. The Web-based reporting system for the project allows the user to zoom in on subregions of particular interest.

Although these static displays are of limited use, they become more interesting when run in real time or, for retrospective analysis, as a time-lapse film. More sophisticated smoothing methods, including covariate adjustment, could be applied by using a space–time generalized additive model (Hastie and Tibshirani, 1990; Kelsall and Diggle, 1998). However, our view is that nonparametric smoothing methods require a higher rate of occurrence of cases than applies in the AEGISS project and that a parametric modeling approach will be more effective. In particular, the very wide vari-

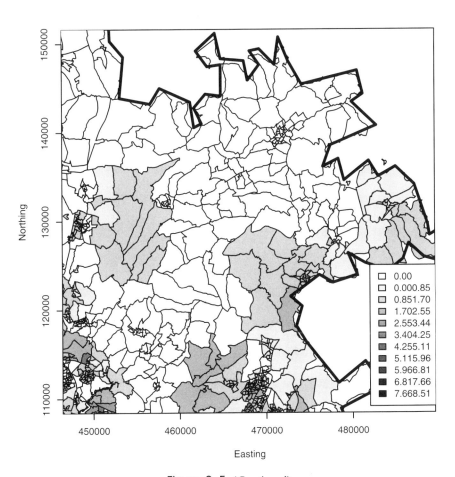

Figure 9–5 (*Continued*).

ation in the ED-level risk estimates reflects the sparseness of the data at this level (Fig. 9–5). For surveillance of more common diseases, or in applications where fine spatial and temporal resolution is considered less important, nonparametric approaches may be more effective.

Web-Based Reporting

An integral part of the AEGISS project is to develop a Web-based reporting system in which analyses are updated whenever new incident data are obtained. The results are posted to a Web page giving a combination of numerical and graphical summaries.

Every working day, the GP-reported data are sent by e-mail from Southampton to Lancaster. The data file is sent as an encrypted, compressed attachment for security and speed. When the message arrives, it is automatically decrypted and decompressed, and the data are stored in a PostgreSQL data base (http://www.postgresql.org/) table. This data base table is the point of access to the data for local researchers and the Web-based reporting system, ensuring that everyone has the latest data.

Another daily task, scheduled to occur after the data arrive, runs statistical analyses and updates files that are required for the Web-based presentation. The task involves generating HTML code for tables to be displayed on the Web site, producing a graphic image for the time series plot, and creating data files for the embedded mapping application. The actual analyses of the data are carried out using C programs with an interface to the R system (http://www.r-project.org/).

The machine that performs all of these tasks is a standard PC with dual Pentium III 933MHz processors, 512Mb of memory, and 30Gb of disk storage. It runs the RedHat (http://www.redhat.com/) distribution of the GNU/Linux (http://www.linux.org/) operating system, and the Apache web server (http://www.apache.org). This combination of hardware and software enables us to build a flexible, programmable web site using off-the-shelf hardware and free software. Access to the web page is restricted by a username–password pair. An initial request for pages in the system causes the user's browser to ask for a username and password before the page is returned.

At the time of writing, the Web updating process applies simple exploratory methods to the GP-reported data. In due course, the results of hierarchical model-based analyses at individual level, the small-area level, and GP level or any combination of these will be added. A screen-dump of the current implementation, which divides the page into three sections, is shown in Figure 9–6.

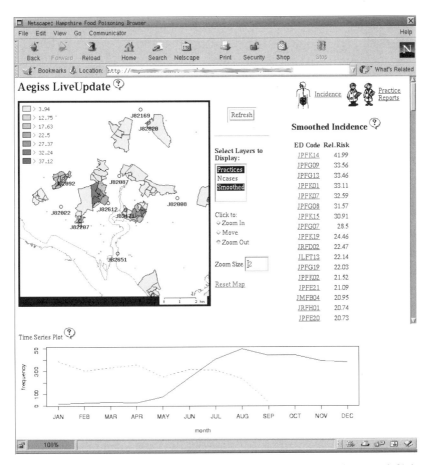

Figure 9–6 A screen-dump of the AEGISS Web-page. The mapping section (top left) is created by the MapServer (http://mapserver.gis.umn.edu/) application from a configuration file, some web page templates, and several data sets. These data sets are created for the current analysis during the daily update step from the primary care reporting database. The MapServer application displays the results as shaded polygons, based on the exploratory spatial analysis at the ED level, as described in the text. A color extends from white (and hence invisible) indicating negligible estimated risk, to red, indicating high relative risk areas (top left corner of the map). The user can zoom in on and move over the study area. The "layers" selection box allows the user to add data layers or remove them from the map; for example, a layer can be added that displays GP locations or the actual case locations plotted by post-code. In due course, additional layers of spatial predictions derived from the point process or discrete spatial modeling approaches will be added. A table (right-side) gives direct access to individual ED risk estimates or GP information. It displays either a list of EDs sorted by decreasing relative risk or a list of GP identifiers sorted by decreasing number of reported cases. Clicking on an ED or GP in this list zooms the map to that point. A time-trend graph (bottom), showing the number of cases reported in time, is based on a full calendar year display, using 2001 and 2002 as previous and current years. The data from 2001 are represented by a black line, and data from 2002 by a red line. The rising trend during 2001 reflects progressive recruitment of GPs to the project during that year, rather than a genuine underlying trend in disease incidence. On each web page section a small "Help" icon pops up a short summary of the information displayed in that section. On this web page, the user has zoomed in on part of Southampton and has activated the "Smoothed" layer, to display the current relative risk map, and the "Practices" layer, to show the GP locations. GP locations that have submitted cases contributing to the current risk estimates are shown as blue circles with "J-number" labels; other GP locations are shown as small blue dots.

POINT PROCESS MODELS

Model Formulation

Our point process model assumes that cases form an inhomogeneous Poisson point process with intensity $\lambda(x,t)$ which we express as

$$\lambda(x,\ t) = \lambda_0(x,\ t)\rho(x,t) \qquad (9\text{--}3)$$

In Eq. 9–3, $\lambda_0(x,t)$ represents the space–time intensity of the population at risk, which in practice may be assumed to be time-constant. The risk surface, $\rho(x,t)$, may exhibit space–time variations for either or both of two reasons: natural variation from known causes (e.g., spatial variation in the local age-profile of the population, or long-term seasonal or day-of-the-week effects) and anomalous variation representing outbreaks. Our objective is to identify the latter while allowing for the former. To achieve this aim, we further decompose $\rho(x,t)$ into

$$\rho(x,t) = \exp\{d(x,t)'\beta + S(x,t)\} \qquad (9\text{--}4)$$

where $d(x,t)$ denotes a vector of known, measured risk factors, β is the associated vector of regression parameters and $S(x,t)$ represents anomalous variation in risk. The elements of $d(x,t)$ may be of two distinct kinds: inherent properties of location, x, or time, t; and properties of the individual patient resident at location x who presents at time t. The distinction may be important in practice, even if both can be subsumed in the same formal model. For example, we may choose to absorb effects of the first kind into the specification of $\lambda_0(x,t)$, based on contextual knowledge.

   At first sight, the Poisson process assumption is questionable as a model for infectious diseases. However, because of the duality between clustering and heterogeneity of risk (Bartlett, 1964), a sufficiently flexible inhomogeneous Poisson model can describe clustered patterns of incidence empirically by ascribing local spatial temporal concentrations of cases to peaks in the risk surface $\rho(x,t)$. Also, it is arguable whether a patient's residential address is the most relevant spatial reference point for exposure to disease risk.

   Given the model specification, the formal solution of the surveillance problem is to develop a predictive inference for the space–time surface $S(x,t)$. The output from the model would then be a continuously updated map of the relevant predictive probabilities. For example, to monitor departures from a known, constant level of risk, an appropriate quantity to map would be $P\{S(x,t) > c|\text{data up to time } t\}$, where c is an agreed threshold level at which intervention by public health authorities would be considered appropriate. This quantity is identifiable because $\lambda_0(x,t)$ is either known or can be estimated independently of the data on incident cases. Another possibility would be to monitor changes in the risk surface, in which case quantities of the form $P\{S(x,t) - S(x,t - u) > c|\text{data up to}$ time $t\}$ should be mapped for an agreed threshold level c and time lag u. If the population at risk can be assumed to be constant over a time period of up to k days, then for all (x,t) and any $u \leq k$, $\lambda_0(x,t) = \lambda_0(x,t - u)$ and under the model in Eq. 9–3,

$$\lambda(x,t)/\lambda(x,t - u) = \rho(x,t)/\rho(x,t - u)$$

Hence, changes in risk can be monitored by changes in incidence, without explicit reference to the spatial distribution of the population at risk. Of course, inferences about $S(x,t) - S(x,t - u)$ which assume only that $\lambda_0(x,t)$ is time-constant but otherwise arbitrary will be less sensitive than inferences about $S(x,t)$, which assume that $\lambda_0(x,t)$ is known.

Brix and Diggle (2001) specify a model of the form $\rho(x,t) = \exp\{S(x,t)\}$ where $S(x,t)$ is a stationary space–time Gaussian process. This model corresponds to a special case of Eq. 9–4, in which there are no relevant explanatory variables. The resulting model is an example of a log-Gaussian Cox process, as introduced by Møller et al. (1998).

To complete the specification of a log-Gaussian Cox process model, we need only to specify the mean and covariance structure of $S(x,t)$. In the absence of explanatory variables, we follow Brix and Diggle (2001) in specifying a constant mean, μ, and variance, σ^2, for $S(x,t)$, and a separable space–time correlation structure $r(u,v) = r_x(u)r_t(v)$ for the correlation between $S(x,t)$ and $S(x - u,t - v)$. Brix and Diggle (2001) allow $r_x(u)$ to be arbitrary but assume that $r_t(v) = \exp(-|v|/\alpha)$, which is computationally convenient because it makes the process Markov in time. In practice, the model is implemented in discrete space–time, with space represented by a fine regular lattice and time represented as discrete calendar dates. In the temporal dimension, this model relies on the approximation

$$\int_{t-\delta}^{t} \exp\{S(x,u)\}\,du \approx \delta\exp\{S(x,t)\}$$

where $\delta = 1$ day, together with an analogous two-dimensional integral approximation in the spatial dimension.

Let $\mathbf{S}_t$ denote the vector of values of $S(x,t)$ at the discrete set of lattice-points x on day t. Let N_t denote the locations of all incident cases up to and including time t. Suppose that $\lambda_0(x,t)$ and all model parameters are known or can be estimated with high precision under the assumed model.

Brix and Diggle (2001) propose simple, moment-based estimators for the model parameters and a Markov chain Monte Carlo algorithm to generate samples from the conditional distribution of $\mathbf{S}_t$ given N_t. Appropriate summaries of these empirical samples can be used to make predictions about the underlying realizations of the space–time surfaces $\mathbf{S}_t$. In particular, the predictive probabilities of pointwise exceedances, $P(S(x,t) > c|N_t)$, or day-to-day changes, $P(S(x,t) - S(x,t-1) > c|N_t)$, can be calculated as simple proportions and displayed on maps.

Although S_t is Markov in time, N_t is not, and the predictive distribution of $S(x,t)$ strictly depends on the complete history of N_t. In practice, events from the remote past have a vanishing influence on the predictive distribution of $S(x,t)$. To avoid storing infeasible amounts of historical data, Brix and Diggle (2001) applied a 5-day cutoff, determined experimentally as the point beyond which, in their illustrative example, retention of historical data had essentially no effect on the predictive distribution. The appropriate choice of cutoff will be application-specific, depending on the abundance of the data and the pattern of temporal correlation.

Analysis of National Health Service Direct Data

The first stage in analyzing NHS Direct data is to estimate $\lambda_0(x)$ and other model parameters. Our approach is to divide the data into two time periods. We use the $n = 2401$ incident cases between August 1, 2000 and May 6, 2001 (279 days) to estimate the average intensity of cases per day as a function of location, x, which we take to be proportional to the effective population at risk, $\lambda_0(x)$, as discussed in Data Sources and Limitations, above. We then use the 973 cases between May 14, 2001 and August 26, 2001 (105 days) to estimate parameters of the latent process $S(x,t)$.

To estimate $\lambda_0(x)$, we use a kernel smoothing method, with a Gaussian kernel $\phi(x) = (2\pi h^2)^{-1} \exp\{-0.5\|x\|^2/h^2\}$ and bandwidth $h = 3$ km. Hence,

$$\hat{\lambda}_0(x) = \sum_{i=1}^{n} \phi(x - x_i)$$

where $x_i : i = 1, \ldots, n$ are the locations of the n incident cases in the first time period (Fig. 9–7).

To estimate parameters of $S(x,t)$, we use the moment-based methods of Brix and Diggle (2001), which operate by matching empirical and theoretical descriptors of the spatial and temporal covariance structure of the point process model. For the spatial correlation structure of $S(x,t)$, we assume a simple exponential, $r_x(u) = \exp(-|u|/\theta)$. Then, the pair correlation function of the point process N_t is $g(u) = \exp\{\sigma^2 \exp(-|u|/\theta)\}$, and we estimate σ^2 and θ to minimize the criterion

$$\int_0^{u_0} [\{\log \hat{g}(u)\}^{0.5} - \{\log g(u)\}^{0.5}]^2 du \qquad (9\text{–}5)$$

where $u_0 = 2$ kilometers and $\hat{g}(u)$ is the empirical pair correlation function. The resulting fitted and empirical functions $\log g(u)$ are compared in Figure 9–8A.

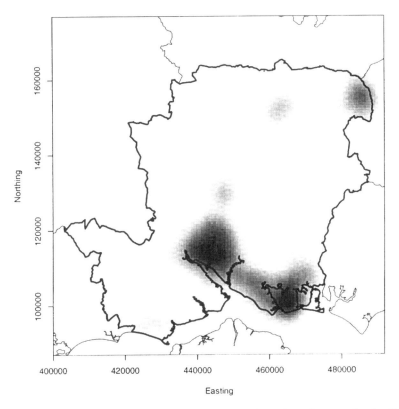

Figure 9–7 Kernel estimate of $\lambda_0(x)$ for the NHS Direct data. See text for detailed explanation.

For the temporal correlation structure of $S(x,t)$, we again assume a simple exponential form, $\rho_t(v) = \exp(-|v|/\alpha)$, and estimate α and μ by matching empirical and theoretical temporal covariances of the observed numbers of incident cases per day, N_t say. The expression for $\text{Cov}(N_t, N_{t-v})$ in Brix and Diggle (2001) is incorrect. The correct expression is

$$\text{Cov}(N_t, N_{t-v}) = \exp(2\mu + \sigma^2)\int_W \int_W \lambda_0(x)\lambda_0(x')[\exp\{\sigma^2\rho(\|x - x'\|,v)\} - 1]dxdx'$$

The estimation criterion is now

$$\int_0^{v_0} \{\hat{C}(v) - C(v; \alpha)\}^2 \, dv$$

where $v_0 = 7$ days, $\hat{C}(v)$ is the empirical autocovariance function of the daily incident counts and $C(v;\alpha) = \text{Cov}(N_t, N_{t-v})$. For each value of α we estimate μ by matching the theoretical and empirical autocovariances at lag $v = 0$, and the remaining parameters σ^2 and θ are fixed at the values

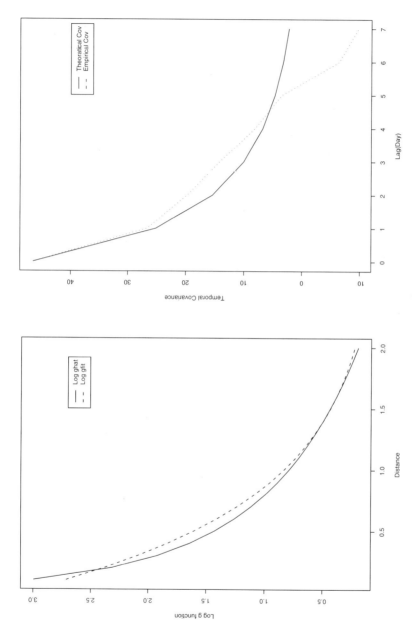

Figure 9–8 A. Empirical (solid line) and fitted (dashed line) log-pair correlation functions for the NHS Direct data. B. Empirical (dashed line) and fitted (solid line) autocovariance functions for the NHS Direct data. See text for detailed explanation.

estimated by minimization of the right side of Eq. 9–5. The resulting fitted and empirical autocovariance functions are compared in Figure 9–8B.
The resulting set of parameter estimates is $\hat{\mu} = -1.466$, $\hat{\sigma}^2 = 3.091$, $\hat{\alpha} =$
3.070, $\hat{\theta} = 0.764$. These parameter values are used to generate samples
from the predictive distribution of $S(x,t)$ given N_t, using the Metropolis-
adjusted Langevin algorithm (MALA) of Brix and Diggle (2001). At any
time point t, the MALA generates samples from the posterior distribution
of the surface $S(x,t)$, conditional on the observed pattern of incident cases
up to and including time t. From the simulated samples, observed proportions of exceedances are used to calculate an estimate of the surface
$p(x,t) = P[\exp\{S(x,t) - \mu\} > c]$ for any chosen threshold, c. The resulting
surfaces for $c = 2$ and $c = 4$, at a time when the daily incidence is about 3
times higher than average, are shown in Figure 9–9. The shading distinguishes posterior probabilities $p(x,t) < 0.5$, $0.5 \leq p(x,t) < 0.9$, $0.9 \leq$
$p(x,t) < 0.99$ and $p(x,t) \geq 0.99$, estimated from 10,000 simulated samples
from the predictive distribution. The small, dark patches corresponding to
large values of $p(x,t)$ represent potential outbreaks, whose provenance (or
not) would need to be established by detailed follow-up investigation of
cases in their immediate vicinity. In practice, the choice of which value
of c defines an appropriate threshold for intervention is context-dependent.

Discussion

Point process modeling has the advantage of imposing no artificial, discrete
spatial or temporal units on the underlying risk surface. Specifically, the
scales of stochastic dependence in space and in time are determined by the
data, and these estimated scales are then reflected in the extents of the spatial and temporal smoothing that are applied to the data to construct the
predicted risk surfaces. Against this, the approach assumes the substantive
relevance of the residential location of each case, whereas in practice an individual's exposure to risk is determined by a complex combination of their
residential, working and leisure locations and activities.

To apply the point process methodology to the GP-reported data, some
allowance would need to be made for variation in reporting rates between
GPs. As noted in Brix and Diggle (2001), an allowance can be made by
extending the basic model, Eq. 9–4, to

$$\rho(x,t) = \exp\{d(x,t)\beta + U_{i(x,t)} + S(x,t)\} \tag{9–6}$$

where $i(x,t)$ identifies the reporting GP for the (unique) case at location x
and at time t, and the U_i are a set of random effects corresponding to the
variable overall reporting rates of individual GPs. As noted earlier, this

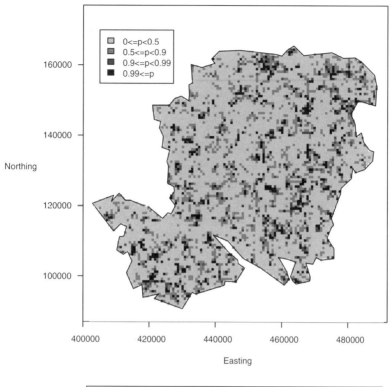

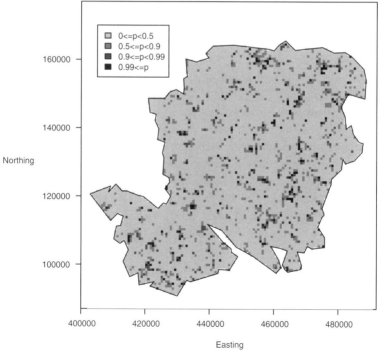

model assumes that an individual GP's reporting rate is consistent over time; if the U_i were replaced by time-varying random effects $U_i(t)$, they would be confounded with the latent process $S(x,t)$.

DISCRETE SPATIAL MODELS

Model Formulation

We now discuss two formulations for data aggregated not only by day $t = 1, \ldots, T$ but also by spatial units, $i = 1, \ldots, I$, defined using area aggregations (e.g., EDs), or individual GPs. Both formulations require specifying for each spatial unit i all of its geographically neighboring units. For example, two EDs could be considered to be neighbors if they share a common boundary, or two GPs could be considered to be neighbors if they are within a given distance of each other. The approach also allows neighboring pairs to be differentially weighted to reflect assumptions about the way in which the strength of the conditional spatial dependence between a pair of units is affected by their relative locations.

Throughout the modeling process, the number of incident cases y_{it} in unit i on day t is assumed to be binomially distributed, with the corresponding known denominators n_{it} and an unknown disease risk probability π_{it}. For area-based analyses, the denominators would be obtained from census information, whereas for GP-based analyses they correspond to practice capitation counts. Given the rareness of the disease, we could use a Poisson approximation to the binomial, which then corresponds to a discrete version of the Poisson process model, Eq. 9–3, in which y_{it} is Poisson distributed with rate $n_{it}\pi_{it}$. In this formulation, n_{it} in the discrete spatial model corresponds to $\lambda_0(x,t)$ in the Poisson process model, and π_{it} corresponds to $\rho(x,t)$.

We first discuss a baseline model, which will be suitable if the space–time pattern of the disease can be separated into spatial and temporal trends. We then describe two ways to extend this formulation, with a view to early

---

Figure 9–9 Posterior exceedance probabilities, $p(x,t) = P[\exp\{S(x,t) - \mu\} > c]$, for $c = 2$ (upper panel) and $c = 4$ (lower panel). The shading distinguishes posterior probabilities $p(x,t) < 0.5$, $0.5 \leq p(x,t) < 0.9$, $0.9 \leq p(x,t) < 0.99$ and $p(x,t) \geq 0.99$, estimated from 10,000 simulated samples from the predictive distribution. The small, dark patches corresponding to large values of $p(x,t)$ represent potential outbreaks, whose provenance (or not) would need to be established by detailed follow-up investigation of cases in their immediate vicinity. In practice, the choice of which value of c defines an appropriate threshold for intervention is context-dependent.

detection of local outbreaks. These extensions are based on the formulations proposed by Knorr-Held (2000) and Knorr-Held and Richardson (2003). Both formulations could easily be extended further by including additional covariate information, if available.

In our baseline model, we decompose the log odds additively into temporal (short-term), seasonal and spatial effects; hence,

$$\eta_{it} = \log(\pi_{it}/(1 - \pi_{it})) = T_t + D_t + U_i \qquad (9\text{--}7)$$

The temporal effects T_t describe smooth long-term trends in overall incidence and are modeled as a second order Gaussian random walk. The effects D_t describe a 7-day seasonality resulting from day-of-the-week effects. More specifically, the parameters are assumed to add up to Gaussian white noise over a moving window that has a length of 7 days. Such a formulation allows the seasonal pattern to change over time, in contrast to other modeling approaches, in which the components must sum exactly to zero. Finally, the spatial effects U_i represent time-constant variation among the spatial units and are modeled as an intrinsic Gaussian Markov random field (MRF). Additional effects representing unstructured heterogeneity amongst the spatial units (Besag et al., 1991) could also be included, if necessary. For each of the three components in Eq. 9–7, a hyperprior is assigned to an additional smoothing (or precision) parameter, which is to be estimated from the data.

This baseline formulation, Eq. 9–7, can now be extended to

$$S_{it} = T_t + D_t + U_i + W_{it}$$

where W_{it} follows a MRF on the space $\times$ time domain. A similar framework was proposed in Knorr-Held (2000) for application to chronic disease data. The W_{it} term allows for space-time variation that cannot be attributed to the spatial or temporal main effects. We follow Clayton (1996) and define the precision matrix of the interaction term W_{it} as the direct product of the precision matrices of the temporal second-order random walk and the intrinsic autoregression. This formulation results in a prior in which the contrasts

$$(W_{it} - 2W_{i,t-1} + W_{i,t-2}) - (W_{jt} - 2W_{j,t-1} + W_{j,t-2}) : t = 1, \dots, T - 1$$

for all pairs of adjacent spatial units $i \sim j$ are independent Gaussian random variables. This result implies that the W_{it} are dependent in space and in time. Again, an additional unknown smoothing parameter will be associated with the W_{it} term. Such a prior model seems most suitable for modeling infectious disease outbreaks, assuming that local temporal trends (represented by the second differences $W_{it} - 2W_{i,t-1} + W_{i,t-2}$) are different among the spatial units but are more likely to be similar for adjacent units. For identifiability, sum-to-zero constraints must be imposed on the W_{it}. We can now monitor the posterior distribution of W_{it} and the corresponding posterior probabilities $P(W_{it} > 0 | \text{data})$ to quantify the size and the significance of potential localized outbreaks. An essential difference between the Knorr-Held model and the point process model described in Point Process Models, above is that space–time anomalies W_{it} are defined only after adjusting for arbitrary spatial and temporal trends; the corresponding feature for the point process model would require a decomposition of the process $S(x,t)$ of the form $S(x,t) = T(t) + U(x) + W(x,t)$. Alternatively, a MRF could be specified directly on the η_{it} term, but this process would require a specification that takes into account the different scales of the spatial and temporal domains (Gössl et al. 2001) Such an approach has been described in Gössl et al. (2001) in the context of spatial temporal functional magnetic resonance imaging. A second way of extending Eq. 9–7 to incorporate space–time interaction, described by Knorr-Held and Richardson (2003), is to include additional autoregressive terms on the number of cases at time $t - 1$ in the linear predictor; hence,

$$\eta_{it} = T_t + D_t + U_i + X_{it} f_i (Y_{t-1}, \beta)$$

Here, $f_i (Y_{t-1}, \beta)$ denotes a deterministic function of the number of cases, Y_{t-1}, incident at time $t - 1$, and unknown parameters β, with the implication that the occurrence of a case at time $t - 1$ directly increases the probability of an additional case at time t. In contrast, X_{it} are a set of binary indicators, with zero and one corresponding respectively to nonepidemic and epidemic states in unit i at time t. Terms of this kind of capture, at least qualitatively, the epidemic nature of infectious disease incidence patterns. The indicators X_{it} determine whether or not the autoregressive term, $f_i(\cdot)$, is active in unit i on day t. For each spatial unit, the X_{it} are assumed to follow a simple binary Markov model. The transition matrix of the binary Markov model and the autoregressive parameter β are treated as unknown. The autoregressive term $f_i(\cdot)$ may include information on the number of cases in the same unit as well as in neighboring units, if appropriate; specific functional forms are discussed in Knorr-Held and Richardson (2003). The posterior probability that the indicators are in an epidemic state, that is $P(X_{it} = 1 | \text{data})$, can now be used to quantify the evidence for local outbreaks.

This formulation is somewhat in the spirit of so-called "switching" regression models that are popular in econometrics. However, these econometric models typically assume a Gaussian response variable, whereas we

have a binomial (or Poisson) response and an additional spatial component to describe dependence between neighboring spatial units.

Analysis of General Practice–Reported Data

As an illustration, results from an analysis based on the Knorr-Held-
Richardson model is reported. All 2758 cases diagnosed between August 1,
2001 and February 28, 2002 are included, and the spatial units are defined
as the individual GPs; 134 of these cases were resident outside the study
area, and were excluded from the exploratory ED-level analysis reported in
Exploratory Analysis of the General Practice–Reported Data, above. Practice capitation numbers for the 99 GPs reporting cases ranged from 1656
to 20,911 and have been used for the denominators $n_{it} = n_i$. For each GP,
the three closest GPs (based on Euclidian distance) were first defined to be
neighbors. However, this definition does not ensure the symmetry required
by Markov random field models, and the adjacencies have been correspondingly adjusted, resulting in a median number of four neighbors (range,
3 to 7) for each GP.

The six different choices for the autoregressive term $f_i(Y_{t-1}, \beta)$ described
in detail in Knorr-Held and Richardson (2001) were tried. Here only results from the preferred model in which $f_i(Y_{t-1}, \beta) = \beta I(Y_{i,t-1} > 0$ or
$Y_{j,t-1} > 0$ for at least 1 $j \sim i$), where $I(\cdot)$ denotes the indicator function, is
discussed. The basic idea of this formulation is that, in the epidemic state,
$X_{it} = 1$, risk π_{it} will be increased if *at least one case at time $t - 1$ is from the
same GP or from neighboring GPs*.

A smooth time trend $\hat{T}_t$ with 80% credibility intervals, the estimated
seasonal pattern $\hat{D}_t$ (without credibility intervals for reasons of presentation), and the sum of the two (again without credibility intervals) are presented in Figure 9–10. The seasonal effect appears to be rather large but
also rather unstable over the time domain. Interestingly, the seasonal pattern peaks on December 24, Christmas Eve.

Averaged weekday effects, again with 80% credibility intervals were
also computed (Fig. 9–11). The estimated effects agree with the corresponding descriptive figures reported in Exploratory Analysis of the General Practice–Reported Data, above, with highest averaged weekday effects
on Sunday and Monday. All weekdays between Tuesday and Saturday have
consistently lower values. Somewhat surprising is the relatively high value
on a Friday.

The estimated GP effects $\hat{U}_i$ show a 70-fold variation between the low-
est and the highest estimated relative risks. This result is no surprise, because the GP-specific numbers of total cases per capitation range between

Trend Parameter

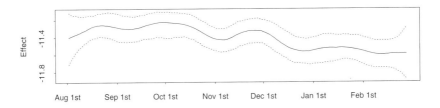

Seasonal Parameter

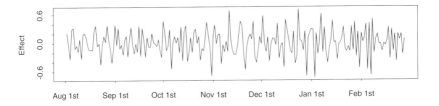

Trend + Seasonal Parameter

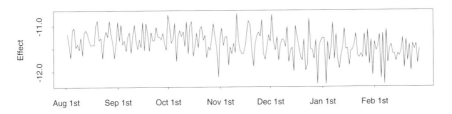

Figure 9–10 Estimated temporal trends of baseline formulation.

0.0001 and 0.025. The scale of this variation underlines the importance of including GP effects in the model.

Turning now to the epidemic part of the formulation, Figures 9–12 and 9–13 display observed counts y_{it}, fitted rates $n_{it}\hat{\pi}_{it}$ and the corresponding posterior probabilities for an epidemic state for four selected GPs. These figures illustrate the potential of the proposed approach to detect anomalies in disease incidence. For example, there is some evidence for an outbreak shortly before New Year 2002 for the first GP (Fig. 9–12, lower left panel) with a posterior probability close to unity. This apparent outbreak would be difficult to detect from the raw counts, particularly because the posterior probabilities are adjusted for global temporal trends and GP ef-

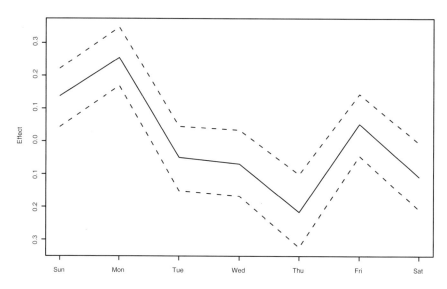

Figure 9–11 Estimated average weekday effects. Posterior median with 80% credible intervals.

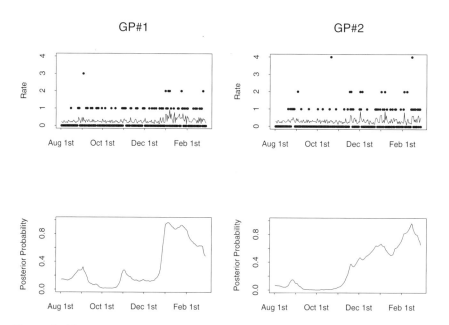

Figure 9–12 The observed counts and the fitted rate for 2 selected GPs (top) and the corresponding posterior probabilities for an epidemic state (bottom).

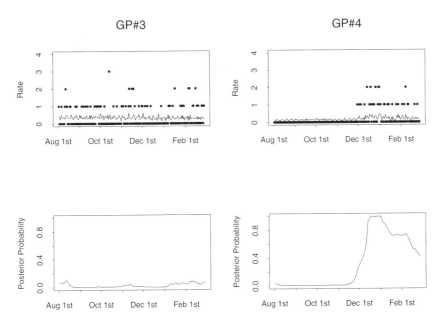

Figure 9–13 The observed counts and the fitted rates for the other 2 selected GPs (top) and the corresponding posterior probabilities for an epidemic state (bottom).

fects, while also incorporating the number of cases at time $t - 1$ in neighboring GPs. A somewhat similar pattern can be seen for the second GP (Fig. 9–12, right panels); however, the posterior probabilities peak here about 1 month later.

The left panels in Figure 9–13 gives an example of a GP with relatively high but stable incidence pattern, with no indication of an epidemic at any time. Finally, the right panels give an example in which the method fails. This failure relates to a GP who reported no cases at all in the first half of the study period. The cases reported in the second half are then classified by the model as epidemic, because GP reporting rates are assumed to be time constant in the baseline model. This artificial phenomenon occurs because the data-collection protocol was unable to distinguish between a nil return and a failure to report. If GP reporting rates do change with time, separating epidemic trends from simple changes in reporting rates is impossible.

This section closes with some details about estimated hyperparameters in this model. The entries in the transition matrix of the latent Markov models are estimated as 0.007 for a change from nonepidemic to epidemic, and 0.041 for the reverse step (posterior medians). The stationary probability for an epidemic state is estimated as 0.148, which seems high. However, this estimate will be biased upwards through nonconstant GP reporting rates. Similar comments apply to the estimated expected duration time in an epidemic state $1/0.041 \approx 24$ days, which seems too long. Finally, if a GP is in an epidemic state, the presence of at least one case at time $t - 1$ is estimated to increase the incidence by a factor of $\exp(\hat{\beta}) \approx 3.17$.

Discussion

The application of discrete spatial models requires a definition of spatial units and of a neighborhood relationship between them. These choices contain some level of arbitrariness and will affect the resulting inference, at least to some extent. However, the GPs seem to represent a natural choice for the spatial units, and analysis suggests that ignoring GP effects will result in strongly misleading results. The need to define neighborhood relationships between GPs seems nevertheless slightly odd. An alternative approach would be to analyze the data on a truly spatial resolution, for example on ED or ward level, while including additional (unstructured) GP effects in the formulation, similar to the extended point process model, Eq. 9–6.

There are several aspects of the two models that need elaboration. Further stratification (e.g., by age) could be interesting and could easily be done by including covariate terms explicitly in the formulation, or by using a Poisson framework with expected numbers precalculated based on some age-standardization method. Also, the autoregressive part of the second model could be refined; in particular, the inclusion of cases at time $t - 2$ may be worthwhile. However, such extensions may not be needed for this application, given the sparseness of the data; nearly 90% of the daily incidence counts y_{it} are zero.

CONCLUSION

This chapter has illustrated how spatial statistical methods can be used to help develop on-line surveillance systems for common diseases. The spatial statistical analyses are intended to supplement, rather than to replace, existing protocols. Their aim is to identify, as quickly as possible, statistical anomalies in the space–time pattern of incident cases, which would be followed up by other means. In some cases, the anomalies will be transient features of no particular public health significance. In others, the statistical early warning should help to ensure timely intervention to minimize the public health consequences; for example, when follow-up of cases in an area with a significantly elevated risk shows exposure to common risk factors or infection with a common pathogen.

The choice of a statistical modeling framework is informed by the nature of the data; the use of discrete spatial modeling for the GP-reported data, and point process modeling for the NHS Direct data. Rather than formally integrating the two approaches into a single analysis, we envisage running them in parallel and reporting the results from both approaches simultaneously in the Web-reporting framework.

A final, cautionary remark is that the most critical element in the success or failure of a surveillance system is the quality of its input data. High adherence rates and consistent reporting over time are vital. Given these prerequisites, real-time spatial statistical analyses of the kind illustrated here can add substantial value to traditional methods based on population-level summary statistics.

ACKNOWLEDGMENTS

Project AEGISS is supported by a grant from the Food Standards Agency, United Kingdom, and from the National Health Service Executive Research and Knowledge Management Directorate. We also thank NHS Direct, Hampshire and Isle of Wight, participating general practices and their staff, and collaborating laboratories for their input to AEGISS. AEGISS website: www.aegiss.soton.ac.uk

REFERENCES

Bartlett, M.S. (1964). The spectral analysis of two-dimensional point processes. *Biometrika* **51**, 299–311.

Besag, J.E., York, J.C., and Mollié, A. (1991). Bayesian image restoration with two applications in spatial statistics (with discussion). *Annals of the Institute of Statistical Mathematics* **43**, 1–59.

Best, N.G., Ickstadt, K., and Wolpert, R.L. (2000). Spatial Poisson regression for health and exposure data measured at disparate resolutions. *Journal of the American Statistical Association* **95**, 1076–1088.

Brix, A. and Diggle, P.J. (2001). Spatiotemporal prediction for log-Gaussian Cox processes. *Journal of the Royal Statistical Society, Series B* **63**, 823–841.

Clayton, D.G. (1996). Generalized linear mixed models. In Gilks, W.R., Richardson, S. and Spiegelhalter, D.J., eds. *Markov Chain Monte Carlo in Practice*. London: Chapman & Hall, pp. 275–301.

Cox, D.R. (1955). Some statistical methods related with series of events (with Discussion). *Journal of the Royal Statistical Society, Series B* **17**, 129–157.

Food Standards Agency. (2000). *A Report of the Study of Infectious Intestinal Disease in England*. London: Food Standards Agency.

Gössl, C., Auer, D.P., and Fahrmeir, L. (2001). Bayesian spatiotemporal inference in functional magnatic resonance imaging. *Biometrics* **57**, 554–562.

Hastie, T. and Tibshirani, R. (1990). *Generalized Additive Models*. London: Chapman & Hall.

Joint FAO/WHO Expert Committee on Food Safety (1984). *The Role of Food Safety in Health and Development: Report of a Joint FAO/WHO Expert Committee on Food Safety.* Technical Report Series 705. Geneva: WHO.

Kelsall, J.E. and Diggle, P.J. (1998). Spatial variation in risk of disease: a nonparametric binary regression approach. *Journal of the Royal Statistical Society Series C (Applied Statistics)* **47,** 559–573.

Knorr-Held, L. (2000). Bayesian modeling of inseparable space-time variation in disease risk. *Statistics in Medicine* **19,** 2555–2567.

Knorr-Held, L. and Richardson, S. (2003). A hierarchical model for space-time surveillance data on meningococcal disease incidence. Applied Statistics *Journal of the Royal Statistical Society, Series C* **52** (in press).

Møller, J., Syversveen, A., and Waagepetersen, R. (1998). Log Gaussian Cox processes. *Scandinavian Journal of Statistics* **25,** 451–482.

Turner, A.M. (2000). *Infectious Intestinal Disease Surveillance in Wessex Data Review and the Role of the General Practitioner.* MPH dissertation, University of Wales College of Medicine, Cardiff.

10

Bayesian Hierarchical Modeling of Public Health Surveillance Data: A Case Study of Air Pollution and Mortality

SCOTT L. ZEGER, FRANCESCA DOMINICI,
AIDAN MCDERMOTT, JONATHAN M. SAMET

Exposure to environmental pollutants likely contributes to morbidity and mortality around the world. An important question is how many persons in a given population suffer adverse health effects from environmental exposures. To address this question and others like it, U.S. government agencies, including the National Center for Health Statistics and Environmental Protection Agency, regularly collect monitoring data on health outcomes and pollutant levels. These data must be carefully analyzed in order to quantify health risks.

One example of a potentially important exposure in United States urban populations is particulate air pollution (Dockery et al., 1993; Pope et al., 1995a; American Thoracic Society, 1996; National Research Council, 1998; Pope and Dockery, 1999). The evidence for an association between particulate pollution concentrations and mortality and morbidity is strong (Lipfert and Wyzga, 1993; Pope et al., 1995a; Schwartz, 1995). Hence, public health and government officials seek to determine whether air pollution causes premature illness and death and, if so, to quantify the magnitude of the problem (Environmental Protection Agency, 1995; National Research Council, 1998).

This chapter presents statistical approaches for estimating the risk of death as a function of the concentration of particulate air pollution, a key component of risk analysis. It focuses on multistage models of daily mortality data in the 88 largest cities in the United States to illustrate the main ideas. These models have been used to quantify the risks of shorter-term exposure to particulate pollution and to address key causal questions (Samet et al., 2000a; Dominici et al., 2000a, 2002a).

The air pollution mortality association has received much attention over the last decade since the publication of articles by Schwartz and Marcus (1990), Dockery et al. (1993), and Pope et al. (1995b). That high levels of particulate pollution can cause illness and death has been generally accepted since the 1952 London smog episode caused thousands of excess deaths in a short time (Logan and Glasg, 1953; Bell and Davis, 2001). Governments in North America and Europe initiated large pollution-control programs in the 1970s as a result. Schwartz and Marcus (1990), however, presented evidence from time series studies in selected U.S. cities to support the hypothesis that daily fluctuations in particulate levels within a population, well within current federal standards, continue to cause hospitalizations and premature deaths. Dockery et al. (1993) and Pope et al. (1995b) showed that persons living in cities with higher particulate levels suffer higher mortality risks than those living in less polluted cities, even after controlling for many important individual confounding variables such as smoking, socioeconomic status and education.

The evidence for an association between particulate air pollution concentration and mortality derived from time series is different from that derived from cohort studies. The time series studies (Schwartz and Marcus, 1990; Schwartz, 1995; Kelsall et al., 1997; Smith et al., 2000) rely on variations over time within a population, and compare the number of deaths on more-to-less polluted days. They depend on statistical control for within-population confounders including secular trends in mortality attributable to changing health practice and risk behaviors; effects of weather; and seasonal influenza epidemics. Even the multicity studies (Katsouyanni et al., 1997; Samet et al., 2000c; Dominici et al., 2000a, 2002a; Hwang and Chan, 2001) rely entirely on within-population comparisons; they increase power and possibly robustness by pooling relative risks across many cities. Time series models estimate the health risk associated with shorter-term exposures, on the order of days or weeks. Thus time series studies provide little evidence on the health effects of more chronic exposures. Kelsall et al. (1999), Zeger et al. (1999), Schwartz (2000) and Dominici et al. (2002d) have discussed how to estimate pollution relative risks at different time scales using time series data.

The cohort studies (Dockery et al., 1993; Pope et al., 1995b; Krewski et al., 2000) compare mortality risks across distinct populations rather than over time for a population. They have shown that persons living in more-polluted cities are at higher risk for mortality than otherwise similar persons in less polluted cities. Here, "otherwise similar" refers to a population in which age, gender, socioeconomic factors, smoking, and additional person-level confounding variables have been adjusted statistically. The cohort studies estimate the association of daily mortality with longer-term exposure. For example, Pope et al. (1995b) used average concentration for the past year as the predictor of mortality.

To date, the cohort studies have indicated larger relative risk than the time series studies. For example Pope et al. (1995b) in the American Cancer Society (ACS) Study report a 6.4% increase in mortality per $10\mu g/m^3$ increase in particulate matter less than 2.5 microns ($PM_{2.5}$) while Dominici et al. (2002a) in the National Morbidity and Mortality Air Pollution Study (NMMAPS) multisite time series study report a 0.41% per $10\mu g/m^3$ increase in particulate matter less than 10 microns (PM_{10}). Recent reanalyses of the NMMAPS study have lowered this estimate to 0.21% per $10\mu g/m^3$ increase in PM_{10} (Dominici et al., 2002,b,d).

The difference between time series and cohort studies results likely reflects one or more factors, including the possibility that longer-term exposures have greater health consequences than do shorter-term exposures (Zeger et al., 1999; Schwartz, 2000; Dominici et al., 2002c), or that the cohort study estimates are confounded by unmeasured differences among the populations compared (Guttorp et al., 2001).

This chapter provides an overview of the time series approach to estimating the relative risk of mortality from particulate air pollution. How time series models might be used to partially address the possible difference in the mortality effects from shorter- to moderate-term variations of exposures is discussed.

The following section 2 reviews the NMMAPS data base that comprises a time series of daily mortality, air pollution, and weather variables between 1987 and 1994 for the 88 largest cities in the United States. The next section presents several models for time series data and describes the time series approach to estimating a pollution relative risk while controlling for likely confounders for a single city. We summarize the models used to characterize the variability in relative risks among cities within and across regions and also to produce a pooled estimate across all 88 cities and we report the pooled estimate. Then we decompose the pollution time series into multiple predictors to estimate the relative risk of acute and more chronic exposures. We illustrate the difficulty of using time series models to estimate chronic health effects in four cities with daily particulate pollution data over 8 years. Finally, we offer an approach for future analyses that might combine cohort and time series information.

NATIONAL MORBIDITY AND MORTALITY
AIR POLLUTION STUDY DATA

The National Morbidity and Mortality Air Pollution Study was a systematic investigation of the dependence of daily hospitalization and mortality counts on particulate and other air pollutants. Its data base includes mortality, weather, and air pollution data for the 88 largest metropolitan areas in the United States for the years 1987 through 1994. Since its inception, the NMMAPS has contributed information relevant to air quality policy, including:

- national, regional, and city estimates of the relative risk of mortality associated with concentrations of PM_{10} and other pollutants for the 88 urban centers (Samet et al., 2000a,b,c; Dominici et al., 2000a, 2002a)
- a critical review of the impact of measurement error on time series estimates of relative risks and an estimate of the PM_{10} relative risk that is corrected for measurement error (Dominici et al., 2000b; Zeger et al., 2000)
- evidence that contradicts the harvesting hypothesis that the apparent association is attributable to the frail who die days earlier than they would have otherwise, absent air pollution (Zeger et al., 1999; Dominici et al., 2002c)
- evidence that contradicts the threshold hypothesis that particles and mortality are not associated except above a threshold concentration (Daniels et al., 2000; Schwartz, 2000; Dominici et al., 2002a)

The daily time series of PM_{10}, O_3, mortality, temperature, and dew point for one NMMAPS urban center, Pittsburgh, Pennsylvania, is illustrated in Figure 10–1. The data on mortality, air pollution, and weather, were drawn from public sources. The cause-specific mortality data at the county level were obtained from the National Center for Health Statistics. The focus was on daily death counts for each site, excluding accidental deaths and deaths of nonresidents. Mortality information was available at the county level but not at a smaller geographic unit to protect confidentiality. All predictor variables were therefore also aggregated at the county level.

Hourly temperature and dew point data were obtained from the National Climatic Data Center, specifically the EarthInfo CD data base (http://www.sni.net/earthinfo/cdroms/). After extensive preliminary analyses that considered various daily summaries of temperature and dew point as predictors, we chose the 24-hour mean to characterize each day. If a county had more than one weather station, the average of the measurements from all stations was used.

The daily time series of PM_{10} and other pollutants for each city were obtained from the Aerometric Information Retrieval Service data base maintained by the U.S. Environmental Protection Agency (http://www.wpa. gov/airs/airs.html). The pollutant data were also averaged over all monitors

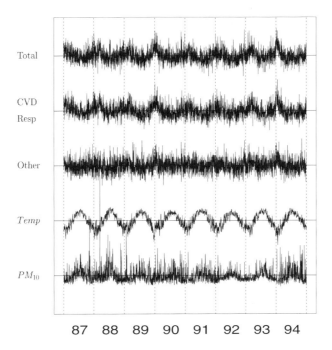

Figure 10–1 Total, cardiovascular-respiratory (CVD RESP), and other causes mortality daily counts. Temperature (Temp) and PM_{10} $\mu g/m^3$ daily time series. Data for Pittsburgh, Pennsylvania, for 1987 through 1994.

in a county. To protect against outlying observations and instrument drift, a 10% trimmed mean was used to average across monitors after correcting for each monitors yearly average. Information on several city-specific characteristics from the 1990 Census CD (email:info@censuscd.com) was also collected. A more detailed description of the data base is provided in NMMAPS reports (Samet et al., 2000b,c).

STATISTICAL MODELS FOR TIME SERIES DATA

Time Series Model for a Single Location

In this section, we specify the model for estimating air pollution-mortality relative risk separately for each location, accounting for age-specific longer-term trends, weather, and day of the week as potential confounding variables. The core analysis for each city is a log-linear generalized additive model (GAM) (Hastie and Tibshirani, 1990) with smoothing splines or a

Poisson model with regression splines (McCullagh and Nelder, 1989). Smoothing splines or natural cubic splines of time are included in the model to account for smooth fluctuations in mortality caused by nonpollution mechanisms that potentially confound estimates of the pollution effect, introduce autocorrelation in mortality series, or both.

We model daily expected deaths as a function of the pollution levels on the same or immediately preceding days, and not the average exposure for the preceding month, season, or year as might be done in a study of chronic effects. We use models that include smooth functions of time as predictors to control for possible confounding by seasonal influenza epidemics and by other longer-term changes in the population, demographic composition, personal behaviors (including smoking), and access to, and quality of, medical services.

To specify our approach, let y_{at}^c be the observed mortality for age group $a = (\leq 65, 65\text{--}75, \geq 75$ years) on day t at location c, and $\boldsymbol{x}_{at}^c$ be a $p \times 1$ vector of air pollution variables. Let $\lambda_{at}^c = E(y_{at}^c)$ be the expected number of deaths and $v_{at}^c = \text{var}(y_{at}^c)$. We use a log-linear model

$$\log \lambda_{at}^c = \boldsymbol{x}_{at}^{c\prime} \beta^c + \text{confounders} \qquad (10\text{--}1)$$

$$v_{at}^c = \phi^c \lambda_{at}^c, \; c = 1, \ldots, C$$

that allows the mortality counts to have variances v_{at}^c that may exceed their means (i.e., be overdispersed) with the overdispersion parameter ϕ^c also varying by location.

To protect the pollution relative risks β^c from confounding by longer-term trends, and to account for any additional temporal correlation in the count time series, we estimate the pollution effect using only shorter-term variations in mortality and air pollution. To do so, we partial out the smooth, i.e., longer-term fluctuations in the mortality over time by including a smooth function (smoothing splines or natural cubic spline) of the calendar time $S^c(\text{time}, \nu)$ for each city. Here, ν is a smoothness parameter that we specify, from epidemiologic knowledge of the time scale of the major possible confounders to have 7 degrees of freedom per year of data so that little information from time-scales longer than approximately 2 months is included when β^c is estimated. We believe this choice substantially reduces confounding from seasonal influenza epidemics and from longer-term trends resulting from changing medical practice and health behaviors. We also control for age-specific longer-term and seasonal variations in mortality by adding a separate smooth function of time with 1 additional degree of freedom per year (8 total) for each age group.

To control for weather, we fit smooth functions of the same-day temperature (temp$_0$), average temperature for the 3 previous days (temp$_{1\text{--}3}$), each with 6 degrees of freedom, and the analogous functions for dew point (dew$_0$, dew$_{1-3}$), each with 3 degrees of freedom. In U.S. cities, mortality decreases smoothly with increasing temperature until reaching a relative minimum and then increases quite sharply at higher temperature (Curriero et al., 2002). We choose 6 degrees of freedom to capture this highly non-linear bend near the relative minimum as well as possible. Because there are missing values in air pollution concentration, and occasionally in other variables, we restricted analyses to days with no missing values across the full set of predictors.

In summary, we fit the following log-linear model to obtain the estimated pollution log-relative risk $\hat{\beta}^c$ and the sample covariance matrix V^c at each location:

$$\log \lambda_{at}^c = \boldsymbol{x}_{at}^{c'} \beta^c + \gamma^c \mathrm{DOW}_t + S_1^c(t, 7/\mathrm{year}) +$$

$$+ S_2^c(\mathrm{temp}_{0t}, 6) + S_3^c(\mathrm{temp}_{1-3t}, 6) + S_4^c(\mathrm{dew}_{0t}, 3) + S_5^c(\mathrm{dew}_{1-3t}, 3)$$

$$+ \text{intercept for age group } a$$

$$+ \text{separate smooth functions of time 1 df/year for age group } a$$

$$(10\text{–}2)$$

where DOW_t are indicator variables for day of week. Samet et al. (1999) and Kelsall et al. (1997) have given additional details about functions used to control for longer-term trends and weather. Alternative modeling approaches that consider different lag structures of the pollutants, and of the meteorological variables, have also been studied (Smith et al., 1997, 2000; Zanobetti et al., 2000) More general approaches that consider nonlinear modeling of the pollutant variables have been discussed by Smith et al. (1997) and by Daniels et al. (2000).

Model for Multisite Time Series Studies

In this section, a hierarchical regression model designed to estimate city-specific pollution relative risks, pooled national relative risk, and within- and between-region variances of the city-specific values is presented. As discussed in National Morbidity and Mortality Air Pollution Study, above, even the pooled time-series estimates derive entirely from within-population comparisons of shorter-term effects. A three-stage hierarchical model is assumed with the following structure:

Stage I: City
Given a time series of daily mortality counts at a given city (actually counties containing the city), the association between air pollution and health

within the site is described using the regression model defined in Equation 10-2. Among the output of the stage-I analysis are the point estimate $(\hat{\beta}_r^c)$ and the statistical variance (v_r^c) of the relative mortality risk (β_r^c) associated with each air pollutant within site c belonging to the geographical region r.

Stage II: Geographical Region

The information across cities within a region is combined by using a linear regression model in which the outcome variable is the log pollution relative risk for each city, and the explanatory variables (X_j^c) are site-specific characteristics, such as population density, yearly averages of the pollutants, and temperature. Formally:

$$\beta_r^c = \alpha_{0r} + \sum_{j=1}^{p} \alpha_j^c X_j^c + error_r.$$

If the predictors X_j^c are centered about their means, the intercept (α_{0r}) is interpreted as the pooled regional effect for a city with mean predictors. The regression coefficients (α_j^c) indicate the change in the relative risk of mortality associated with a unit change in the corresponding site-specific variable.

Stage III: Country

The information across regions is combined by using a linear regression model in which the outcome variable is α_{0r} the true average regional relative mortality risk, and the explanatory variables (W_{jr}) are the region-specific characteristics (toxic composition of air pollution, climate variables). Formally:

$$\alpha_{0r} = \alpha_0 + \sum_{j=1}^{p} \alpha_j W_{jr} + error.$$

As in Stage II, if the predictors W_{jr} are centered about their means, the intercept α_0 is the pooled national effect for a region with mean values of the predictors. The regression coefficients (α_j) measure the change in true regional relative risk of mortality associated with a unit change in the corresponding region-specific variable.

The sources of variation in estimating of health effects of air pollution are specified by the levels of the hierarchical model. Under a three-stage model, the difference between the estimated site-specific relative risk $(\hat{\beta}_r^c)$ and the true pooled relative risk (α_0) can be decomposed as:

$$(\hat{\beta}_r^c - \alpha_0) = (\hat{\beta}_r^c - \beta_r^c) + (\beta_r^c - \alpha_{0r}) + (\alpha_{0r} - \alpha_0).$$

The variation of $(\hat{\beta}_r^c)$ about β_r^c is measured by the within-site statistical variance (v_r^c), which depends on the number of days with air pollution data and on the predictive power of the site-specific regression model. The variation of β_r^c about α_{0r} is described by the between-site variance (τ^2), which measures the heterogeneity of the true air pollution effects across cities within a region. We assume τ^2 is constant across regions. Finally, the variance of α_{0r} about α_0 (σ^2) measures the heterogeneity of the true regional air pollution effects across regions.

A Bayesian hierarchical model is specified by selecting the prior distributions for the parameters at the top level of the hierarchy. If there is no desire to incorporate prior information into the analysis, then conjugate priors with large variances are often used. However, sensitivity of the substantive findings to the prior distributions should be investigated. Complex hierarchical models can be fit using simulation-based methods (Tierney, 1994; Gilks et al., 1996) that provide samples from the posterior distributions of all parameters of interest. Several software packages are now available (see for example http://www.mrc-bsu.cam.ac.uk/bugs/).

Results for National Morbidity, Mortality, Air Pollution Study

Dominici et al. (2002a) estimated city-specific air pollution effects by applying a GAM to each city, and approximated posterior distributions of regional, and national air pollution effects by applying a Bayesian three-stage hierarchical model to the NMMAPS data base. Results are reported for 88 of the largest metropolitan areas in the United States from 1987 to 1994.

Recently, Dominici et al. (2002c) discovered that when GAM is applied to time-series analyses of contemporary data on air pollution and mortality, the defaults in the S-PLUS software (Version 3.4) package gam do not assure convergence of its iterative estimation procedure, and can provide biased estimates of the regression coefficients and standard errors. Thus the NMMAPS data base has been recently reanalyzed by using Poisson regression models with parametric nonlinear adjustments for confounding factors (natural cubic splines) (Dominici et al., 2002b,d). The revised maximum likelihood estimates and 95% confidence intervals (CI) of the log-relative risks of mortality per 10 $\mu g/m^3$ increase in PM_{10} for each location are shown in Figure 10–2.

The estimate of the national pooled relative risk was a 0.22% increase in mortality per $10\mu g/m^3$ increase in PM_{10}, with a 95% posterior interval between 0.03 and 0.42. The pooled regional estimates of the PM_{10} effects vary across the regions; the estimated relative risk was greatest in the Northeast, with a value of 0.41% per $10\mu g/m^3$ (95% CI 0.12, 0.85).

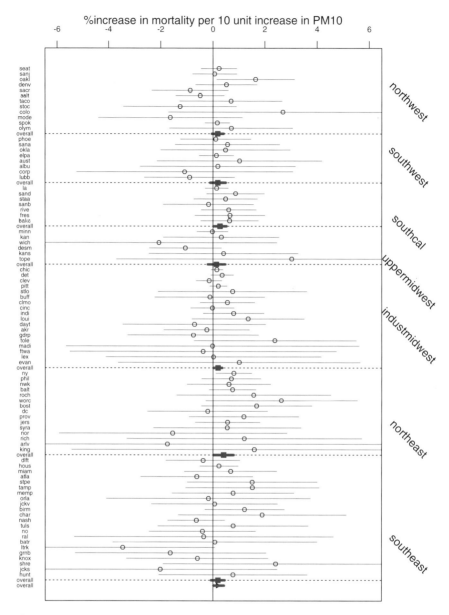

Figure 10–2 Maximum likelihood estimates and 95% confidence intervals of the log-relative risks of mortality per $10\mu g/m^3$ increase in PM_{10} for each location. The solid circles with the bold segments denote the posterior means and 95% posterior intervals of the pooled regional effects. At the bottom, marked with a triangle and a bold segment, is the overall effects for PM_{10} for all the cities.

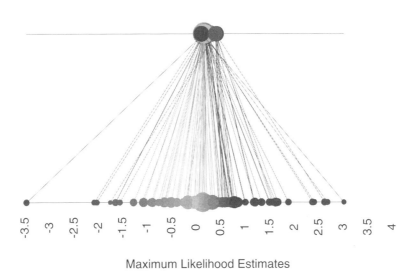

Figure 10–3 Maximum likelihood (bottom) and Bayesian posterior estimates (top) of the relative risks of mortality for the 88 U.S. largest cities. Size of the circle is proportional to the statistical precisions.

Figure 10–3 shows the maximum likelihood estimates (bottom) and the Bayesian estimates (top) of the relative risks of mortality for the largest 88 cities. Sizes of the circles are proportional to the statistical precisions. The Bayesian estimates of the city-specific air pollution effects are shrunk toward the pooled estimate. The shrinkage factor is proportional to the statistical uncertainty of the maximum likelihood estimates, but inversely proportional to the degree of heterogeneity of the city-specific relative risks. In other words, imprecise maximum likelihood estimates (smaller dots) are shrunk toward the pooled estimate more heavily than precise maximum likelihood estimates (larger dots), and the shrinkage is more substantial when the between-city variance of the true relative risks is small.

HEALTH EFFECTS OF EXPOSURE OVER DIFFERENT TIME PERIODS

The previous section discussed the use of time-series data to quantify the association of mortality with short-term exposure to particulate pollution. As mentioned in the Introduction, short-term effects from time series studies appear to be smaller than long-term effects from chronic studies. In this section we discuss how within-city time series comparisons might be used to estimate the effects of exposures of different periods ranging from 1 day to 1 month. The effects of exposures on longer time scales are confounded in time series studies by other causes of seasonal and long-term fluctuations in mortality.

To start, we consider the log-linear distributed lags model for one city:

$$E(y_t) = \exp\left(\eta + \sum_{u=0}^{U} \theta_u x_{t-u}\right)$$

where x_{t-u} is the pollution concentration u days before day t (lag u). Under this model, a unit increase in exposure on day t produces an increase of θ_0 in the linear predictor; an increase of 1 unit for 3 consecutive days, t, $t-1$, and $t-2$ causes an increase of $\theta_0 + \theta_1 + \theta_2$, and so forth. The lagged exposure series are highly colinear, so it is desirable to constrain θ_u to a lower-dimensional subspace. It is common to assume the θ_u form a polynomial or spline function of u (Judge, 1985; Davidson and MacKinnon, 1993; Zanobetti et al., 2000). More generally, we can let $\theta_u = \sum_{j=1}^{p} A_j(u)\beta_j$, so that the distributed lag models above become

$$
\begin{aligned}
Ey_t &= \exp\left(\eta + \sum_{u=0}^{U} \theta_u x_{t-u}\right) \\
&= \exp\left\{\eta + \sum_{j=0}^{p} \beta_j \left(\sum_{u=0}^{U} A_j(u)x_{t-u}\right)\right\} \\
&= \exp\left\{\eta + \sum_{j=1}^{p} \beta_j x_{jt}\right\}
\end{aligned}
\tag{10-3}
$$

where $x_{jt} = \sum_{u=0}^{U} A_j(u)x_{t-u}$ is a linear combination of past exposures.

Kelsall et al. (1999), Zeger et al. (1999), Schwartz (2000), and Dominici et al. (2002d) defined the $A_j(u)$ to obtain a Fourier decomposition or moving average of the exposure time series, so that each x_{jt}, $j = 1, \ldots, p$ represents exposures at different time scales.

Here we define the x_{jt} as follows:

$$x_{1t} = x_t \qquad\qquad x_{4t} = (x_{t-7} + \ldots + x_{t-29})/23$$

$$x_{2t} = (x_{t-1} + x_{t-2})/2 \qquad\qquad x_{5t} = (x_{t-30} + \ldots + x_{t-59})/30$$

$$x_{3t} = (x_{t-3} + \ldots + x_{t-6})/4$$

The β_1 is the log relative rate of mortality of current-day exposure; $\beta_1 + \beta_2$ is the log relative rate of mortality of exposure over the last 3 days, and $\beta_1 + \beta_2 + \beta_3$ is the log relative rate of mortality for the past week exposure.

Figure 10–4 shows the decomposition of the PM_{10} and the temperature time series for Pittsburgh. The component series become smoother at the longer time scales, Also, the PM_{10} series at the longer time scales (30 to 60 days) and the temperature are highly correlated. This correlation reveals the potential for weather and or seasonality to confound the estimates of the chronic exposure effects.

Setting aside this concern temporarily, we estimated model 2 including all of the component PM_{10} series. Figure 10–5 displays the estimated rel-

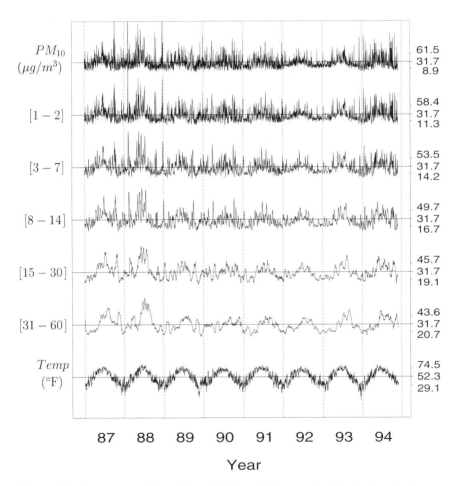

Figure 10–4 Decomposition of the PM10 $\mu g/m^3$ time series for Pittsburgh, Pennsylvania for 1987 through 1994 into 6 average past exposures, as defined in the text. Numbers on the left indicate past days included in each average. Numbers on the right the 10 and 90 percentiles of PM_{10} (Temp).

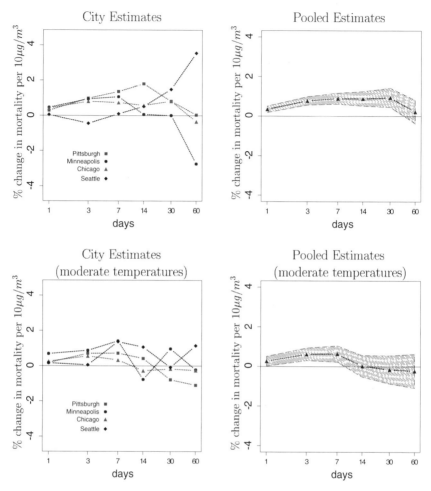

Figure 10–5 Left panels: at the top estimates of the log relative risks of mortality per $10\mu g/m^3$ change in average PM_{10} exposure for the period indicated on the horizontal axis (logarithm scale); at the bottom, estimates of the log relative risks of mortality are obtained by including days with moderate temperatures (e.g., days in the winter season and days with temperatures lower than 40° and higher than 70° Fahrenheit are excluded.) Right panels: pooled estimates of the log relative risk of mortality per $10\mu g/m^3$ change in average reexposure for the period indicated on the horizontal axis (logarithm scale). These results combine the results in the left panels for four cities (Pittsburgh, Minneapolis, Chicago, and Seattle) by taking weighted averages. The shading indicates ± standard errors of the pooled estimates.

ative risk of mortality associated with a 10 $\mu g/m^3$ increase in PM_{10}, for each of the 4 cities with daily PM_{10} data, for the time period indicated on the abscissa for each city (left top panel) and pooled across cities (right top panel). These estimates are just the cumulative sum of the regression coefficients for the components at time scales up to and including the indicated period.

Note that the Seattle results are distinct from those for Pittsburgh, Minneapolis, and Chicago. In Seattle, the relative risk depends on length of exposure: longer exposure has a greater estimated effect on mortality. Instead, in Chicago and Pittsburgh, longer exposure to increased levels of PM_{10} is associated with lower mortality.

These divergent patterns indicate that, at longer time scales, weather and/or seasonality might confound the air pollution mortality association. In Pittsburgh, Minneapolis, and Chicago, PM_{10} has a summer maximum, as does temperature. But mortality is highest in the winter because of weather and influenza epidemics. Hence, both temperature and the slowly varying components of PM_{10} are negatively correlated with mortality. Failure to completely control for weather, season, or both, would therefore bias the coefficients for longer-term components of PM_{10} to more negative values.

Because of use of wood stoves, in Seattle PM_{10} has a winter maximum instead. Hence, it has the opposite relationship to temperature. Here, failure to completely control for weather and season will tend to bias the coefficients at the longer time scales to more positive values. In summary, it is expected that confounding would produce the pattern seen here. In addition, the degree of separation in patterns between Seattle and the other cities changes with the numbers degrees of freedom in the spline function of time, further indicating that the pattern is the result of confounding.

To simplify the problem of completely controlling for weather and seasonality, we repeated the analysis above restricting our attention to the non-winter days with temperatures in the temperate range 40–70° Fahrenheit. Figure 10–5 shows the new estimates of the period-specific relative risks for the four cities and pooled across cities. The difference between Seattle and the other cities has been reduced but not entirely eliminated. This analysis demonstrates the difficulty of using time series data to estimate health effects of chronic exposures in the presence of other confounding variables at longer time scales.

JOINT ANALYSIS OF COHORT AND TIME SERIES DATA

As is discussed in Health Effects of Exposure over Different Time Periods, above, the health effects of long-term exposure to air pollution cannot be estimated unless risks are compared across populations, in this case cities. This problem arises because long-term exposure varies a little within a city in long-term exposure and because of confounding by influenza and other trends represented by S^c(time) in model 10-2.

In this section, we briefly discuss a model for simultaneously estimating the effects of chronic and acute exposures on mortality. We envision a data set that consists of the mortality data, daily pollution concentrations, and personal risk factors for a population living in a large number of distinct geographic regions. Such data are available for the Medicare and veteran populations, for example.

The basic model for λ_{it}^c, the risk for an individual i living in county c on day t, is

$$\lambda_{it}^c = \lambda_{0it}^c \exp\left(\sum_{j=0}^{p} x_{jt}^c \beta_j^c + z_{it}^c \alpha^c\right)$$

where λ_{0it}^c is the baseline risk without pollution exposure, x_{jt}^c is the j-th exposure variable in city c on day t, as discussed in Health Effects of Exposure over Different Time Periods, above, and z_{it}^c is a vector of personal characteristics centered at their average value. To combine the cohort and time series analyses under a common umbrella, we define the first exposure $x_{0t}^c = \bar{x}^c$ to be the average exposure values for a prior extended period and center the remaining exposure variables about $\bar{x}^c$; that is, replace x_{jt}^c by $x_{jt}^c - \bar{x}^c$. To compare persons across cities, we must further assume that z_{it}^c includes all relevant person- and city-level confounders so that $\lambda_{0it}^c = \lambda_{0t}^c$. Then, we have

$$\lambda_{it}^c = \lambda_{0t}^c \exp\left(\bar{x}^c \beta_C + \sum_{j=1}^{p} x_{jt}^c \beta_{T_j}^c + z_{it}^c \alpha^c\right) \tag{10-4}$$

This model is the basis for simultaneous inference about both the "cohort" β_C and the "time series" $\beta_{T_j}^c$ relative risks. As discussed above, the x_{jt}^c that represent long-term exposures are confounded by components in z_{it}^c at similar time scales (e.g., seasonality), necessitating comparisons across cities. We would again use $\beta_{T_j}^c$ in a two- or three-level hierarchical model to pool the time series relative risks for different exposure periods across cites and regions. By formulating the model to include both β_C and $\beta_{T_j}^c$, we can estimate and test the difference between β_C and the $\sum_{j=1}^{p} \beta_{T_j}^c$.

Estimating the parameters in Eq. 10-4 is computationally intensive. At one extreme, this estimation can be treated as a very large parametric survival analysis with possibly millions of persons at risk and many time-varying predictor variables. But, the analyses can be simplified because z_{it}^c

contains two kinds of predictor variables: those such as smoking or socioeconomic factors that vary across individuals but not across time (z_{1i}); and others such as temperature and season, that vary across time but not across individuals within a city (z_{2t}^c). We write $z_{it}^c \alpha^c = z_{1i} \alpha_1^c + z_{2t}^c \alpha_2^c$. Then, if we sum Eq. 10–4 across individuals within a city, we have

$$\mathrm{E}(y_t^c) \simeq \exp\left(S^c(t) + \sum_{j=1}^{p} x_{jt}^c \beta_{T_j}^c + z_{2t}^c \alpha_2^c \right)$$

where $S^c(t) = \log\lambda_{0t} + \bar{x}^c \beta_C + \bar{z}_1 \alpha_1^c$. This is the usual time series model discussed in Statistical Models for Time Series Data, above.

The likelihood function for $S^c(t)$, λ_{0t}, β_C, α_1^c, $\beta_{T_j}^c$, and α_2^c can be jointly maximized. Alternatively, a simpler algorithm might involve two steps: use standard semiparametric log-linear regression to estimate $\beta_{T_j}^c$ and α_2^c, removing information about $S^c(t)$, and regressing $\hat{S}^c(t)$ on a smooth function of time common to all cities to estimate $\log \lambda_{0t}$, and on $\bar{x}^c$ and $\bar{z}_1$ to estimate β_C and α_1^c. Interesting methodological questions include how to formulate the joint estimation of β_C and $\beta_{T_j}^c$, in the hierarchical extension of Eq. 10–4; whether the simpler two-stage algorithm is nearly efficient; and how to extend Eq. 10–4 to use cohort and time series information to estimate some of the $\beta_{T_j}^c$s for x_{jt}s that vary at longer time scales.

CONCLUSION

This chapter illustrates the use of log-linear regression and hierarchical models to estimate the association of daily mortality with acute exposure to particulate air pollution. We used daily time series data for the 88 largest cities in the United States from 1987 to 1994 obtained from NMMAPS. Time series analyses such as those ones illustrated here rely entirely on comparisons of mortality across days within a population. They therefore have the advantage of avoiding confounding by unmeasured differences among populations, as may occur in cohort studies. They have the disadvantage of only providing evidence about the health effects of shorter-term acute exposures. The reason is that longer-term exposures hardly vary within a population. Also processes such as influenza epidemics or changes in health behaviors are difficult to quantify, occur at these longer time scales, and will likely confound estimates from time series studies of the effects of chronic exposures. We chose to control for longer-term confounders by using models that partial out the variation in exposure and mortality at longer time scales. We achieved this control by including spline functions of time with 7 degrees of freedom per year and spline functions of temperature and dew point temperature to control for weather (smoothing splines or natural cubic splines). We checked whether using half or twice as many degrees of freedom quantitatively change the results and found that it does not. The possibility remains, however, that the effects of confounders are not totally controlled by these statistical adjustments.

We fit a separate log-linear regression for each of the 88 cities and conducted a second-stage analysis to estimate the variability in the pollution relative risk among cities within a region and among regions; to obtain empirical Bayes estimates of each city's relative risk, and to estimate the average relative risk across the 88 cities. As did others (Smith et al., 1997, 2000; Clyde, 2000), we found that the exact specification of the log-linear regression (e.g., the choice of the number of degrees of freedom in the smoothing splines or the number and location of knots in the regression splines), can substantially affect the estimated pollution relative risk for a particular city. However, we found that variations in the specification tend to have little effect on the pooled estimate or on the empirical Bayes estimates for that city. Hence, pooling information across a large number of cities provides a more robust model. The details of such investigations have been provided by Dominici et al. (2000a).

A Bayesian hierarchical model to pool information across 88 cities was used. This model requires specifying prior distributions. Here, the key priors are for the within- and among-region variances of the true relative risks. We assumed half-normal priors with large variances instead of the more traditional conjugate inverse gamma prior. In our experience, the inverse gamma prior implicitly rules out the possibility of no variability in the relative risks and produces posterior distributions with more mass at larger values. The result is to borrow less strength across cities when estimating the risk for one city and wider confidence intervals for the estimated average coefficient across cities. The posterior distribution obtained, assuming a half-normal prior, is more similar to the likelihood function and hence we prefer it in this application. Sensitivity analyses of the posterior distribution of the pooled air pollution effect, under four specifications of the prior distributions for the within- and among-region variances of the true relative risks in alternative to the half-normal, have been discussed by Dominici et al. (2002a).

We used the time series data from four cities with more complete particulate pollution records to estimate a distributed lags model. We then estimated the mortality relative risk associated with a 10 $\mu g/m^3$ increase in PM_{10} for 1, 3, 7, 30, and 60 days. We found evidence of possibly substantial confounding by seasonality and weather at the longer time scales. In fact, the longer-term variation in PM_{10} is highly correlated with temperature. To overcome this problem, we restricted the analyses to nonwinter days with moderate temperature. In this subset of the data, we found that the mortality relative risk increases with the duration of exposure up to approximately 7 to 14 days but not beyond. The total effect sizes are still much smaller than those seen in the cohort studies. The evidence of confounding of the longer-term components of PM_{10} shows the limitations of time series models for estimating the health effects of chronic exposure to pollutants.

Finally, we briefly outlined an approach to jointly estimate the cohort and time series relative risks from a single, large data base. Several such data bases exist, including the Medicare Cohort from the National Claims History File. This data base includes all mortality, morbidity, and basic demographic information on more than 2 million persons per year. In addition, the Medicare Current Beneficiary Survey provides detailed personal information on a representative subsample of roughly 13,000 persons per year. If these data were merged with weather and pollution time series for each person, chronic and acute effects could be estimated from a common data source. The differences in the current estimates of the particulate air pollution relative risks deriving from cohort and time series studies must be better understood. When these are obtained from different sources of data with different protocols, it is unclear whether the differences reflect greater effects of chronic exposure or biases from one or both of the studies. The proposed approach can address some of these issues using a refined version of the analyses discussed here.

REFERENCES

American Thoracic Society, Basom, R. (1996). Health effects of outdoor air pollution, Part 2. *American Journal of Respiratory and Critical Care Medicine* **153,** 477–498.

Bell, M. and Davis, D. (2001). Reassessment of the lethal london fog of 1952: novel indicators of acute and chronic consequences of acute exposure to air pollution. *Environmental Health Perspective* **109,** 389–394.

Clyde, M. (2000). Model uncertainty and health effect studies for particulate matter environmetrics. *Environmetrics* **11,** 745–763.

Curriero, F., Heiner, K., Samet, J., Zeger, S., Strug, L., and Patz, J. (2002). Temperature and mortality in 11 cities of the eastern United States. *American Journal of Epidemiology* **155,** 80–87.

Daniels, M., Dominici, F., Samet, J.M., and Zeger, S.L. (2000). Estimating PM10-mortality dose-response curves and threshold levels: an analysis of daily time-series for the 20 largest US cities. *American Journal of Epidemiology* **152,** 397–412.

Davidson, R. and MacKinnon, J. (1993). *Estimation and Inference in Econometrics.* New York: Oxford University Press.

Dockery, D., Pope, C.A., Xu, X., Spengler, J., Ware, J., Fay, M., Ferris, B., and Speizer, F. (1993). An association between air pollution and mortality in six U.S. cities. *New England Journal of Medicine* **329**, 1753–1759.

Dominici, F., Daniels, M., Zeger, S.L., and Samet, J.M. (2002a). Air pollution and mortality: Estimating regional and national dose-response relationships. *Journal of the American Statistical Association* **97**, 100–111.

Dominici, F., McDermott, A., Zeger, S.L., and Samet, J.M. (2002b). On the use of generalized additive models in time series studies of air pollution and health. *American Journal of Epidemiology* **156**, 1–11.

Dominici, F., McDermott, A., Zeger, S.L., and Samet, J.M. (2003c). Airborne particulate matter and mortality: time-scale effects in four US cities. *American Journal of Epidemiology (in press)*.

Dominici, F., McDermott, A., Zeger, S.L., and Samet, J.M. (2002d). *A Report to the Health Effects Institute on Reanalyses of the NMMAPS Database*. Cambridge, MA: The Health Effects Institute.

Dominici, F., Samet, J.M., and Zeger, S.L. (2000a). Combining evidence on air pollution and daily mortality from the twenty largest US cities: a hierarchical modeling strategy (with discussion). *Royal Statistical Society, Series A* **163**, 263–303.

Dominici, F., Zeger, S.L., and Samet, J.M. (2000b). A measurement error correction model for time-series studies of air pollution and mortality. *Biostatistics* **2**, 157–175.

Environmental Protection Agency (1995). Proposed guidelines for neurotoxicity risk assessment. *Environmental Protection Agency*.

Gilks, W.R., Richardson, S., and Spiegelhalter, D.J., eds. (1996). *Markov Chain Monte Carlo in Practice*. London: Chapman and Hall.

Guttorp, P., Sheppard, L., and Smith, R. (2001). *Comments on the PM Criteria Document*. Technical report, University of Washington, Seattle, Washington.

Hastie, T.J. and Tibshirani, R.J. (1990). *Generalized additive models*. New York: Chapman and Hall.

Hwang, J. and Chan, C. (2002). Air pollution effects on daily clinic visits for lower respiratory illness. *American Journal of Epidemiology* **155**, 1–10.

Judge, G.G. (1985). *The Theory and Practice of Econometrics, 2nd ed.* New York: Wiley.

Katsouyanni, K., Toulomi, G., Spix, C., Balducci, F., Medina, S., Rossi, G., Wojtyniak, B., Sunyer, J., Bacharova, L., Schouten, J., Ponka, A., and Anderson, H.R. (1997). Short term effects of ambient sulphur dioxide and particulate matter on mortality in 12 european cities: results from time series data from the APHEA project. *British Medical Journal* **314**, 1658–1663.

Kelsall, J., Samet, J.M., and Zeger, S.L. (1997). Air pollution, and mortality in Philadelphia, 1974–1988. *American Journal of Epidemiology* **146**, 750–762.

Kelsall, J., Zeger, S.L., and Samet, J.M. (1999). Frequency domain log-linear models; air pollution and mortality. *The Royal Statistical Society, Series C* **48**, 331–344.

Krewski, D., Burnett, R.T., Goldberg, M.S., Hoover, K., Siemiatycki, J., Jerrett, M., Abrahamowicz, M., and White, W.H. (2000). *Reanalysis of the Harvard Six Cities Study and the American Cancer Society Study of Particulate Air Pollution and Mortality*. Cambridge, MA: Health Effects Institute.

Lipfert, F. and Wyzga, R. (1993). Air pollution and mortality: issues and uncertainty. *Journal of the Air Waste Management Association* **45**, 949–966.

Logan, W. and Glasg, M. (1953). Mortality in London for incident, 1953. *Lancet*
1, 336–338.

McCullagh, P. and Nelder, J.A. (1989). *Generalized Linear Models*, 2ND Ed. London: Chapman & Hall.

National Research Council (1998). Research priorities for airborne particulate matter. part i. immediate priorities and a long-range research portfolio. *Washington, DC: National Academy Press.*

Pope, A.C. and Dockery, D.W. (1999). Epidemiology of particle effects. In: *Air Pollution and Health.* San Diego: Academic Press, pp. 673–705.

Pope, C.A., Dockery, D., and Schwartz, J. (1995a). Review of epidemiological evidence of health effects of particulate air pollution. *Inhalation Toxicology* **47,** 1–18.

Pope, C.A., Thun, M., Namboodiri, M., Dockery, D., Evans, J., Speizer, F., and Heath, C. (1995b). Particulate air pollution as a predictor of mortality in a prospective study of U.S. adults. *American Journal of Respiratory Critical Care Medicine* **151,** 669–674.

Samet, J.M., Dominici, F., Curriero, F., Coursac, I., and Zeger, S.L. (2000a). Fine particulate air pollution and mortality in 20 U.S. cities: 1987–1994 (with discussion). *New England Journal of Medicine* **343,** 1742–1757.

Samet, J.M., Zeger, S.L., Dominici, F., Curriero, F., Coursac, I., Dockery, D., Schwartz, J., and Zanobetti, A. (2000b). *The National Morbidity, Mortality, and Air Pollution Study (HEI Project No. 96-7): Morbidity and Mortality from Air Pollution in the United States.* Cambridge, MA: Health Effects Institute.

Samet, J.M., Zeger, S.L., Dominici, F., Dockery, D., and Schwartz, J. (2000c). *The National Morbidity, Mortality, and Air Pollution Study (HEI Project No. 96-7): Methods and Methodological Issues.* Cambridge, MA: Health Effects Institute.

Schwartz, J. (1995). Air pollution and daily mortality in Birmingham, Alabama. *American Journal of Epidemiology* **137,** 1136–1147.

Schwartz, J. (2000). Harvesting and long term exposure effects in the relation between air pollution and mortality. *American Journal of Epidemiology* **151,** 440–448.

Schwartz, J. and Marcus, A. (1990). Mortality and air pollution in London: a time series analysis. *American Journal of Epidemiology* **131,** 185–194.

Smith, L., Davis, J., Sacks, J., Speckman, P., and Styer, P. (1997). Assessing the human health risk of atmospheric particle. *Proceedings of the American Statistical Association. Section on Environmental Statistics.*

Smith, R., Davis, J., Sacks, J., Speckman, P., and Styer, P. (2000). Regression models for air pollution and daily mortality: analysis of data from Birmingham, Alabama. *Environmetrics* **100,** 719–745.

Tierney, L. (1994). Markov chains for exploring posterior distributions (with discussion). *Annals of Statistics* **22,** 1701–1762.

Zanobetti, A., Wand, M., Schwartz, J., and Ryan, L. (2000). Generalized additive distributed lag models. *Biostatistics* **1,** 279–292.

Zeger, S., Thomas, D., Dominici, F., Cohen, A., Schwartz, J., Dockery, D., and Samet, J. (2000). Measurement error in time-series studies of air pollution: concepts and consequences. *Environmental Health Perspectives* **108,** 419–426.

Zeger, S.L., Dominici, F., and Samet, J.M. (1999). Harvesting-resistant estimates of pollution effects on mortality. *Epidemiology* **89,** 171–175.

11

Some Considerations in Spatial-Temporal Analysis of Public Health Surveillance Data

ANDREW B. LAWSON

This chapter deals with the development and use of statistical methods for geographic disease surveillance. Where appropriate, it refers to temporal aspects of surveillance that have been developed and raises the possibilities for spatiotemporal disease surveillance. Surveillance has an implicit temporal dimension, that is, populations are often monitored over time to assess changes that may warrant action.

The following section discusses some ideas that are commonly used in statistical process control (SPC) and considers their relevance to disease surveillance. The third section addresses the three areas to which the study of the distribution of disease can be applied: disease mapping, disease clustering, and ecological analysis. The fourth section presents models for spatial surveillance of disease maps and considers disease clustering. The fifth section describes monitoring in a fixed time period and in an evolving time frame. The sixth section reviews disease surveillance modeling and present a simple example of a spatial temporal disease map analysis. Finally the software available for spatial temporal map surveillance is described.

STATISTICAL PROCESS CONTROL AND SURVEILLANCE

Surveillance of the health of populations is fundamental to public health intervention, yet statistical approaches to temporal, and especially, spatial epidemiology are underdeveloped. Although temporal cluster alarm monitoring has received some attention in disease surveillance (see for example Chen et al. [1993, 1997]) few attempts have been made to examine spatiotemporal problems. Rogerson (1997) made one such attempt by examining changes in spatial clustering over time for noninfectious diseases.

Surveillance data can be used to set limits on the acceptable incidence of disease in a temporal or spatial domain and on actions taken if these limits are passed. Limits may be based on a single observed disease pattern or on the outcomes of many ancillary variables. For example, outbreaks of acute intestinal disease could be accompanied by increased sales of diarrhea remedies, and thus monitoring of the disease and pharmaceutical sales may form the basis of a surveillance system. This is the basis of syndromic health surveillance.

Several methods have been developed for detecting changes in populations over time. These methods involve estimating changepoints in a sequence of disease events or a time series of population rates (Lai [1995]), or determining or applying control limits to the behavior of a system. Simple methods can assist in assessing change or "in control" behavior. Some methods are derived from SPC, which was developed in manufacturing for the monitoring of industrial processes over time and could be applied in a disease surveillance program with due care. For example, the temporal variation in count data can be monitored by using a Poisson control chart (C or U chart), upon which can be plotted specific limits, beyond which corrective action should be taken. These charts are based on normal pivotal approximations.

An exact interval could be constructed for independent Poisson counts in an attempt to use SPC methods in disease surveillance. However, if the counts were correlated even under the null hypothesis, some allowance must be made for this correlation in the chart. A further issue in the use of such methods in disease monitoring, is incorporating any changes in the background at-risk population. One possibility, in the temporal domain, is to employ relative risk estimates. An example is the use of standardized ratios, for example y_i/e_i, where y_i is the count of disease within the ith time period, and e_i is the expected count for the same period. The expected count could be calculated from a standard population. A commonly used ratio of this form is the standardized mortality ratio (SMR), and y_i would be the count of deaths from the disease of interest. An appropriate sampling distribution could be used to provide control limits. One simple possibility might be to use a log transformation of the SMR (possibly with a correction factor) and to assume an approximate Gaussian sampling distribution. However, the SMR at a given time point is a saturated estimate, and, to avoid instabilities related to the ratio form, it may be better to monitor sample averages of SMRs (or transformations of averages) over time periods. Incorporating correlation or correlated heterogeneity should also be considered. For large aggregation scales, time series methods that allow temporal dependence have been used (Farrington and Beale, 1998; see also Chapters 8 and 9).

In addition, special charts (cusum charts) have been developed specifically to detect changes in patterns over time (changepoints). Cusum charts are constructed by recording events cumulatively over time; the accumulation is sensitive to changepoints in the process under consideration. Frisen and co-workers and others (Frisen and Mare, 1991; Frisen, 1992; Lai, 1995; Wessman, 1998) have applied these ideas in medical surveillance and monitoring. These methods must be specially adapted to deal with the spatial and spatiotemporal nature of geographic surveillance.

The main issues in temporal surveillance that affect spatial and spatiotemporal surveillance fall into three categories. (1) detecting changepoints (mean level, variance), (2) detecting clusters, and (3) detecting overall process change. Conventional SPC would use control limits to detect shifts in single or multiple parameters in situations where the target parameters are usually constant. However any monitoring system must allow for natural variations in disease incidence, especially when the population at risk varies. Particular departures from the normal variation are often of greater interest than simple shifts of parameters. Changepoints, which indicate jumps in incidence, could be of interest, as could clusters of disease or an overall process change, wherein various parameters change. A disease surveillance system is likely to focus on one or all of these changes. Indeed the multiple focus of such a system poses challenges for the development of statistical methodology.

ISSUES IN DISEASE MAPPING

Maps of disease-incidence data are basic tools for assessing regional public health. An early example of disease mapping is the mapping of addresses of cholera in 1854 by John Snow, who recorded victims. addresses and assessed their proximity to putative pollution sources (water supply pumps).

Recent interest in disease mapping (Elliott et al., 2000; Lawson and Williams, 2001; Lawson, 2001a,b) has led to a great use of geographic or spatial statistical tools in analyzing data routinely collected for public health purposes and found in ecologic studies of disease causation. The study of the geographic distribution of disease has many applications, including disease mapping, disease clustering, and ecologic analysis. The main purpose of disease mapping is to estimate the true relative risk of a disease of interest across a geographic study area (map): a process similar to that of processing pixel images to remove noise. Applications lie in health services resource allocation and disease atlas construction (see, for example, Pickle et al. [1999]).

Disease clustering is particularly useful for assessing whether a disease is clustered and where clusters are located (Lawson [2001b]; see also Chapter 6). This may lead to examination of potential environmental hazards. Analyzing disease incidence around a putative source of pollution hazard is a special case of cluster detection (Lawson [2001b]; see also Chapter 7).

Ecologic analysis, is useful in epidemiologic research, because it focusses on the geographic distribution of disease in relation to explanatory covariates, usually at an aggregated spatial level. Many issues in disease mapping apply to ecologic analysis, but in ecologic analysis issues relating to incorporating covariates must also be considered.

SOME MODELS FOR SPATIAL DISEASE SURVEILLANCE

In spatial surveillance, a wide range of methods can be applied to a single map of events within a fixed time frame or period. Many methods in disease mapping, clustering, or ecologic analysis can be used as surveillance tools (Jarpe, 1998). For example, general clustering tests could be applied, or residuals from disease maps fitted in each time period could be examined. Such methods may provide evidence of unusual variation in incidence, unusual clustering, or a spatial trend on the map (e.g., related to a putative source). However, few methods are designed to detect a spatial temporal pattern or change in pattern. As in temporal surveillance (see Statistical Process Control and Surveillance, above), important features to detect in the spatial domain are localized discontinuities in mean level or variance of risk (changepoints), spatial clusters of disease, and overall process change. Standardized mortality ratios for lip cancer in former East Germany for 1980–1989, computed in the 219 municipalities from expected counts based on the age $\times$ sex breakdown of the study region (Eastern Germany) reveal all three forms of change (Fig 11–1): large changes of risk between neighbors can be seen in the north (discontinuities), a cluster of low incidence in the south (spatial clusters), and north–south change in overall level of incidence and variability (process change).

In the spatial domain, disease map variation may be modelled using global models; that is, the overall variation in the map is described by a

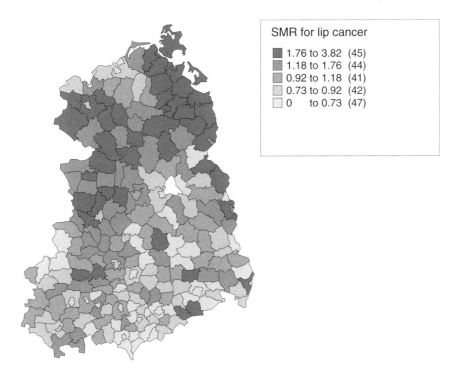

SMR for lip cancer

- ■ 1.76 to 3.82 (45)
- ■ 1.18 to 1.76 (44)
- ▦ 0.92 to 1.18 (41)
- ▧ 0.73 to 0.92 (42)
- □ 0   to 0.73 (47)

Figure 11–1 Standardized mortality ratio (SMR) for lip cancer in 219 municipalities of the former East Germany from 1980 to 1989, expected rates are based on the national rates for 18 age/sex classes. Parenthetical numbers are group counts.

model in which single parameters describe the global characteristics of the map, such as a long range trend, a short-range covariation or a nonspatial variation. One approach to such modeling is to assume a Bayesian model for the variation in incidence in which the features of interest are specified under prior distributions. The full model posterior distribution of relative risk across the map is sampled and typically averaged to give posterior expected values. The Bayesian model fitted to the lip cancer data in Figures 11–1 and 11–2 was a global model (the Besag-York-Mollié (BYM) model [Besag et al., 1991]), that included terms describing nonspatial and spatial heterogeneity. The count, y_j, in each small area, is assumed to follow a Poisson distribution and the expected count under this model is $E(y_j) = e_j\theta_j$ where the standardized rate for the small area is e_j and the relative risk is θ_j. Further the log relative risk is assumed to consist of a sum of components of variation:

$$\log(\theta_j) = u_j + v_j$$

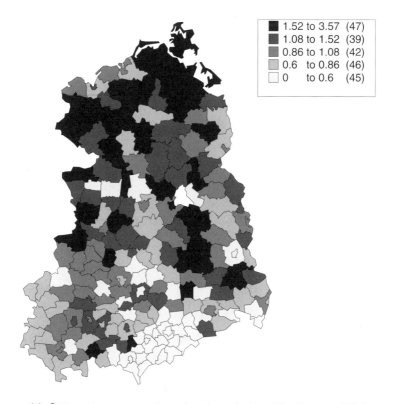

■	1.52 to 3.57	(47)
■	1.08 to 1.52	(39)
■	0.86 to 1.08	(42)
■	0.6 to 0.86	(46)
□	0 to 0.6	(45)

Figure 11–2 Posterior expectations for the relative risks from a full Bayesian (BYM) model fitted with correlated and uncorrelated components of variation.

The u_j term represents spatially correlated extra variation, and the v_j term represents uncorrelated extra variation. The components have prior distributions that define their identifiable role and also allow their proper estimation. The model is designed to address the recovery of true risk by smoothing out noise, and is not specifically designed to detect clusters or localized discontinuities. The resulting relative risk estimates (Fig 11–2) do display some evidence of such features but they are not estimated directly as parameters. Although these models impose global structure on the map, they can also be used informally to assess localized features by residual analysis. Fig 11–3 displays a residual p-value surface that suggests that the southern area of the map contains a cluster of low incidence. Lawson (2001a) discusses in more detail the derivation and use of p-value residual surfaces.

For assessing clustering or localized discontinuities, the use of models that are sensitive to the localized spatial structure of the map, termed specific models, are more appropriate. This is particularly important when spa-

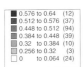

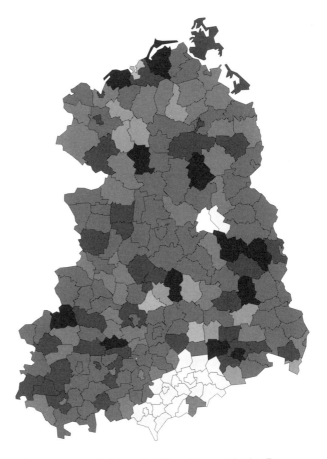

Figure 11–3 P-value surface computed from the Bayesian residuals (Lawson, 2001a) from the BYM model fit in Figure 11–2, based on a parametric bootstrap from the MCMC model fit.

tiotemporal surveillance is envisaged, as it may be the spatial spread of disease over time which is a focus, and this cannot be easily captured by global models. Hence pointwise goodness-of-fit measures from global nonspecific models can be useful. However, specific spatiotemporal models that address features such as discontinuities, clusters and process change are also needed.

SPATIOTEMPORAL MONITORING

Here, I consider two situations in which monitoring or surveillance is carried out: a fixed time period or frame, where all cases of a disease are recorded; and an evolving time frame. In the first situation, a time period, T, say, and a spatial window or frame, W, are specified.

Fixed Spatial and Temporal Frame

Case events

A case event is the residential address of a person (case) with a disease, and is usually unique, because for most noninfectious diseases, multiple cases have little chance of arising in one specific location. The residential address can be an exact street address or a broader location (e.g., a zip code [USA] or a post code unit [UK]).

For m case events in the frame, the location of each event is recorded in space–time coordinates $\{s_i, t_i\}$, $i = 1, \ldots, m$. First consider the simple situation where the time coordinates $\{t_i\}$ are unknown. When location is all that is known only a spatial realization is available, and the spatial structure can only be examined for spatial effects (e.g., spatial clusters or clustering, or association with putative sources, etc.). In principle, any relevant spatial testing or modeling procedure could be applied (see Chapters 3 and 4), and the choice of procedure would depend on the hypotheses to be assessed. For example, monitoring disease clusters in the space–time frame chosen might address a public health concern, and so a cluster model or general clustering test might be performed. This form of surveillance does not explicitly include any temporal comparison, although different time frames, for the same spatial frame, might be informally compared.

When both the spatial and temporal coordinates of case events are available, a temporal component of the analysis can be included. Here, it is assumed that a sequential analysis is precluded, and that the complete realization of events within the space–time frame is to be considered. Including a temporal component considerably widens the scope and potential focus of the surveillance task. For example, it is possible to consider general models for the spatial temporal variation in disease and to estimate spatial, temporal and spatiotemporal aspects of these models for the complete realization of events. The intensity of such a model could be, in its general form:

$$\lambda(\mathbf{s}, t) = p.g(\mathbf{s}, t).f_1(\mathbf{s}; \theta_s).f_2(t; \theta_t).f_3(\mathbf{s}, t; \theta_{st}) \tag{11–1}$$

Here, the parameters are divided into spatial (θ_s), temporal (θ_t), and spatiotemporal (θ_{st}) components, and the model consists of components relating to each of these categories ($\{f_i\}$). If the aim of surveillance is to assess spatiotemporal features of the realization, the θ_{xt} can be the main focus. Focussing on purely temporal and spatial aspects as well may also be of interest. If spatiotemporal clustering is of interest, then $f_3(\mathbf{s}, t; \theta_{st})$ can be structured to include cluster term(s), and the other components can be regarded as nuisance terms. For purely spatial effects, parameters in θ_s must be estimated jointly with other components.

Tract counts

A tract count is a count of cases of disease found in a specific tract or small area. For tract counts in fixed spatial regions, a similar approach may be used when the integrated intensity is adopted:

$$E\{y_{jt}\} = \int_{l_t} \int_{a_j} \lambda(\mathbf{u},v)\,d\mathbf{s}dt \qquad (11\text{--}2)$$

for the time frame T, in which fixed time periods are $\{l_t\}$, t = 1, . . . , T. Here, I assume the complete realization of counts within the time frame T is to be modeled. Again, similar considerations apply when different components of the intensity are the focus. In the spatiotemporal case, clustering or interaction of spatial and temporal random effects may be the main concern, and would be estimated jointly with other components. If the focus is purely temporal, Poisson regression can be used with the decoupling approximation (assumption of constant rates within tracts) to estimate temporal trend and covariate effects. However, Poisson regression usually involves estimation of the spatial and spatiotemporal effects as nuisance effects, and these components are better estimated jointly. Similar considerations apply when a spatial focus is required.

Although a purely parametric approach to surveillance can be used, as described above, an approach that makes few assumptions may also be favored. When little is known about the cause of a disease, a nonparametric approach might be suitable. In that case, the methods used depend on the focus of the inquiry. For example, if the purpose is to examine the space–time variation in disease to, say, isolate areas of elevated risk (possible clusters), smoothing techniques may be best, and nonparametric density estimation or kernel regression could be used. The approach of Kelsall and Diggle (1995) and Lawson and Williams (1993) in estimating relative risk surfaces could be extended to the space-time framework and could lead to the construction of p value surfaces based on simulation. The main drawback of these methods is that they do not use probability models for the data likelihood and so may not correctly represent the underlying true risk. This problem was found in simulation studies which evaluated a variety of purely spatial methods (Lawson et al., 2000). Thus the use of empirical Bayes methods of smoothing based on relatively simple probability models for the random variation, may be preferable. Alternatively, the relative risk generalized additive models (GAMs) of Kelsall and Diggle (1998) may be extended.

Fixed Spatial Frame and Dynamic Temporal Frame

Here I consider two scenarios: monitoring continues until the next event (either a case event with known location in space-time or one known only to reside in a particular census tract), or monitoring is carried out in specific sequential time periods. In the former, a new event activates the examination of the map. In the latter, the end of a time period allows the map to be evaluated retrospectively. Retrospective evaluation is the simplest method of surveillance for routinely collected health data. For example, yearly recordings of mortality counts in small areas are commonly available in many countries.

Case events

Time to next event monitoring.

When locations of cases in space–time are available, developing a "time-to-event" monitoring system can be considered. An early example of a sequential method for examining point events, in strictly temporal monitoring, was proposed by Bartholomew (1956). More recently, Chen (1978) and Chen et al. (1993) proposed a method of temporal surveillance based on the assumption that times between events have a simple exponential distribution with a fixed mean μ, and the authors developed a method of detecting sequences of short times. If the assumptions made for spatial case event intensities are mirrored, a basic assumption of the case event temporal distribution would be that

$$\lambda(t) = g(t).f(t) \qquad (11\text{--}3)$$

where it may be possible to assume that $g(t) \equiv g$, a constant for certain time periods. In that case, $y \sim Pois\{g.\int_0^T f(u)du\}$ in a time period T.

In spatial temporal monitoring, the joint space–time intensity of an event at $\{\mathbf{s},t\}$ is specified as $\lambda(\mathbf{s},t;\theta)$, where θ is a parameter vector. In the context of optimal surveillance, an alarm function could be constructed for this situation as

$$p_n = \sum_{k=1}^{n} \pi_k \sum_{u=k}^{n} \left\{ \frac{\lambda(\mathbf{s}_u,t_u;\theta_1)}{\lambda(\mathbf{s}_u,t_u;\theta_0)} \right\} \exp\{-\Lambda_{\theta_1} + \Lambda_{\theta_0}\} / \sum_{k=1}^{n} \pi_k, \qquad (11\text{--}4)$$

where $\Lambda_\theta = \int_0^{t_n} \int_W \lambda(\mathbf{s},t;\theta)d\mathbf{s}dt$, t_n is the time of the nth event, and the probability of an alarm at the kth event is π_k.

Tests may be constructed that are sequential but exploit Markov chain-Monte Carlo (MCMC) methods whereby the null distribution of the test is the equilibrium distribution of the chain, and the chain is run from the current observed data in specified directions toward the equilibrium distribution. For example, to test for spatial temporal correlation in case events, a test statistic could be calculated from the existing data, and a birth death algorithm could be used that has as its equilibrium distribution complete spatial temporal randomness (conditional on nuisance parameters). Besag and Clifford (1991) discussed the sequential implementation of such procedures.

Extending these procedures to models wherein prior distributions are admitted would typically require the deployment of Bayesian methodology. Several approaches might be fruitful. Bayes factors could be examined to detect changes in overall pattern in space–time. In spatial temporal models it may be possible to examine two different situations: use the predictive distribution of future events to examine the distribution of the next case, or compare a model for the current realization of cases with a model fitted to the current realization and the new case. The first option may require a formulation that is akin to the updating methods of Kong et al. (1994) and Berzuini et al. (1997), which were originally applied to fixed-time-frame examples.

Some hypotheses in spatial temporal studies may require specific models or test procedures to be developed. For example, although examining global clustering by sequential or other methods may be beneficial, devising methods for examining the local variation in clustering in subsections of space or time may also be useful. To this end, models or tests that monitor localized aggregations of events (which may be aggregated to assess global features) may be a fruitful avenue for further development.

Fixed-time-period monitoring.   The evolution of mapped case event data in fixed time periods can be regarded as a special case of the situation described in Case Events, above, wherein the spatial distribution of cases is to be examined and compared between time slices. In this situation, the cumulative realization of events (up to the current period) may be examined, either by sequentially examining the cumulative effects of time progression or by a comparing the current complete realization of events to the previous one. Further, a sequential procedure can be constructed that would detect changes in the spatial temporal distribution of events by adding each time frame. These methods could also be adapted to this situation.

Tract counts

Time-to-next-event monitoring.   Rogerson (1997) proposed a method of monitoring that involves computing a cusum of standardized deviation from expectation whenever a new case arises in a tract. This method relies on computing a global clustering measure (in Rogerson, 1997), Tango's general clustering test C_G is used) and its comparison with the expected value conditional on the measure computed at the time of the previous case event. The statistic used is:

$$Z_i = \frac{C_{G,i} - E(C_{G,i}|C_{G,i-1})}{\sigma_{C_{G,i}|C_{G,i-1}}} \tag{11-5}$$

where subscript i denotes the current event, $i - 1$ denotes the previous event, and $\sigma_{C_{G,i}|C_{G,i-1}}$ is the standard error of the difference. The conditional expectation is defined by computing a function of the clustering measure, with a single case added to the $i - 1$th counts in each of the m tracts in turn. The $\{Z_i\}$ will not be normally distributed and the author recommended that batches of these measures be averaged. Process control methods are used to monitor these batch means. In principle this method could be used with a range of possible general tests for spatial pattern as long as the expectations and variances could be computed within Z_i. The method can also be specified for surveillance around putative sources of hazard. A recent reference to this approach is Rogerson (2001).

This approach to space–time surveillance has several limitations. First, the procedure has no explicit mechanism for incorporation of changes in expected counts or in the spatial covariance matrix (assumed to be fixed) within C_G. Features of these parameters could also evolve with time. Second, the time to the new event is not explicitly measured and temporal effects are not modelled. The correlation induced in the $\{Z_i\}$ by this approach should also be considered. Further, the approach is defined for global measures of spatial structure, and, as mentioned above, designing a monitoring procedure for localized detection of changes may be more appropriate, whether these changes are clusters or individual areas of excess risk.

A testing procedure akin to the alarm function defined in Eq. 11–4 could be proposed for the tract count case. There, the Poisson process likelihood is replaced by a Poisson count likelihood and a sequential sampling procedure could be used.

Fixed-time-period monitoring.   Updating algorithms could be applied in fixed-time-period monitoring. Moreover, the imputation methods, possibly based on sampling-importance resampling (SIR) (Carlin and Louis, 1996) could be used to update of model parameters faster. Methods similar to those discussed for case events could be developed. Some methods have been considered for fixed lattice data (Jarpe, 1998).

BUILDING DISEASE SURVEILLANCE MODELS

I have focused on the use of hypothesis testing in surveillance, because these methods are most fully developed. However in many statistical applications, especially those in observational studies, restricting the analysis to simple hypotheses would not be considered appropriate. Instead, a variety of influences can more easily be assessed within a modelling framework. Parameters that describe particular features of interest can be estimated. In disease mapping, parameters can represent spatial or temporal effects on disease maps, or both. For example, in the BYM model in Some Models for Spatial Disease Surveillance, above, the two heterogeneity terms, u_j and v_j, have prior distributions that control their form. The forms of these distributions are functions of single parameters (β, τ, say) that control the global form of the map. Estimating these parameters allows their importance in describing the mapped distribution to be assessed. Modeling also provides estimates of the variability of parameters. For spatial temporal modeling, a more complex model is needed to capture the possible spatial, temporal, and spatial temporal effects.

In model-based surveillance, the monitoring of parameters must naturally be considered. In spatiotemporal surveillance, a model must be chosen that can describe the overall behavior of disease in space and time (i.e., that can capture spatial and temporal effects and spatial temporal interaction effects). The model must also allow for, and be sensitive to, temporal changes in the spatial temporal structure and be flexible enough to include multiple foci (i.e., a variety of behaviors). This goal may be achieved by maintaining a relatively simple model that allows important deviations to be detected.

Particular problems arise in spatial temporal applications, because both spatial effects and temporal effects could be present. Also, various interaction may occur (e.g., between clustering effects, between main effects and variance effects, and between main effects).

A possible simple model for disease count data surveillance, defined for a fixed time period and spatial frame, could consist of the following components. To examine a change in a fixed time period t and spatial unit j, assume the following model for the count of disease in the j, tth unit:

$$y_{jt} \sim Poisson(e_{jt}.\theta_{jt})$$

where y_{jt} is the observed number of cases in the jth region in time period t, e_{jt} is the expected number of cases in the jth region in time period t, and θ_{jt} is the relative risk in the jth region in time period t. A model could be assumed for the relative risk of the form:

$$\ln \theta_{jt} = \lambda_{jt} = \rho + \varphi_t + \phi_j + \tau_j + \gamma_{jt} \tag{11-6}$$

where ρ is an intercept term defining the overall level of the relative risk, φ_t is a component describing the temporal variation, and ϕ_j, τ_j are components describing the spatial extravariation, as described in Some Models for Spatial Disease Surveillance, above. The component ϕ_j is the correlated component, and τ_j the uncorrelated component. The final term, γ_{jt}, represents the interaction between spatial and temporal effects in the maps. In this form, independent temporal and spatial terms are used, and the relation between them is assumed to be included in the γ_{jt} term. This model is relatively simple compared with that needed to take into account the large number of possible effects. For example, in some studies, ϕ_j and τ_j are regarded as time-dependent also, and terms such as ϕ_{jt} and τ_{jt} appear Xia and Carlin (1998). Other studies include simple time trends Bernardinelli et al. (1995), and spatial trends may also be included.

For the model in Eq. 11–6, prior distributions for the parameters can be specified. These distributions help to define the role of the parameters in the relative risk and make them easier to estimate. The prior distributional specifications assumed are as follows. The temporal effect distribution is defined as:

$$\varphi_t|\varphi_{t-1} \sim N(\nu\varphi_{t-1}, K_1.\sigma_t^2) \qquad (11\text{–}7)$$

where ν is an autoregressive parameter and σ_t^2 is the variance. This distribution allows a smooth time-on-time variation in risk at any spatial site. The spatial components are specified as

$$\phi|\phi_{-j} \sim N\left(\overline{\phi}_{\delta_j}, K_2.\frac{\sigma_{ss}^2}{m_j}\right) \qquad (11\text{–}8)$$

where m_j is the number of spatial neighbors of the j th region, δ_j is the set of neighbors of the jth region, ϕ_{-j} is the parameter set excluding ϕ_j; σ_{ss}^2 is the correlated spatial component variance and

$$\tau_j \sim N(0, K_3.\sigma_{us}^2) \qquad (11\text{–}9)$$

where σ_{us}^2 is the uncorrelated spatial component variance. These components are not dependent on time and are estimated for the complete data available at any given time. The spatial temporal effect is defined as

$$\gamma_{jt} \sim N(0, K_4.\sigma_{st}^2) \qquad (11\text{–}10)$$

where σ_{st}^2 is the spatial temporal component variance. This component is estimated for each site at each period. The K_* parameters are scaling constants that will be used in the surveillance exercise.

In space–time surveillance, changes to a process must be monitored via changes in parameter values. A variety of changes can be monitored by examining changes in K_1, K_2, K_3, K_4. If the process is in control, $K_1 = K_2 = K_3 = K_4 = 1$. If $K_1 > 1$, a sharp jump in the risk occurs in time, $K_2 > 1$ is a change in the global spatial correlation structure, $K_3 > 1$ suggests a change in variability across the map, and $K_4 > 1$ is a change in the risk at a particular space–time location. Hence, the basic procedure involves examining changes to global model parameters by sequentially fitting a global model.

Variants of this model were examined by Knorr-Held (2000), who fitted them to complete space–time sequences of lung cancer in Ohio. He found that a variant of the above model fits the complete 21-year sequence well. The variant specifies the interaction prior distribution as:

$$\gamma_{jt} \sim N(\gamma_{jt-1}, K_4.\sigma_{st}^2) \qquad (11\text{--}11)$$

where the interaction has a random walk dependence, as opposed to a zero-mean prior distribution. However, Knorr-Held did not examine the surveillance of the sequence of maps of lung cancer as they arose. The following section examines the difference in these two interaction models by applying them to the surveillance of the Ohio lung cancer example.

Ohio Lung Cancer Example

Here, a simple example of a spatiotemporal disease map analysis, with a multiple focus on global parameter changes and jump assessment is presented. Also discussed is a surveillance model based on the mapping models discussed earlier (Eqs. 11–6–11).

The Ohio lung cancer data set, described by Carlin and Louis (1996), among others, consists of lung cancer counts for 88 counties of Ohio for 21 1-year time periods from 1968 to 1988. The surveillance of the 21 years of the map sequence is examined. Fitting a complex Bayesian model to space–time data, typically requires using simulation algorithms such as Markov chain Monte Carlo methods to provide samples of the posterior distribution of the parameters. Estimates of these parameters are based on functions of the posterior sample, such as the sample mean or variance. These algorithms are not readily available for use by nonspecialists, although the package WinBUGS (see Software for Spatiotemporal Map Surveillance, below) provides an environment in which spatiotemporal models can be fitted to complete sequences of maps. Currently, maps cannot be sequentially analyzed in WinBUGS. In the models presented here, the posterior sampling was custom-programmed in Visual Fortran. The models fitted were sampled using Metropolis-Hastings steps. Although these steps are easy to implement, sequentially refitting of the models is difficult because a new set of data is added and a new set of parameters is included at each new time period. Some solutions to this problem are discussed in The Role of Resampling Methods. A simple approach to the problem is to adopt a sliding window of time units within which the effects are estimated. This approach is an approximate procedure, because temporal effects lasting longer than the window will not be properly estimated. Here, such a moving window, of length 3 periods, is used to reduce the computational time (see, for example, Berzuini et al., 1997 and Doucet et al., 2001). Each model fit was monitored for convergence using a range of diagnostics that included posterior convergence plotting and variance comparisons.

The output from the fitted models included the posterior samples of variance parameters and their associated K_* parameters. For simplicity, I estimated the K_* parameters as ratios of current to lag-one variances. I examine the multiple time series of K_1, K_2, K_3, K_4 and the corresponding variances. Figures 11–4 to 11–7, show the SMRs for lung cancer for 1968, 1969 and 1988, 1989, based on an Ohio state yearly rate for each 1-year period (Figs. 11–4–11–7). Two basic models are examined: the models with independent space-time interaction (Eq. 11–10) and the dependence model (Eq. 11–11). Figures 11–8 and 11–9 display the time series for the four K_* parameters for the two models fitted.

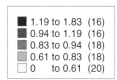

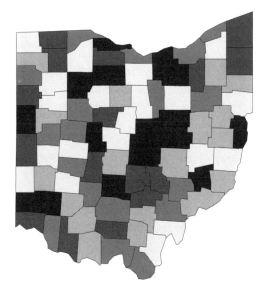

Figure 11–4 Standardized Mortality Ratio map for the Ohio lung cancer data for 1968, based on the yearly standardized rate across all population subgroups. Parenthetical numbers are group counts.

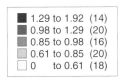
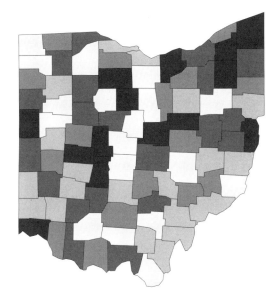

Figure 11–5 Standardized Mortality Ratio map for the Ohio lung cancer data for 1969, based on the yearly standardized rate across all population subgroups. Parenthetical numbers are group counts.

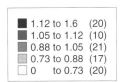
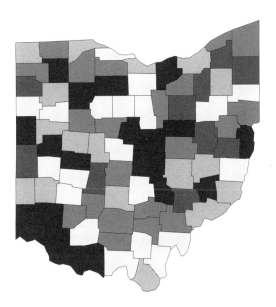

Figure 11–6 Standardized Mortality Ratio map for the Ohio lung cancer data for 1987, based on the yearly standardized rate across all population subgroups. Parenthetical numbers are group counts.

305

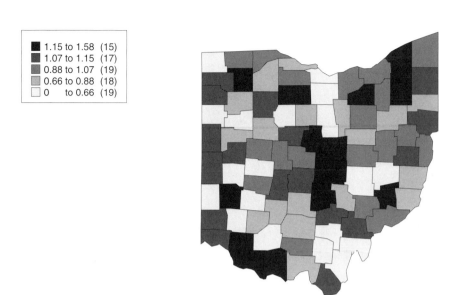

Figure 11–7 Standardized Mortality Ratio map for the Ohio Lung cancer data for 1988, based on the yearly standardized rate across all population subgroups. Parenthetical numbers are group counts.

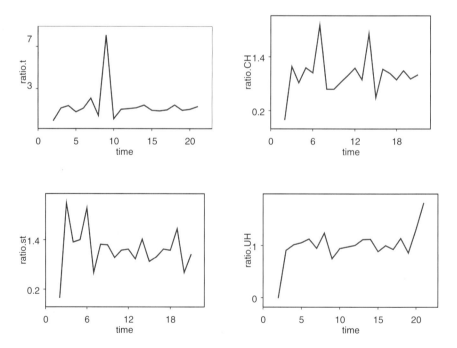

Figure 11–8 Empirical lag-one ratios of variance parameters for the independence spatiotemporal interaction model; top left: time; bottom left: space-time; right panels: spatial correlated (top) and uncorrelated (bottom) ratios.

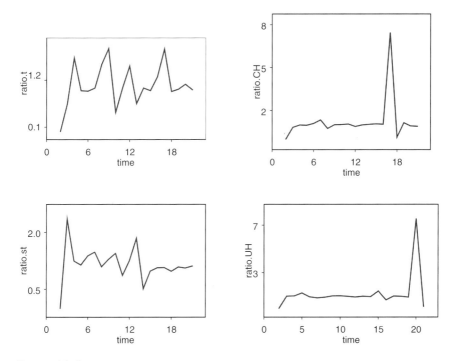

Figure 11–9 Empirical lag-one ratios of variance parameters for the random walk spatiotemporal interaction model: top left: time; bottom left: space-time; right panels: spatial correlated (top) and uncorrelated (bottom) ratios.

DISCUSSION

Only empirical ratios of variances as crude estimates of the K_* parameters have been reported because there is some indeterminacy in this parameterization. Further hyperpriors could be used to distinguish the parameters, but the need for parsimony deters such steps. The variance parameters display a variety of differences. The spatial parameters are similar between models and show a few isolated peaks, particularly near the end of the period, and ratios close to one, except near the period end. These findings suggest short-term changes in variability of the Ohio counties and possibly some clustering.

The time variances show an increasing trend in both models. The spatial temporal increase suggests that, as time proceeds, changes occur in localized incidence. Some interaction between the unstructured spatial component and time parameters is evident, and may be related to the spatiotemporal interaction effects.

Other studies of the Ohio data set found considerable upward trend overall in the study region, along with localized differences in pattern.

Here, the existence of jumps or changepoints in the temporal increases and in the interactions is reported, which suggest clustering changes. Carlin and Louis (1996) found marked positive temporal trends for the study area and also marked increases in the southwest counties, Hamilton, Clermont, Butler, and Warren. In Hamilton there is a large urban area (Cincinnati). Neither analysis provided the temporal measure of parameter change provided in this chapter. Although the spatial distribution of the parameter change results is not examined in depth, note the importance of being able to flag, in real time, any changes in pattern and to examine quickly the corresponding spatial distribution of changes.

The sequential approach could be used to isolate forms of variation in trend, s–t clustering, and global changes in the spatial structure. Bayesian alarm monitoring could form the next extension to this study.

Another feature of this approach is the examination of overall goodness-of-fit over time. As time proceeds, it can be assessed whether the model fits the data well or if it diverges globally in its goodness-of-fit. Being not in a control system and not able to adjust the behavior of the system immediately, it is desirable to alter the model if the global goodness-of-fit suggested a serious lack of fit. To this end here is displayed the sequential Bayesian Information Criterion (BIC) for the interaction dependence model. The Bayesian Information Criterion is based on the difference between a function of the log-likelihood for the given model and a penalty term, which is a function of the number of parameters used in the model:

$$\frac{2}{B} \sum_{b=1}^{B} \log L(\theta^{(b)}) - p \log n$$

where B is the number in the posterior sample, and $\theta^{(b)}$ is the vector of parameter values for the b th sample value, p is the number of parameters (in the vector θ) and n is the number of data points. As time proceeds the number of parameters and the number of data points also increase and so the balance between the likelihood and penalty could change. When a sliding scan window is used then this effect should be reduced.

Figure 11–10 displays the successive BIC values for this model. The overall reduction in validity of the model over time may suggest that a more flexible modelling strategy should be envisaged. One possibility would be to include a general first order autoregressive (AR1) prior specification for

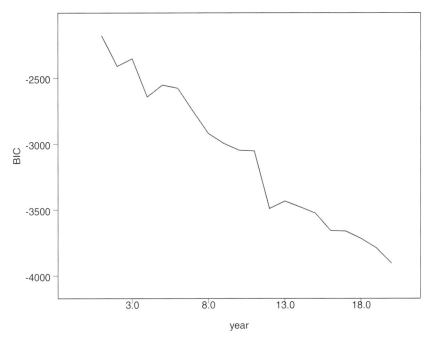

Figure 11–10 Successive BIC values for the interaction dependence model.

the interaction component, thereby allowing a range of models within one prior:

$$\gamma_{jt} \sim N(\alpha \gamma_{jt-1}, K_4.\sigma_{st}^2) \qquad (11\text{--}12)$$

Separating nonstationary components would require care, and raises the question of how to determine which components of the model are lacking in goodness-of-fit, and how to allow for this lack of fit in an active sequential surveillance system.

The Role of Resampling Methods

For any sequential model analysis of disease data, the size of the data, and possibly the parameter space associated with the problem, will expand with each new observation. In the Ohio data example, the amount of data increases as data from the new year for each county are added, and the parameter space is also increases if there are any global time-specific or county-specific time-specific parameters. For example, the spatial CH term fitted might be made time-dependent as in Zia et al. (1997). If the models fitted were relatively complex and required considerable computation during fitting (such as MCMC algorithms), the fitting time would also increase as the series of observations expanded. This possibility has been discussed by Kong et al. (1994), and Berzuini et al. (1997) in the context of Bayesian modeling. This development led to the use of importance sampling to resample the past realizations from the posterior distribution, rather than the complete sampling of the new data sets. These resampling methods have been pursued in other areas such as optimal control, and much of the literature on particle filtering addresses these concerns. Recent reviews are cited in Doucet et al. (2001). Resampling the past is one approach to this problem. Another possible approach is to use a temporal moving window to allow the admission of data between the $t - p$ th and t-th time period. The choice of p would crucially affect the ability to estimate temporal interaction effects but would allow for a localized smoothing in time.

SOFTWARE FOR SPATIAL TEMPORAL MAP SURVEILLANCE

The development of software for analyzing disease maps has been sporadic and uneven. For example, software exists for certain types of analysis of simple disease maps, but only limited facilities are available for more advanced spatial or spatiotemporal analyses. Geographic Information Systems (GIS), which can manipulate and display spatial data and can provide a useful presentational tool for disease maps, has undergone considerable development. Such packages as ArcView (www.esri.com/software/arcview) or MapInfo (www.mapinfo.com) provide packaged GIS capability. Both these commercially available packages allow count data from administrative regions to be manipulated. They can also handle data measurements on networks where contour maps of interpolated values are of interest.

Common end products of this type of analysis are thematic maps of relative risk estimates (for example SMRs), such as those shown in Figures 11–4 and 11–5. However, these packages have severely limited statistical capabilities. ArcView has a link to the statistical package S-Plus, but specialized methods for analyzing count data in small areas are not available. The Environmental Systems Research Institute has produced a module called ArcGIS Geostatistical Analyst, which allows the geostatistical modeling of data measured on spatial networks. A similar development is anticipated for small area health data but is not yet available.

Although no commercial GIS with appropriate packaged statistical capabilities currently exists, the results of statistical calculations can be transported into a GIS system. Simple SMR maps can be produced easily in GIS systems, as long as the observed and expected counts are available in the MapInfo table or .mid file, or in the shape file in ArcView. In Map-Info, once a table that can be mapped has been obtained (i.e., the small areas of the map are held as polygons in a mappable table), columns of results (e.g., from an Excel worksheet or a text file), can be copied into a table in the GIS system and linked with the mappable table of small areas. In ArcView, once a shape file for the small areas has been obtained, similar procedures can add information to the mappable shape file. Interchange facilities allow the conversion of file formats between the two main GIS systems. The boundary files that delimit small areas are often available from government agencies. For example, in the United Kingdom, boundary files for a range of postal areas or census tracts may be downloaded from a central agency (http://edina.ac.uk/ukborders/data). In the United States, county and state boundary files are found in standard GIS packages, and some are held in the map library of the statistical package S-Plus.

Although not directly available in current GIS systems, the statistical procedures for producing smoothed disease maps, can be found in many statistical packages. Log linear regression can be used to examine the relation between small area counts and explanatory variables, such as deprivation scores or urbanicity indices, or even spatial variables describing long-range trends (see for example, Lawson, 1993). Packages such as R, S-Plus, or SAS provide such model fitting. The fitted values from such analyses provide estimates of relative risk under the model fitted. The S-Plus ArcView link can be used for this approach. In addition, the availability of generalized additive modelling in S-Plus allows more flexible models to be used.

Specialist Bayesian modeling of disease maps is aided by the use of WinBUGS and GeoBUGS, which are available free from www.mrc-bsu.cam.ac.uk/bugs/winbugs/. WinBUGS is a menued version of BUGS that was developed to allow full Bayesian models to be fitted to a wide range of data. For non-specialist users, the programming for implementing procedures in the system is possibly daunting, because no simple menu-based analysis options are provided. Tutorial help is available on the website, however. GeoBUGS is intended to provide a GIS-style presentation of output from spatial analysis in the WinBUGS program. In the newest version (1.4), the importation of MapInfo or ArcView files has been implemented. The WinBUGS manual available from the website contains examples of possible analyses, including the full Bayesian analysis of the Scottish Lip Cancer data, a well-known and often used data set. The analysis typically produces posterior expected relative risks, as derived for the East German example in Figure 11–2. If suitably programmed, it can also be used to produce the output in Figure 11–3.

WinBUGS also allows space–time analysis of a complete temporal set of disease maps (see for example Xia and Carlin, 1998). However, a sequential analysis of the kind suggested here, cannot be implemented, because the data set and parameters increase with each new time period, so a static model definition is not possible.

No software is readily available for modeling disease maps that focus on clustering, as opposed to global incidence changes. However, hypothesis testing in this area has been rapidly developed and software is available for test-based surveillance (e.g., Rogerson's surveillance test and Kulldorf's scan tests). One source is ClusterSeer (www.terraseer.com/) a commercial product produced by BioMedware Inc. The Kulldorf Scan statistic package (SaTScan) is available free from www.cancer.gov/prevention/bb/SaTScan.

CONCLUSIONS

Considerable opportunities exist for developing new methods for surveillance of disease maps. Although methods developed in other areas are useful in surveillance systems, spatial methods must be developed that are sensitive to the sequential nature of the surveillance task. Possibilities include updating algorithms or using sequential methods, such as those discussed here. Methods that can be used easily and routinely in public health surveillance must be developed if they are to be adopted by public health analysts.

REFERENCES

Bartholomew, D.J. (1956). A sequential test of randomness for events occurring in time and space. *Biometrika* **43**, 64–78.

Bernardinelli, L., Clayton, D., Pascutto, C., Montomoli, C., Ghislandi, M., and Songini, M. (1995). Bayesian analysis of space-time variation in disease risk. *Statistics in Medicine* **14**, 2433–2443.

Berzuini, C., Best, N., Gilks, W., and Larissa, C. (1997). Dynamic conditional independence models and markov chain monte carlo methods. *Journal of the American Statistical Association* **92**, 1403–1412.

Besag, J., and Clifford, P. (1991). Sequential monte carlo p-values. *Biometrika* **78**, 301–304.

Besag, J., York, J., and Mollié, A. (1991). Bayesian image restoration with two applications in spatial statistics. *Annals of the Institute of Statistical Mathematics* **43**, 1–59.

Carlin, B.P., and Louis, T.A. (1996). *Bayes and Empircal Bayes Methods for Data Analysis*. London: Chapman and Hall.

Chen, R. (1978). A surveillance system for congenital abnormalities. *Journal of the American Statistical Association* **73**, 323–327.

Chen, R., Connelly, R., and Mantel, N. (1993). Analysing post alarm data in a monitoring system, in order to accept or reject the alarm. *Statistics in Medicine*, **12**, 1807–1812.

Chen, R., Iscovich, J., and Goldbourt, U. (1997). Clustering of leukaemia cases in a city in Israel. *Statistics in Medicine* **16**, 1873–1887.

Doucet, A., de Freitas, and Gordon, N. (Eds.) (2001). *Sequential Monte Carlo Methods in Practice*. New York: Springer Verlag.

Elliott, P., Wakefield, J.C., Best, N.G., and Briggs, D.J. (Eds.) (2000). *Spatial Epidemiology: Methods and Applications*. London: Oxford University Press.

Farrington, C.P., and Beale, A.D. (1998). The detection of outbreaks of infectious disease. In Gierl, L., Cliff, A., Valleron, A.-J., Farrington, P., and Bull, M., eds. *Geomed '97: Proceedings of the International Workshop on Geomedical Systems*. Leipzig: Teubner Verlag, pp. 97–117.

Frisen, M. (1992). Evaluations of methods for statistical surveillance. *Statistics in Medicine* **11**, 1489–1502.

Frisen, M. and Mare, J.D. (1991). Optimal surveillance. *Biometrika* **78**, 271–280.

Jarpe, E. (1998). Surveillance of spatial patterns. Technical Report 3, Department of Statistics, Goteborg University, Sweden.

Kelsall, J. and Diggle, P. (1995). Non-parametric estimation of spatial variation in relative risk. *Statistics in Medicine* **14**, 2335–2342.

Kelsall, J. and Diggle P. (1998). Spatial variation in risk of disease: a nonparametric binary regression approach. *Applied Statistics* **47**, 559–573.

Knorr-Held, L. (2000). Bayesian modeling of inseparable space-time variation in disease risk. *Statistics in Medicine* **19**, 2555–2567.

Kong, A., Lai, J., and Wong, W. (1994). Sequential imputations and Bayesian missing data problems. *Journal of the American Statistical Association* **89**, 278–288.

Lai, T.L. (1995). Sequential changepoint detetion in quality control and dynamical systems. *Journal of the Royal Statistical Society B* **57**, 613–658.

Lawson, A.B. (1993). On the analysis of mortality events around a prespecified fixed point. *Journal of the Royal Statistical Society A* **156**, 363–377.

Lawson, A.B. (2001a). Disease map reconstruction: a tutorial. *Statistics in Medicine* **20**, 2183–2204.

Lawson, A.B. (2001b). *Statistical Methods in Spatial Epidemiology*. New York: Wiley.

Lawson, A.B., Biggeri, A., Boehning, D., Lesaffre, E., Viel, J.-F., Clark, A., Schlattmann, P., and Divino, F. (2000). Disease mapping models: an empirical evaluation. *Statistics in Medicine* **19**, 2217–2242. Special Issue: Disease Mapping with Emphasis on Evaluation of Methods.

Lawson, A.B. and Williams, F. (1993). Applications of extraction mapping in environmental epidemiology. *Statistics in Medicine* **12**, 1249–1258.

Lawson, A.B. and Williams, F.L.R. (2001). *An Introductory Guide to Disease Mapping*. New York: Wiley.

Pickle, L., Mungiole, M., Jones, G., and White, A. (1999). Exploring spatial patterns of mortality: the new atlas of united states mortality. *Statistics in Medicine* **18**, 3211–3220.

Rogerson, P. (1997). Surveillance systems for monitoring the development of spatial patterns. *Statistics in Medicine* **16**, 2081–2093.

Rogerson, P. (2001). Monitoring point patterns for the development of space-time clusters. *Journal of the Royal Statistical Society* **164,** 87–96.

Wessman, P. (1998). Some principles for surveillance adopted for multivariate processes with a common change point. *Communications in Statistics, Theory and Methods* **27,** 1143–1161.

Xia, H. and Carlin, B. (1998). Spatio-temporal models with errors in covariates: mapping Ohio lung cancer mortality. *Statistics in Medicine* **17,** 2025–2043.

Zia, H., Carlin, B.P., and Waller, L.A. (1997). Hierarchical models for mapping Ohio lung cancer rates. *Environmetrics* **8,** 107–120.

12

Ecologic Inference Problems in the Analysis of Surveillance Data

SANDER GREENLAND

Surveillance data (e.g., vital statistics and registry data) are often collected at great expense and therefore should be exploited fully. They are useful in preliminary searches for disease risk factors, and they often describe outcomes across a much broader spectrum of exposures than is found in typical cohort or case-control studies. This breadth suggests that the power to detect effects in surveillance data would be greater than in cohort or case-control studies, if biases could be controlled. However, surveillance data on risk factors and outcomes are usually unlinked on the individual level and thus allow only ecologic (group-level) associations to be examined.

The limitations of surveillance data are illustrated in the often-cited characteristic of Florida's population, where people are "born Hispanic and die Jewish." These average characteristics of the state's population tell little about the reality of individuals living in Florida because the birth and death rates are group averages and are not even derived from the same individuals. Linked birth and death data would show little or no change in ethnic identity over a lifetime. Unlinked data allow only ecologic (group-level) associations to be examined; attempts to draw individual-level inferences or causal inferences (whether individual or group level) may suffer from problems subsumed under the topic of ecologic bias and ecologic fallacies. This chapter reviews the theory needed to understand these problems. It emphasizes the nonseparability of contextual (group-level) effects from individual-level effects that is due to the multilevel causal structure of ecologic (aggregate) data. Contrary to common misperceptions, this problem afflicts ecologic studies in which the sole objective is to estimate contextual effects, as well as studies in which the objective is to estimate individual effects. Multilevel effects also severely complicate causal interpretations of model coefficients.

The terms *ecologic inference* and *ecologic analysis* refer to any analysis based on data that are limited to characteristics of groups (aggregates) of individuals (Langbein and Lichtman, 1978). Typically, these aggregates are geographically defined populations, such as counties, provinces, or countries. An enormous body of literature on ecologic inference extends at least as far back as the early twentieth century. See, for example, Iversen (1991) and Achen and Shively (1995) for reviews of the social science literature, and Morgenstern (1998) for a review of the health-sciences literature.

The objectives of ecologic analyses may be roughly classified into two broad categories: individual objectives, which examine relations of group and individual characteristics to the outcomes of the individuals in the groups, and purely contextual objectives, to examine relations of group characteristics to group outcomes. A study may have both objectives. Most authors have focused on studies with only individual-level objectives and have emphasized the obstacles to cross-level inference from group-level (ecologic) observations to individual-level relationships. This focus has led to a common misperception that individual-level relationships can be safely ignored if contextual objectives are the only interest. Several authors have also criticized the common practice of using strong (and sometimes implausible) modeling assumptions to generate cross-level inferences (Iversen, 1991; Achen and Shively, 1995; Morgenstern, 1998; Greenland, 2001).

The following section is an overview of the literature surrounding these problems and the controversy they generate. The third section provides some basic multilevel (hierarchical) structural-model theory to define the problems ("structural" here means the underlying regression structure), apart from issues of random error or sampling variation; further statistical theory, including fitting methods, can be found in Navidi et al. (1994), Guthrie and Sheppard (2001), Wakefield and Salway (2001) and Sheppard (2003)). The fourth section describes multilevel studies that combine data from individual and ecologic (aggregate) levels. The fifth section briefly describes other special problems of inference from ecologic data and discusses some difficulties in causally interpreting the coefficients of contextual variables in multilevel models.

ECOLOGIC VERSUS INDIVIDUAL-LEVEL SOURCES OF BIAS

Introduction

Studies limited to characteristics of aggregates are usually termed ecologic studies (Langbein and Lichtman, 1978; Piantadosi et al., 1988; Cleave et al., 1995; Plummer and Clayton, 1996; Morgenstern, 1998). This term is perhaps unfortunate because the word ecologic suggests that such studies are especially appropriate for examining the impact of environmental factors, including societal characteristics, and invites confusion between an ecologic perspective (addressing relations at the environmental or social level) and an ecologic study. As many authors have pointed out (Firebaugh, 1980; Von Korff et al., 1992; Navidi et al., 1994; Susser and Susser, 1996; Duncan et al., 1996, 1998; Greenland, 2001, 2002), overcoming this confusion requires adopting a multilevel perspective, which allows theory and observations to be integrated on all levels: physiologic (exposures and responses of systems within individuals), individual (exposures and responses of individuals), and aggregate or contextual (exposures and responses of aggregates or clusters of individuals, such as locales or societies).

Defenders of ecologic studies argue (correctly) that many critics have presumed individual-level relationships are the ultimate target of inference of all ecologic studies, when this is not always so (Schwartz, 1994; Pearce, 1996; Susser and Susser, 1996), and that contagious outcomes necessitate group-level considerations in modeling, regardless of the target level (Koopman and Longini, 1994). They also point out that an ecologic summary may have its own direct effects on individual risk, beyond that conferred by the contributing individual values. For example, the average economic status of an area can have effects on an individual over and above the effects of the individual's economic status (Firebaugh, 1978; Hakama et al., 1982). Unfortunately, some defenders make implicit assumptions to prove that entire classes of ecologic studies are valid, or at least no less valid than individual-level analyses. (See Greenland and Robins, 1994a,b; Morgenstern, 1998; and Naylor, 1999 for critical commentaries against such arguments in the health sciences.) Some ecologic researchers are well aware of these problems and so explain their assumptions (King, 1997, 1999), but they still draw criticism because inferences are sensitive to those assumptions (Rivers, 1998; Freedman et al., 1998a, 1999).

In the present section, some controversial assumptions in ecologic analyses of surveillance data are reviewed and then multilevel methods that represent individual-level and ecologic data in a single model are discussed briefly. Simple illustrations are used to make the points transparent to nonmathematical readers, problems of confounding and specification bias are highlighted, and an overview of the underlying mathematical theory is provided. Researchers have raised many other issues in the ongoing ecologic study controversy; see the references for details, especially those in Other Special Problems of Ecologic Analysis.

Aggregate-Level Confounding due to Individual-Level Effects

Two major types of measurements are used to describe aggregated data: summaries of distributions of individuals within the aggregates, such as mean age or percent female, and purely ecologic (contextual) variables that are defined directly on the aggregate, such as whether there is a needle-exchange program in an area. The causal effects of the purely contextual variables are the focus of much social and epidemiologic research (Schwartz, 1994; Susser and Susser, 1996; Duncan et al., 1996; Borgatta and Jackson, 1980; Iversen, 1991). Nonetheless, most outcome variables of public-health importance are summaries of individual-level distributions, such as prevalence, incidence, mortality, and life expectancy, all of which can be expressed in terms of average individual outcomes (Rothman and Greenland, 1998). Furthermore, many contextual variables are surrogates that summarize individual data; for example, neighborhood social class is often measured by average income and average education.

The use of summary measures in an ecologic analysis introduces a major source of uncertainty in ecologic inference. Summary measures depend on the joint individual-level distributions within aggregates, but distributional summaries do not fully determine (and sometimes do not seriously constrain) those joint distributions. This problem corresponds to the concept of information lost to aggregation, and is a key source of controversy about ecologic studies (Achen and Shively, 1995).

The confounding of contextual and individual effects is illustrated in Table 12–1. For simplicity, just two areas are used, but examples with many areas are available (Greenland and Robins, 1994a). Suppose we wish to assess a contextual effect, such as the impact of an ecologic difference between areas A and B (such as a difference in laws or social programs) on the rate of a health outcome. We measure this effect by the amount RR_A that this difference multiplies the rate (the true effect of being in A versus being in B). One potential risk factor, X, differs in distribution between the areas; an effect of X (measured by the rate ratio RR_X comparing $X = 1$ to $X = 0$ within areas) may be present, but we observe no difference in rates between the areas.

Do the ecologic data in Panel 1a of Table 12–1 show no contextual effect? That is, do they correspond best with $RR_A = 1$? Unfortunately, the

Table 12-1 Example demonstrating the confounding of both contextual and individual effects in ecologic data

1A. ECOLOGIC (MARGINAL) DATA:

	Group A			Group B		
	X = 1	X = 0	Total	X = 1	X = 0	Total
Y = 1	?	?	560	?	?	560
N	60	40	100	40	60	100
Rate	?	?	5.6	?	?	5.6

1B. POSSIBILITY 1 ($RR_X = 2$, $RR_A = 7/8$):

Y = 1	420	140	560	320	240	560
N	60	40	100	40	60	100
Rate	7.0	3.5	5.6	8.0	4.0	5.6

1C. POSSIBILITY 2 ($RR_X = 1/2$, $RR_A = 8/7$):

Y = 1	240	320	560	140	420	560
N	60	40	100	40	60	100
Rate	4.0	8.0	5.6	3.5	7.0	5.6

The ecologic data cannot identify the effect of group (A versus B) on the rate of the outcome Y = 1 when only a marginal summary of the individual-level covariate X is available. Panels 1b and 1c show how within-group differences in outcome rates can affect inferences based on the ecologic data in Panel 1a. N = denominator (in thousands of person-years); RR_A and RR_X are the rate ratios for the true effects of A versus B and of X = 1 versus X = 0, respectively.

ecologic (marginal) data on X distributions and the outcome rates are mathematically equally compatible with a broad spectrum of possibilities, two of which are given in Panels 1b and 1c of Table 12–1. In the first possibility, area A has benefited from the contextual difference ($RR_A < 1$), but this fact has been obscured by area A's higher prevalence of X, which is harmful ($RR_X > 1$). In the second possibility, area A has been harmed by the contextual difference ($RR_A > 1$), but this fact has been obscured by area A's higher prevalence of X, which is beneficial ($RR_X < 1$). The correct answers in either possibility could be obtained by comparing the area rates after they have been standardized directly to a common X distribution; however, such standardization would require knowing the X-specific rates *within* the areas, which are not available in the example. Furthermore, an ecologic regression could not solve the problem because it would only regress the crude area rates on the proportion with X = 1 in each area: Because both crude area rates are 5.6, the ecologic X-coefficient would be zero, hence the regression would produce no X-adjustment of the area rates.

Lacking within-area data on the joint distribution of X and the outcome, an ecologic analysis must necessarily rely on external (prior) information to provide inferences about the contextual effect, although the margins may impose some bounds on the possibilities (Duncan and Davis, 1953; Achen and Shively, 1995; King, 1997). If the X-specific rates in each area were assumed to be proportional to those in some external reference population with known X-specific rates, those external rates could be used to construct and compare standardized morbidity ratios for the areas (indirect adjustment). Unfortunately, such external rates are rarely available for all important covariates, and so other external (prior) information must be used to estimate the effect.

The results of such an analysis can be disappointing if the prior information is ambiguous. If X indicates, say, regular cigarette use, and the outcome is total mortality, we might be confident that RR_X is well above 1 and, hence, that the contextual effect (i.e., the A–B rate ratio) is protective. However, if X indicates regular alcohol consumption, we might feel justified in ruling out scenarios involving values for the rate ratio RR_X that are very far from 1. Nonetheless, because alcohol may be protective at moderate levels and causative at higher levels, we could not be sure of the direction of RR_X; that would depend on the relative proportion of moderate and heavy drinkers in the areas. As a consequence, we could not be sure of the direction (let alone degree) of confounding in the ecologic estimate of the contextual effect (i.e., the ecologic A/B rate ratio of 5.6/5.6 = 1).

The problem of cross-level confounding just illustrated has been discussed extensively since the early twentieth century (see Achen and Shively, 1995) and is a mathematically trivial consequence of the fact that marginals do not determine joint distributions. Yet this logical problem, which differentiates ecologic from and individual-level studies, continues to be misunderstood or ignored by many ecologic researchers, so much that Achen and Shively (1995) remarked:

A cynic might conclude that social scientists tend to ignore logical problems and contradictions in their methods if they do not see anything to be done about them.

Their remark applies to the health sciences as well, as illustrated by this quote:

In practice, it may be that confounding usually poses a more intractable problem for ecological than for individual-level studies. But this is due to the greater reliance on secondary data and proxy measures in ecological studies, *not to any problem inherent in ecological studies*

Schwartz, 1994 [emphasis added]

Although ecologic studies do suffer from greater reliance on secondary data and proxy measures, this passage is typical of defenses that overlook the aspects of confounding that *are* inherent in ecologic studies. Other examples of such defenses are Cohen (1990, 1994, 2000), Susser (1994), and

Pearce (1996). A point illustrated in Table 12–1 is that, given confounding by a measured risk factor X, the individual-level data allow one to control the confounding in the most straightforward way possible: stratify on X. In contrast, confounding by X cannot be controlled by using only the ecologic data, despite the fact that the effect under study is contextual (the effect of the social differences between areas A and B on outcome rates). Because contextual and individual effects are completely confounded in ecologic data (Firebaugh, 1980; Greenland, 2001, 2002), the only solutions to this problem are to obtain individual data within the ecologic units or to use assumptions that are untestable with the ecologic data (Greenland and Robins, 1994a,b; Achen and Shively, 1995).

Another fallacy in some defenses of ecologic studies is the claim that individual-level information is not needed if one is interested only in contextual (ecologic) effects. Examples such as that in Table 12–1 show that such "holistic" arguments are incorrect, especially in health studies in which the outcome measure is an individual-level summary, because individual-level factors can confound the ecologic results even if the study factor is contextual (Firebaugh, 1980; Greenland, 2001, 2002). Holistic arguments also tend to overlook the fact that ecologic data usually refer to arbitrary administrative groupings, such as counties, that are often poor proxies for social context or environmental exposures (Achen and Shively, 1995), and that ecologic relations can be extremely sensitive to the degree of grouping (Openshaw and Taylor, 1981).

The problem illustrated in Table 12–1 also applies to ecologic estimates of average individual-level effects (cross-level inferences from the ecologic to the individual level) (Achen and Shively, 1995; Greenland, 2002; Sheppard, 2003). For example, if the illustration in Table 12–1 represented a contrast of two areas, A and B, with the goal of estimating the impact of differences in the X distribution, we would see very small contextual effects obscure substantial X effects in the ecologic data.

To summarize, observational ecologic data alone tell us little about either contextual or individual-level effects on summary measures of population health because they are compatible with a broad range of individual-level associations. Even if the overall goal is to estimate contextual effects, ecologic manifestations of those effects (Panel 1a of Table 12–1) can be confounded by individual-level relations and are not estimable without information about those relations. Thus, methods that purport to adjust ecologic results for the confounding problem just described either must employ external data about individual relations, or they must make assumptions about those relations. The unobserved nature of the individual relations means that neither approach can be fully tested (validated) against the ecologic data.

Some Assumptions and Fallacies in Ecologic Analyses

All too often, identification is forced by making arbitrary modeling assumptions. Controversy then surrounds the credibility or strength of the assumptions used to derive effect estimates from ecologic data, the sensitivity of those estimates to changes in assumptions, and failures of proposed methods in real or simulated data. For examples, compare Freedman et al. (1998b) with their discussants; compare Greenland and Morgenstern (1989, 1991), Richardson and Hémon (1990), Greenland (1992, 1995), Greenland and Robins (1994a, b), Piantadosi (1994), Stidley and Samet (1994), and Lagarde and Pershagen (1999, 2000) with Cohen (1990, 1994, 1995, 2000); compare King (1997, 1999) with Rivers (1998), Cho (1998), Freedman et al. (1998a, 1999), and the example in Stoto (1998); and compare Wen and Kramer (1999) with Naylor (1999).

All causal inferences from observational epidemiologic data must rely on restrictive assumptions about the distributions of errors and background causes. Most estimates also rely on parametric models for effects. Thus, the validity of inferences depends on examining the sensitivity of the estimates to violations of the underlying assumptions and models.

Randomization assumptions

Interpreting an association as a causal effect depends on some sort of non-confounding or ignorability assumption, which in statistical methodology becomes operationalized as a covariate-specific randomization assumption (Greenland, 1990; Greenland et al., 1999; Rubin, 1990). Such causal inferences are usually sensitive to violations of those assumptions, and this sensitivity is a major source of controversy in most nonexperimental research.

Suppose we are to study K communities. The distinction between ecologic and individual-level confounding may become clearer if we contrast two levels of randomized intervention to reduce sexually transmitted diseases (STDs):

(C) A community-health program (e.g., establishment of free STD clinics) is provided at random to half of the communities (K is assumed to be even).

(W) Within community k, a treatment (e.g., a series of free STD-clinic visits) is randomly provided to a proportion p_k of individuals, and p_k varies across communities.

Trial C is a cluster-randomized design. In this trial, the ecologic data would comprise a community treatment-status indicator plus the outcome measures (e.g., subsequent STD rates). These data would support randomization-based inferences about what the average causal effect of the program would be for the K communities (the communities would be the analysis units, and the sample size for the inferences would be K). Nonetheless, analyzing the individual-level data from trial C as a K-stratum study (the usual individual-level analysis) would support no inferences at all about treatment effects because each stratum (community) would have a zero margin. Put another way, community and treatment effects would be completely confounded in the standard individual-level model. Analyzing the individual-level data would instead require methods for cluster-randomized trials.

In trial W, the ecologic data consist of the proportion treated (p_k) in each community, along with outcome measures. Unless the p_k had been randomly assigned across communities (as in trial C, in which $p_k = 0$ or 1), the ecologic data would *not* support randomization-based inferences about treatment effects. If the p_k were constant, there would be no data for such an analysis; if the p_k varied, the community and treatment effects would be confounded. (This observation is essentially a contrapositive version of Goodman's identification condition for ecologic regression [Goodman, 1959], translated to the present causal setting.) Nonetheless, the individual-level data from any of or all the communities with $0 < p_k < 1$ would support the usual randomization-based inferences (e.g., exact tests stratified on community). Taking X as the treatment indicator and k = A, B, the information in Table 1 can be used as an example of trial W with $p_A = 0.6$ and $p_B = 0.4$. The example then exhibits confounding of the ecologic data with no confounding of the individual-level data within community.

To summarize, different randomization assumptions underlie causal inferences from individual-level and ecologic studies; consequently, valid inferences from these two study types may require controlling for different (although possibly overlapping) sets of covariates (Greenland and Robins, 1994a).

Observational studies

Causal interpretations of associations in observational data have a fundamental weakness: The validity of such interpretations depends on the assumptions that natural or social circumstances have miraculously randomized the study exposure (e.g., by carrying out trial C or W for us). The number of individuals in an individual-level study tells us nothing about the validity of this or other such "no-confounding" assumptions. Larger size only increases the precision of randomization-based inferences by reducing the chance that randomization left large imbalances of uncontrollable covariates across treatment groups. This benefit of size stems from, and depends on, an assumption of exposure randomization, as in trial W.

Systematic (nonrandom) imbalances within groups by definition violate that assumption.

The same argument applies to ecologic studies. The number of ecologic groups involved tells us nothing about the validity of an assumption that the exposure distribution (p_k in the above binary-treatment trials) was randomized across the groups. The benefit of a large number of groups stems from and depends on the assumption that those distributions were randomized, as in trial C. Again, systematic imbalances across groups by definition violate that assumption. Despite these facts, some defenses of ecologic studies have based on the circular argument that large numbers of areas would reduce the chance of ecologic confounding (Cohen, 1990); this circularity arises because the large-number effect assumes randomization across areas, which is precisely the assumption in doubt.

Covariate control

To achieve some plausibility in causal inferences from observational data, researchers attempt to control for covariates that affect the outcome but that are not affected by the exposure (potential confounders). In individual-level studies, the traditional means of control is to stratify the data on these covariates, because within such strata the exposed and unexposed units cannot have any imbalance on the covariates beyond the stratum boundaries; e.g., within a 65- to 74-year-old age stratum, the exposed and unexposed could not be more than 10 years apart in age. Causal inferences then proceed by assuming randomization *within* these strata. However implausible this assumption may be, in the face of observed imbalances it is always more plausible than the assumption of simple (unstratified) randomization.

Ecologic data can be stratified, but with few exceptions, the ecologic exposures and covariates in public-use databases are insufficient in detail and accuracy to create strata with assured balance on key covariates. For example, in ecologic studies of radon levels and lung cancer rates across U.S. counties, the key covariates are the county-specific distributions of age, sex, race, and smoking habits. To address concerns about bias from possible relationships of these strong lung cancer risk factors to radon exposure, the county data would have to be stratified by age, sex, race, and smoking behavior (smoking behavior is multidimensional: it includes intensity, duration, and type of cigarette use). The relationship of radon distributions to lung-cancer rates would then be examined across the stratum-specific county data. This stratified analysis requires the county-specific joint distributions of age, sex, race, smoking behavior, and radon, and age, sex, race, smoking behavior, and lung cancer. Unfortunately, to date no such data have been available. Although data on the age-sex-race-lung cancer distributions in counties are published, their joint distributions with radon and smoking are unobserved. Only marginal distributions of radon are surveyed, and only crude summaries of cigarette sales are available.

The limitations of ecologic stratification data may be better appreciated by considering an analogous problem in an individual-level study of residential radon and lung cancer. One might attempt to control for smoking by using cigarette sales in a subject's county of residence as a surrogate for smoking behavior (as in Cohen, 1990). Presumably, few epidemiologists would regard this strategy as adequately controlling for smoking, especially considering that it would impute an identical smoking level to every subject in the county, regardless of age, sex, or lung cancer status. The shortcomings of this strategy arise precisely because smoking behavior varies greatly among individuals in a county, much more so than average smoking behavior varies across counties (Greenland and Robins, 1994a).

Modeling assumptions

To circumvent the inherent limitations of ecologic studies, investigators have employed models in which ecologic data (simple marginal summaries of crude exposure and covariate measures) are sufficient for causal inference. As mentioned earlier, these models are restrictive and are no more supported by ecologic data than randomization assumptions. For example, a common assumption in ecologic analyses is that effects follow a multiple-linear regression model. This assumption is both natural and somewhat misleading: a multiple-linear model for individual-level effects induces a multiple-linear ecologic model, but this parallel relation between the individual and ecologic regressions fails in the presence of nonadditive or nonlinear effects in the ecologic groups (Vaupel et al., 1979; Richardson et al., 1987; Dobson, 1988; Greenland and Robins, 1994a; Prentice and Sheppard, 1995; Lasserre et al., 2000).

Not even the functional form of individual-level effects (which can confound ecologic associations, as in Table 12–1) is identified by the marginal data in ecologic studies. For example, suppose individual risk R depends on the covariate vector X (which may contain contextual variables) via $R = f(X)$, and A indicates a context (such as geographic area). The ecologic observations identify only relations of average risks $E_A(R)$ to average covariate levels $E_A(X)$ across contexts. These ecologic relationships generally do not follow the same functional form as the individual relationships because $E_A(R) = E_A[f(X)] \neq f[E_A(X)]$, except in very special cases, chiefly those in which f is additive and linear in all the X components.

To prevent negative rate estimates, most analyses of individual-level epidemiologic studies assume a multiplicative (loglinear) model for the regression of the outcome rate on exposure and analysis covariates, in which f(X) = exp(Xβ). Such nonlinearities in individual regressions virtually guarantee that simple ecologic models will be misspecified. These nonlinearities further diminish the effectiveness of controlling ecologic confounding, although the problem can be mitigated somewhat by expanding the ecologic model to include more detailed covariate summaries, if available (Greenland and Robins, 1994a; Guthrie and Sheppard, 2001), and by including higher-order covariate terms (Richardson et al., 1987; Richardson and Hémon, 1990; Lasserre et al., 2000).

Unfortunately, some authors have denied the misspecification problem by claiming that a linear regression is justified by Taylor's theorem (Cohen, 1990). This justification is circular because approximate linearity of f(X) over the within-context (area-specific) range of X is required for a first-order Taylor approximation of f(X) to be accurate (Dobson, 1988; Greenland and Robins, 1994a). Furthermore, in most applications, this requirement is known to be violated. For example, the dependence of risk on age is highly nonlinear for nearly all cancers. Attempts to circumvent this nonlinearity by using age-specific outcomes encounter a lack of age-context-specific measures of potential confounders, such as smoking. Using age-standardized rates also fails to solve the problem because it requires use of age-standardized measures of the covariates in the regression model (see Other Special Problems of Ecologic Analysis, below), and such measures are rarely available.

MULTILEVEL MODEL THEORY FOR ECOLOGIC INFERENCE

Most of the points discussed in this section are consequences of standard multilevel modeling theory (Goldstein, 1995). Suppose Y and X are an outcome (response) variate and a covariate vector defined on individuals, and R and Z are an outcome and covariate vector defined directly on aggregates (clusters); X may contain products among individual and aggregate covariates. For example, Y could be an indicator of being robbed within a given year; X could contain age, income, and other variables. With state as the aggregate, R could be the proportion robbed in the state over the year (which is just the average Y in the state), and Z could contain state average age and income and an indicator of whether hypodermic needles are available without prescription in the state.

Let μ_{ik} and x_{ik} be the expected outcome and X-value of individual i in aggregate k, with $\overline{\mu}_k$ and $\overline{x}_k$ their averages and z_k the Z-value for aggregate k, k = 1, . . . , K. One generalized-linear model (GLM) for individuals is

$$\mu_{ik} = f(\alpha + x_{ik}\beta + z_k\gamma) \qquad (12–1)$$

If $R = \overline{Y}$, as when R is a rate, proportion, or average lifespan, Model 1 induces the aggregate-outcome model

$$E_k(R) = \overline{\mu}_k = \sum_{i=1}^{N_k} f(\alpha + x_{ik}\beta + z_k\gamma)/N_k \qquad (12\text{-}2)$$

where N_k is the size of aggregate k (Prentice and Sheppard, 1995; Sheppard and Prentice, 1995). If $\beta \neq 0$, $\overline{\mu}_k$ will depend on the within-aggregate X-distribution as well as on the individual-specific effects β and the contextual effects γ.

Special Cases

If the individual model is linear (so that $f(u) = u$), and if $Z = \overline{X}$, models 1 and 2 become

$$\mu_{ik} = \alpha + x_{ik}\beta + \overline{x}_k\gamma \qquad (12\text{-}3)$$

and $$\overline{\mu}_k = \alpha + \overline{x}_k(\beta + \gamma) \qquad (12\text{-}4)$$

Model 12–4 exhibits the complete confounding of the individual effects β and the aggregate (contextual) effects γ in ecologic data (Firebaugh, 1978, 1980). Although the induced regression is linear and can be fit with ecologic data, the identified coefficient $\beta + \gamma$ represents a blend of individual and contextual effects, rather than just contextual effects, as often supposed. To see this point, let Y again be a robbery indicator, let X be income (in thousands of dollars), and let k index states. Then β represents the difference in individual robbery risks associated with a $1000 increase in individual income X within a given state; γ represents the difference in individual robbery risks associated with a $1000 increase in state-average income $\overline{X}$ among individuals of a given income X; and $\beta + \gamma$ represents the unconditional difference in average state risk associated with a $1000 increase in average state income. In other words, β represents an intrastate association of personal income with personal robbery risk; γ represents an interstate association of average (contextual) state income with personal robbery risk within personal-income strata; and $\beta + \gamma$ represents an unconditional interstate association of average income with average risk, blending the conditional associations with robbery risk of personal and state-average income differences.

Linear models usually poorly represent risk and rate outcomes because of their failure to constrain predicted outcomes to nonnegative values. If we drop the linearity requirement but maintain $Z = \overline{X}$, model 1 can be rewritten

$$\mu_{ik} = f[\alpha + (x_{ik} - \overline{x}_k)\beta + \overline{x}_k(\beta + \gamma)] \qquad (12\text{-}5)$$

showing that β may also be interpreted as the within-aggregate (intracluster) association of the transformed individual expected outcome $f^{-1}(\mu)$ with departures of X from the aggregate-specific average $\overline{X}$; $\beta + \gamma$ is then the complementary association of $\overline{X}$ with $\overline{\mu}$ across aggregates (Sheppard, 2003). The departure $X - \overline{X}$ is, however, a contrast of individual and contextual characteristics X and $\overline{X}$, rather than a purely individual characteristic X as in model 1, and $\beta + \gamma$ remains a mixture of individual and contextual effects.

Unfortunately, not even the mixed effect $\beta + \gamma$ can be estimated unbiasedly without further assumptions if the model is nonlinear and if the only available covariates are aggregate means $\overline{X}$ and purely contextual variables. Richardson et al. (1987) and Dobson (1988) discussed assumptions for unbiased ecologic estimation of $\beta + \gamma$ under loglinear models, in which $f(u) = e^u$, although they implicitly assumed $\gamma = 0$ (no contextual effect) and so described them as assumptions for estimating β; see also Sheppard (2003), Prentice and Sheppard (1995), and Greenland (1992). From a scientific perspective these assumptions can appear highly artificial (e.g., X multivariate normal with constant covariance matrix across aggregates, which cannot be satisfied if X has discrete components that vary in distribution across aggregates), although the bias from their violation might not always be large (Richardson et al., 1987; Sheppard and Prentice, 1995; Dobson, 1988). Nonetheless, even if the bias in estimating $\beta + \gamma$ is small, β and γ remain inseparable without further assumptions or individual-level data.

Extensions of the Basic Model

Model 12–1 is a bilevel model, in that it incorporates covariates for individual-level characteristics (the X) and for one level of aggregation (the Z). The model can be extended to incorporate characteristics of multiple levels of aggregation (Goldstein, 1995). For example, the model could include a covariate vector Z_c of census-tract characteristics, such as the average income in the tract, and another vector Z_s of state characteristics, such as the law indicators and enforcement variables (e.g., conviction rates and average time served for various felonies). The above points can be roughly generalized by saying that the absence of data on one level should be expected to limit inferences about effects at other levels. The term *cross-level bias* denotes bias in coefficient estimates on one level that results from incorrect assumptions about effects on other levels (e.g., linearity or absence of effects); similarly, *cross-level confounding* denotes inseparability of different levels of effect, as illustrated above.

An important extension of multilevel models adds between-level co-variate products (interactions) to Model 12–1, thus allowing the individual effects β to vary across groups. Even with correct specification and multilevel data, the number of free parameters that results can be excessive for ordinary methods. One solution is to constrain the variation with hierarchical coefficient models, which induces a mixed model for individual outcomes (Goldstein, 1995). For example, adding products among X and Z to Model 12–1 is a special case of replacing β by θ_k, with θ_k constrained by the second-stage model

$$\theta_k = \beta + A_k \delta \tag{12–6}$$

where A_k is a known fixed matrix function of z_k. The ensemble of estimates of the vectors $\theta_1, \ldots, \theta_K$ can then be shrunk toward a common estimated mean $\tilde{\beta}$ by specifying a mean-zero, variance τ^2 distribution for δ. This process is equivalent to (empirical) Bayesian averaging of Model 12–1 with the expanded model

$$\mu_{ik} = f(\alpha + x_{ik}\beta + z_k\gamma + x_{ik}A_k\delta) \tag{12–7}$$

(Greenland, 1999). Unfortunately, the nonidentifiability and confounding problems of ecologic analysis only worsen in the presence of cross-level interactions (Greenland and Morgenstern, 1989).

Ecologic Regression

Many, if not most, ecologic researchers do not consider the individual or aggregated Models 12–1 or 12–2 but instead directly model the aggregated outcome $\overline{Y}$ with an ecologic regression model. If $Z = \overline{X}$, an ecologic generalized linear model is

$$E_k(\overline{Y}) = \overline{\mu}_k = h(a + \overline{x}_k b) \tag{12–8}$$

With $h(u) = u$ and individual linearity (Model 12–3), the results given above imply that b will be a linear combination of individual and contextual effects. Given individual nonlinearities, Model 12–8 will at best approximate a complex aggregate regression like Model 12–2, and b will represent a correspondingly complex mixture of individual and contextual effects (Sheppard, 2003). These results also apply when purely contextual variables are included with $\overline{X}$ in Z and $\overline{x}_k$ is replaced by z_k in Model 12–8.

The classic ecologic fallacy (perhaps more accurately termed cross-level bias in estimating individual effects from ecologic data) is to identify b in Model 12–8 with β in Model 12–1. This identification is fallacious because unless $\gamma = 0$ (contextual effects absent), even linearity does not guarantee $b = \beta$. With individual-level nonlinearity, even $\gamma = 0$ does not guarantee $b = \beta$. Ecologic researchers interested in estimating contextual effects should note the symmetrical results that apply when estimating contextual effects from ecologic data. Even with linearity, $b = \gamma$ will require $\beta = 0$, which corresponds to no individual-level effects of X, even when the aggregate summaries of X in Z (such as $\overline{X}$) have effects. In other words, for the ecologic coefficient b to correspond to the contextual effect γ, any within-group heterogeneity in individual outcomes must be unrelated to the individual analogues of the contextual covariates. For example, if X is income and Z is mean income $\overline{X}$, $b = \gamma \neq 0$ would require individual incomes to have no effect except as mediated though average area income. Such a condition is rarely, if ever, plausible.

MULTILEVEL STUDIES

Problems arising from within-group heterogeneity should diminish as the aggregates are made more homogeneous on relevant covariates. Heterogeneity of social factors may also decline as the aggregates become more restricted (e.g., census tracts tend to be more homogeneous on income and education than counties). Nonetheless, the benefits of such restriction may be nullified if important covariate measures (e.g., alcohol and tobacco) are available only for the broader aggregates, because confounding by those covariates may remain uncontrollable.

Suppose, however, that within-region, individual-level survey data are available for those covariates. Individual-level risk models may then be applied to within-region survey data and the resulting individual risk estimates aggregated for comparison to observed ecologic rates (Kleinman et al., 1981; Dobson, 1988). For example, suppose we have a covariate vector X measured on N_k surveyed individuals in region k, a rate model $r(x; \beta)$ with a β estimate $\hat{\beta}$ from individual-level studies (e.g., a proportional-hazards model derived from cohort-study data), and the observed rate $\tilde{r}_k$ in region k. We may compare $\tilde{r}_k$ to the area rate predicted from the model applied to the survey data, $\sum_i r(x_i; \hat{\beta})/N_k$, where the sum is over the surveyed individuals $i = 1, \ldots, N_k$ and x_i is the value of X for survey individual i. This approach is a regression analogue of indirect adjustment: $\hat{\beta}$ is the external information and corresponds to the reference rates used to construct expectations in standardized morbidity ratios.

Unfortunately, fitted models generalizable to the regions of interest are rarely available. Thus, starting from the individual-level model $r_k(x; \beta) = r_{0k}\exp(x\beta)$, Prentice and Sheppard (1995) and Sheppard and Prentice (1995) proposed estimating the individual parameters β by directly regressing the $\tilde{r}_k$ on the survey data using the induced aggregate model $r_k = r_{0k}E_k[\exp(x\beta)]$, where $E_k[\exp(x\beta)]$ is the average of $\exp(x\beta)$ over the individuals in region k. Prentice and Sheppard (1995) showed how the observed rates $\tilde{r}_k$ and the survey data (the x_i) can be used to fit this model. As with earlier methods, their method estimates region-specific averages from sample averages, but in the absence of external data on β, it constrains the region-specific baseline rates r_{0k} (e.g., by treating them as random effects); see Cleave et al. (1995) and Wakefield (2003) for related approaches.

Prentice and Sheppard (1995) called their method an "aggregate-data study"; however, much of the social science literature has long used this term as a synonym for "ecologic study" (Firebaugh, 1978; Borgatta and Jackson, 1980), and so I would instead call it an incomplete multilevel study (because, unlike a complete multilevel study, individual-level outcomes are not obtained). Prentice and Sheppard (1995) conceived their approach in the context of cancer research, in which few cases would be found in modest-sized survey samples. For studies of common acute outcomes, Navidi et al. (1994) proposed a complete multilevel strategy in which the within-region surveys obtain outcome as well as covariate data on individuals, which obviates the need for identifying constraints.

Multilevel studies can combine the advantages of both individual-level and ecologic studies, including the confounder control achievable in individual-level studies and the exposure variation and rapid conduct achievable in ecologic studies (Guthrie and Sheppard, 2001). These advantages are subject to many assumptions that must be carefully evaluated (Prentice and Sheppard, 1995). Multilevel studies share several of these assumptions with ecologic studies. For example, multilevel studies based on recent individual surveys must assume stability of exposure and covariate distributions over time to ensure that the survey distributions are representative of the distributions that determined the observed ecologic rates. This assumption will be suspect when individual behavioral trends or important degrees of migration emerge after the exposure period relevant to the observed rates (Stavraky, 1976; Polissar, 1980). Multilevel studies can also suffer from the problem, mentioned earlier, that the aggregate-level (ecologic) data usually concern arbitrary administrative or political units, and so can be poor contextual measures. Furthermore, multilevel studies face a major practical limitation in requiring data from representative samples of individuals within ecologic units, which can be many times more expensive to obtain than the routinely collected data on which most ecologic studies are based.

In the absence of valid individual-level data, multilevel analysis can still be applied to the ecologic data via nonidentified random-coefficient regression. As in applications to individual-level studies (Greenland, 2000a), this approach begins with specifying a hierarchical prior distribution for parameters not identified by available data. The distribution for the effect of interest is then updated by conditioning on the available data. This approach is a multilevel extension of random-effects ecologic regression to allow constraints on β (including a distribution for β) in the aggregate model, in addition to constraints on the r_{0k}. It is essential to recognize that these constraints are what identify exposure effects in ecologic data; hence, as with all ecologic results, a precise estimate should be attributed to the constraints that produced the precision.

OTHER SPECIAL PROBLEMS OF ECOLOGIC ANALYSIS

Thus far, I have focused on problems of confounding and cross-level effects in ecologic studies. These are not the only problems of ecologic studies. Several others are especially noteworthy for their divergence from individual-level study problems or their absence from typical individual-level studies.

Noncomparability Among Ecologic Analysis Variables

The use of noncomparably standardized or restricted covariates in an ecologic model such as 12–8 can lead to considerable bias (Rosenbaum and Rubin, 1984; Greenland, 1992). Typically, this bias occurs when $\overline{Y}$ is age-standardized and specific to sex and race categories but $\overline{X}$ is not. For example, disease rates are routinely published in age-standardized, sex-race specific form, but most summary covariates (e.g., alcohol and tobacco sales) are not. Such noncomparability can lead to bias in the ecologic coefficient b in Model 12–8 as a representation of the mixed effect $\beta + \gamma$, because the coefficients of crude covariate summaries will not capture the rate variation associated with variation in alcohol and tobacco use by age, sex, and race.

Unfortunately, noncomparable restriction and standardization of variables remain common in ecologic analyses. Typical examples involve restricted standardized rates regressed on crude ecologic variables, such as sex-race-specific age-standardized mortality rates regressed on contextual variables (e.g., air-pollution levels) and unrestricted unstandardized summaries (e.g., per capita cigarette sales). If, as is usual, only unrestricted, un-standardized regressor summaries are available, less bias might be incurred by using the crude (rather than the standardized) rates as the outcome and controlling for ecologic demographic differences by entering multiple age-sex-race-distribution summaries in the regression (Rosenbaum and Rubin, 1984) (e.g., proportions in different age-sex-race categories). More work is needed to develop methods for coping with noncomparability.

Measurement Error

The effects of measurement error on ecologic and individual-level analyses can be quite different. For example, Brenner et al. (1992a) found that independent nondifferential misclassification of a binary exposure could produce bias away from the null and even reverse estimates from a standard linear or log-linear ecologic regression analysis, even though the same error would produce only bias toward the null in a standard individual-level analysis. Analogous results were obtained by Carroll (1997) for ecologic probit regression with a continuous measure of exposure. Results of Brenner et al. (1992a) also indicate that ecologic regression estimates can be extraordinarily sensitive to errors in exposure measurement. On the other hand, Brenner et al. (1992b) found that independent nondifferential misclassification of a single binary confounder produced no increase in bias in an ecologic linear regression. Similarly, Prentice and Sheppard (1995) and Sheppard and Prentice (1995) found robustness of their incomplete multilevel analysis to purely random measurement errors.

Besides assuming very simple models for individual-level errors, the foregoing results assume that the ecologic covariates in the analysis are direct summaries of the individual measures. Often, however, the ecologic covariates are subject to errors beyond random survey error or individual-level measurement errors, for example, when per capita sales data are used as a proxy for average individual consumption, and when area measurements such as pollution levels are subject to errors. Some researchers have examined the impact of such ecologic measurement error on cross-level inferences under simple error models (Navidi et al., 1994; Wakefield and Salway, 2001), but more research is needed, especially for the situation in which the grouping variable is an arbitrary administrative unit serving as a proxy for a contextual variable.

Problems in Causal Interpretation

This chapter, like most of the literature, has been rather loose in using the word *effect*. Strictly speaking, the models and results discussed here apply only to interpretations of coefficients as measures of conditional associations. Their interpretation as measures of causal effects in formal causal models such as potential-outcome (counterfactual) models (Greenland and Rothman, 1998; Pearl, 2000; Little and Rubin, 2000; Greenland, 2000b) raises some problems not ordinarily encountered in individual-level modeling.

To avoid technical details, consider the linear-model example. A causal interpretation of β in model 3 is that it represents the change in an individual's risk that would result from increasing that person's income by $1000. Apart from the ambiguity of this intervention (does the money come from a pay raise or direct payment?), one might note that it would also raise the average income value $\bar{x}_k$ by $1000/N_k$ and produce an additional change of γ/N_k in the risk of the individual. This interpretation apparently contradicts the original interpretation of β as *the* change in risk, from whence we see that β must be interpreted carefully as the change in risk given that average income is (somehow) held constant, e.g., by reducing everyone else's income by $1000/(N_k - 1)$ each.

If the size of the aggregate N_k is large, this problem is trivial; if it is small, however (e.g., the aggregate is a census tract), it may be important. One solution with a scientific basis is to recognize $\bar{X}$ as a contextual surrogate for socioeconomic environment, in which case the contextual value $\bar{x}_k$ in Model 12–1 might be better replaced by an individual-level variable $\bar{x}_{(-i)k}$, the average income of persons in aggregate k apart from individual i. Note that the mean of $\bar{x}_{(-i)k}$ is $\bar{x}_k$, and so its effect could not be separated from that of personal income when only aggregate means are available; that is, β and γ remain completely confounded.

Causal interpretation of the contextual coefficient γ is symmetrically problematic. This coefficient represents the change in risk from a $1000 increase in average income $\bar{x}_k$, while keeping the person's income x_{ik} the same. This income can be kept constant in many ways, e.g., by giving everyone but person i a $1000N_k/(N_k - 1)$ raise, or by giving one person other than i a $1000N_k$ raise. The difference between these two interventions is profound and might be resolved by clarifying the variable for which $\bar{X}$ is a surrogate. Similar comments apply to causal interpretation of b in the ecologic model (Model 12–8).

Problems of causal interpretation only add to the difficulties in the analysis of contextual causal effects, but, unlike confounding, they may be as challenging for individual-level and multilevel studies as they are for ecologic studies (Iversen, 1991). Addressing these problems demands that detailed subject-matter considerations be used to construct explicit multilevel causal models in which key variables at any level may be latent (not directly measured).

Problems in Aggregation Level

Another serious and often overlooked conceptual problem involves the special artificiality of typical model specifications above the individual level. Ecologic units are usually arbitrary administrative groupings, such as counties, which may have only weak relations to contextual variables of scientific interest, such as social environment (Achen and Shively, 1995). Compounding this problem is the potentially high sensitivity of aggregate-level relationships to the grouping definitions (Openshaw and Taylor, 1981). In light of these problems it may be more realistic to begin with at least a trilevel specification, in which one aggregate level is of direct scientific interest (e.g., neighborhood or community) and the other (or others) are the aggregates for which data are available (e.g., census tracts or counties). This larger initial specification would at least clarify the proxy-variable (measurement surrogate) issues inherent in most studies of contextual effects.

CONCLUSION

The validity of any inference can only benefit from critical scrutiny of the assumptions on which it is based. Users of surveillance data should be alert to the special assumptions needed to estimate an effect from ecologic data alone, and to the profound sensitivity of inferences to those assumptions (even if the estimate is of a contextual effect). The fact that individual-level studies have complementary limitations does not excuse the failure to consider these assumptions.

Nonetheless, despite the critical tone of the remarks here and elsewhere, ecologic data are worth examining. Their value has been demonstrated by careful ecologic analyses (e.g., Richardson et al., 1987; Prentice and Sheppard, 1989) and by methods that combine individual and ecologic data (Navidi et al., 1994; Prentice and Sheppard, 1995; Sheppard and Prentice, 1995; Künzli and Taeger, 1997; Duncan et al., 1998). Furthermore, the possibility of bias does not prove the presence of bias, and a conflict between ecologic and individual-level estimates does not by itself mean that the ecologic estimates are the more biased (Schwartz, 1994; Greenland and Robins, 1994a,b). The two types of estimates share some biases but not others, making it possible for the individual-level estimates to be the more biased.

The effects measured by the two types of estimates may differ as well; ecologic estimates incorporate a contextual component that is absent from the individual estimates derived from a narrow context. Indeed, the contextual component may be viewed as both a key strength and weakness of ecologic studies, because it is often of greatest importance, although it is especially vulnerable to confounding. Thus, in the absence of good multi-level studies, ecologic studies will no doubt continue to fuel controversy and so inspire the conduct of potentially more informative studies.

ACKNOWLEDGMENT

Most of the material in this chapter was adapted from Greenland, S. (2001). Ecologic versus individual-level sources of bias in ecologic estimates of contextual health effects, *International Journal of Epidemiology*, **30**, (Oxford University Press, used by permission), and Greenland, S. (2002). A review of multilevel theory for ecologic analyses, **21**, 389–395 (John Wiley and Sons, used by permission).

REFERENCES

Achen, C.H. and Shively, W.P. (1995). *Cross-Level Inference*. Chicago: University of Chicago Press.

Borgatta, E.F. and Jackson, D.J., eds. (1980). *Aggregate Data: Analysis and Interpretation*. Beverly Hills: Sage.

Brenner, H., Savitz, D.A., Jöckel, K.-H., and Greenland S. (1992a). Effects of nondifferential exposure misclassification in ecologic studies. *American Journal of Epidemiology* **135**, 85–95.

Brenner, H., Greenland, S., and Savitz, D.A. (1992b). The effects of nondifferential confounder misclassification in ecologic studies. *Epidemiology* **3**, 456–459.

Carroll, R.J. (1997). Some surprising effects of measurement error in an aggregate data estimator. *Biometrika* **84**, 231–234.

Cho, W.T.K. (1998). If the assumption fits: a comment on the King ecologic inference solution. *Political Analysis* **7**, 143–163.

Cleave, N., Brown, P.J., and Payne, C.D. (1995). Evaluation of methods for ecological inference. *Journal of the Royal Statistical Society Series A* **158**, 55–72.

Cohen, B.L. (1990). Ecological versus case-control studies for testing a linear-no-threshold dose-response relationship. *International Journal of Epidemiology* **19**, 680–684.

Cohen, B.L. (1994). In defense of ecological studies for testing a linear no-threshold theory. *American Journal of Epidemiology* **139**, 765–768.

Cohen, B.L. (1995). Letter to the editor. *Statistics in Medicine* **14**, 327–328.

Cohen, B.L. (2000). Re: Parallel analyses of individual and ecologic data on residential radon, cofactors, and lung cancer in Sweden (letter). *American Journal of Epidemiology* **152**, 194–195.

Dobson, A.J. (1988). Proportional hazards models for average data for groups. *Statistics in Medicine* **7**, 613–618.

Duncan, C., Jones, K., and Moon, G. (1996). Health-related behaviour in context: a multilevel modeling approach. *Social Science & Medicine* **42**, 817–830.

Duncan, C., Jones, K., and Moon, G. (1998). Context, composition and heterogeneity: using multilevel models in health research. *Social Science & Medicine* **46,** 97–117.

Duncan, O.D. and Davis, B. (1953). An alternative to ecological correlation. *American Sociological Review* **18,** 665–666.

Firebaugh, G. (1978). A rule for inferring individual-level relationships from aggregate data. *American Sociological Review* **43,** 557–572.

Firebaugh, G. (1980). Assessing group effects. In Borgatta, E.F. and Jackson, D.J. eds. *Aggregate Data:Analysis and Interpretation.* Beverly Hills: Sage, pp. 13–24.

Freedman, D.A., Klein, S.P., Ostland, M., and Roberts, M.R. (1998a). Review of "A solution to the ecological inference problem." *Journal of the American Statistical Association* **93,** 1518–1522.

Freedman, D.A., Klein, S.P., Sacks, J., Smyth, C.A., and Everett, C.G. (1998b). Ecological regression and voting rights (with discussion). *Evaluation Review* **15,** 673–816.

Freedman, D.A., Ostland, M., Roberts, M.R., and Klein, S.P. (1999). Reply to King (letter). *Journal of the American Statistical Association* **94,** 355–357.

Goldstein, H. (1995). *Multilevel Statistical Models,* 2nd ed. New York: Edward Arnold.

Goodman, L.A. (1959). Some alternatives to ecological correlation. *American Journal of Sociology* **64,** 610–625.

Greenland, S. (1990). Randomization, statistics, and causal inference. *Epidemiology* **1,** 421–429.

Greenland, S. (1992). Divergent biases in ecologic and individual-level studies. *Statistics in Medicine* **11,** 1209–1223.

Greenland, S. (1995). Author's Reply. *Statistics in Medicine* **14,** 328–330.

Greenland, S. (1999). Multilevel modeling and model averaging. *Scandinavian Journal of Work Environment and Health* **25,** Supplement 4, 43–48.

Greenland, S. (2000a). When should epidemiologic regressions use random coefficients? *Biometrics* **56,** 915–921.

Greenland, S. (2000b). Causal analysis in the health sciences. *Journal of the American Statistical Association* **95,** 286–289.

Greenland, S. (2001). Ecologic versus individual-level sources of bias in ecologic estimates of contextual health effects. *International Journal of Epidemiology* **30,** 1343–1350.

Greenland, S. (2002). A review of multilevel theory for ecologic analysis. *Statistics in Medicine* **21,** 389–395.

Greenland, S. and Morgenstern, H. (1989). Ecological bias, confounding, and effect modification. *International Journal of Epidemiology* **18,** 269–274.

Greenland, S. and Morgenstern, H. (1991). Neither within-region nor cross-regional independence of covariates prevents ecological bias (letter). *International Journal of Epidemiology* **20,** 816–818.

Greenland, S. and Robins, J. (1994a). Ecologic studies—biases, misconceptions, and counterexamples. *American Journal of Epidemiology* **139,** 747–760.

Greenland, S. and Robins, J.M. (1994b). Accepting the limits of ecologic studies. *American Journal of Epidemiology* **139,** 769–771.

Greenland, S., Robins, J.M., and Pearl, J. (1999). Confounding and collapsibility in causal inference. *Statistical Science* **14,** 29–46.

Greenland, S. and Rothman, K.J. (1998). Measures of effect and measures of association. In Rothman, K.J. and Greenland, S., eds. *Modern Epidemiology*, 2nd ed. Philadelphia: Lippincott, pp. 47–66.

Guthrie, K.A. and Sheppard, L. (2001). Overcoming biases and misconceptions in ecologic studies. *Journal of the Royal Statistical Society Series A* **164,** 141–154.

Hakama, M., Hakulinen, T., Pukkala, E., Saxen, F., and Teppo, L. (1982). Risk indicators of breast and cervical cancer on ecologic and individual levels. *American Journal of Epidemiology* **116,** 990–1000.

Iversen, G.R. (1991). *Contextual Analysis*. Thousand Oaks, CA: Sage.

King, G. (1997). *A Solution to the Ecological Inference Problem*. Princeton: Princeton University Press.

King, G. (1999). The future of ecological inference (letter). *Journal of the American Statistical Association* **94,** 352–354.

Kleinman, J.C., DeGruttola, V.G., Cohen B.B., and Madans J.H. (1981). Regional and urban-suburban differentials in coronary heart disease mortality and risk factor prevalence. *Journal of Chronic Diseases* **34,** 11–19.

Koopman, J.S. and Longini, I.M., Jr. (1994). The ecological effects of individual exposures and nonlinear disease dynamics in populations. *American Journal of Public Health* **84,** 836–842.

Künzli, N. and Tager, J.B. (1997). The semi-individual study in air pollution Epidemiology: a valid design as compared to ecologic studies. *Environmental Health Perspectives* **105,** 1078–1083.

Lagarde, F. and Pershagen, G. (1999). Parallel analyses of individual and ecologic data on residential radon, cofactors, and lung cancer in Sweden. *American Journal of Epidemiology* **149,** 268–274.

Lagarde, F. and Pershagen, G. (2000). The authors reply (letter). *American Journal of Epidemiology* **152,** 195.

Langbein, L.I. and Lichtman, A.J. (1978). *Ecological Inference*. Series/No. 07-010, Thousand Oaks, CA: Sage.

Lasserre, V., Guihenneuc-Jouyaux, C., and Richardson, S. (2000). Biases in ecological studies: utility of including within-area distribution of confounders. *Statistics in Medicine* **19,** 45–59.

Little, R.J.A. and Rubin, D.B. (2000). Causal effects in clinical and epidemiological studies via potential outcomes: concepts and analytical approaches. *Annual Reviews of Public Health* **21,** 121–145.

Künzli, N. and Taeger, I.B. (1997). The semi-individual study in air pollution epidemiology: a valid design as compared to ecologic studies. *Environmental Health Perspectives* **105,** 1078–1083.

Morgenstern, H. (1998). Ecologic studies. In Rothman, K.J. and Greenland, S., eds. *Modern Epidemiology*, 2nd ed. Philadelphia: Lippincott, pp. 459–480.

Navidi, W., Thomas, D., Stram, D., and Peters, J. (1994). Design and analysis of multilevel analytic studies with applications to a study of air pollution. *Environmental Health Perspectives* **102,** Supplement 8, 25–32.

Naylor, C.D. (1999). Ecological analysis of intended treatment effects: Caveat emptor. *Journal of Clinical Epidemiology* **52,** 1–5.

Openshaw, S. and Taylor, P.H. (1981). The modifiable area unit problem. In Wrigley, N. and Bennett, R.J., eds. *Quantitative Geography*. London: Routledge, Ch. 9. p 60–69.

Pearce, N. (1996). Traditional epidemiology, modern epidemiology, and public health. *American Journal of Public Health* **86,** 678–683.

Pearl, J. (2000). *Causality*. New York: Cambridge University Press.

Piantadosi, S. (1994). Ecologic biases. *American Journal of Epidemiology* **139,** 761–764.

Piantadosi, S., Byar, D.P., and Green, S.B. (1988). The ecological fallacy. *American Journal of Epidemiology* **127,** 893–704.

Plummer, M. and Clayton, D. (1996). Estimation of population exposure in ecological studies. *Journal of the Royal Statistical Society Series B* **58,** 113–126.

Polissar, L. (1980). The effect of migration on comparison of disease rates in geographic studies in the United States. *American Journal of Epidemiology* **111,** 175–182.

Prentice, R.L. and Sheppard, L. (1989). Validity of international, time trend, and migrant studies of dietary factors and disease risk. *Preventive Medicine* **18,** 167–179.

Prentice, R.L. and Sheppard, L. (1995). Aggregate data studies of disease risk factors. *Biometrika* **82,** 113–125.

Richardson, S. and Hémon, D. (1990). Ecological bias and confounding (letter). *International Journal of Epidemiology* **19,** 764–766.

Richardson, S., Stücker, I., and Hémon, D. (1987). Comparison of relative risks obtained in ecological and individual studies: some methodological considerations. *International Journal of Epidemiology* **16,** 111–120.

Rivers, D. (1998). Review of "A solution to the ecological inference problem." *American Political Science Review* **92,** 442–443.

Rosenbaum, P. R. and Rubin, D.B. (1984). Difficulties with regression analyses of age-adjusted rates. *Biometrics* **40,** 437–443.

Rothman, K.J. and Greenland, S. (1998). Measures of disease frequency. In Rothman, K.J. and Greenland, S., eds. *Modern Epidemiology*. 2nd ed. Philadelphia: Lippincott. pp 29–46.

Rubin, D.B. (1990). Comment: Neyman (1923) and causal inference in experiments and observational studies. *Statistical Science* **5,** 472–480.

Schwartz, S. (1994). The fallacy of the ecological fallacy: The potential misuse of a concept and the consequences. *American Journal of Public Health* **84,** 819–824.

Sheppard, L. (2003). Insights on bias and information in group-level studies. *Biostatistics* **4,** 265–278.

Sheppard, L. and Prentice R.L. (1995). On the reliability and precision of within- and between-population estimates of relative rate parameters. *Biometrics* **51,** 853–863.

Stavraky, K.M. (1976). The role of ecologic analysis in studies of the etiology of disease: a discussion with reference to large bowel cancer. *Journal of Chronic Diseases* **29,** 435–444.

Stidley, C. and Samet, J.M. (1994). Assessment of ecologic regression in the study of lung cancer and indoor radon. *American Journal of Epidemiology* **139,** 312–322.

Stoto, M.A. (1998). Review of "Ecological inference in public health." *Public Health Reports* **113,** 182–183.

Susser, M. (1994). The logic in ecological. *American Journal of Public Health* **84,** 825–835.

Susser, M. and Susser, E. (1996). Choosing a future for epidemiology: II. from black box to Chinese boxes and eco-epidemiology. *American Journal of Public Health* **86,** 674–677.

Vaupel, J.W., Manton, K.G., and Stallard, E. (1979). The impact of heterogeneity in individual frailty on the dynamics of mortality. *Demography* **16,** 439–454.

Von Korff, M., Koepsell, T., Curry, S., and Diehr, P. (1992). Multi-level analysis in epidemiologic research on health behaviors and outcomes. *American Journal of Epidemiology* **135,** 1077–1082.

Wakefield, J. (2003). Ecological inference for 2 × 2 tables. *Journal of the Royal Statistical Society* **166.**

Wakefield, J. and Salway, R. (2001). A statistical framework for ecological and aggregate studies. *Journal of the Royal Statistical Society Series A* **164,** 119–137.

Wen, S.W. and Kramer, M.S. (1999). Uses of ecologic studies in the assessment of intended treatment effects. *Journal of Clinical Epidemiology* **52,** 7 12.

.

13

Completeness of Reporting: Capture–Recapture Methods in Public Health Surveillance

ERNEST B. HOOK, RONALD R. REGAL

Routine surveillance data on a disorder are often incomplete and seriously undercount the number of affected persons. A possible remedy is to take a complete census of all cases in the community, but this process is often time consuming and expensive. Moreover, census taking always results in uncertainty about whether all cases have been identified. An alternative is the use of capture–recapture methods. As applied in epidemiology, these methods use information from overlapping and incomplete lists, or sources, of diagnosed cases to estimate the prevalence of a disorder in a population. Data from such lists, even if collectively incomplete, may enable the total number of affected persons to be estimated without the expense of a special ad hoc survey.

The term *capture–recapture* comes from ecology and refers to a process in which investigators capture, mark, release, and recapture animals in the wild, perhaps making many recapture attempts in a certain period to estimate the size of the total population. Capture–recapture methods were introduced into epidemiology by Janet Wittes in 1974. (For a general review and history of these methods, see Hook and Regal, 1995 and International Working Group for Disease Monitoring and Forecasting, 1995.) In this field, the name of an affected person in a source, or list of cases, available to an epidemiologist is analogous to the capture of an animal by an ecologist. The number of people in each source used by an epidemiologist is equivalent to the number of animals in a particular population that is captured and subsequently recaptured by an ecologist. The epidemiologist ordinarily must use sources that are available in the community, which are almost always samples of convenience, whereas the ecologist can plan capture attempts in an effort to make the captured animals an unbiased sample. However, the epidemiologist can collapse or pool sources in many more ways than the ecologist, who must respect the temporal ordering of each population capture attempt.

In human studies, each person is already marked with a usually unique, unchanging name and other characteristics, such as date of birth, that allow cases to be matched if a person is listed in more than one source. In most of the comments below, it is presumed that near-perfect matching of records can be obtained. (For implicit or explicit strategies to be used when near-perfect matching is not possible, see Brenner, 1994; Hook and Regal, 1995, 1999.)

It is suggested that epidemiologists use capture–recapture methods in the spirit of the analyses of W.E. Deming (see, for example, Deming, 1938, 1986; Orsini, 1997). Before starting, consider the intended use of the derived estimates, and, by implication, the precision required. Also make the analytic process dynamic by continually checking the methods and results against the indeed use of the data. These considerations are particularly important in surveillance or monitoring.

Epidemiologists have used the terms surveillance and monitoring in different senses (see Hook and Cross, 1982). *Surveillance* is defined the regular review of rates of some type of morbidity or mortality, usually in a large population, to detect nonrandom change in the rates. The definition of *monitoring* is limited to following intensively some subgroup of the population that is already identified as being at high risk for some reason, such as living near a toxic waste site, taking a potent drug, or having a genetic abnormality. Here, we confine our applications to surveillance.

In our opinion, the initial goal of surveillance is to identify in a timely manner a trend of interest, or of concern, in prevalence or incidence that merits further field investigation. (The ultimate public health goal is to identify the cause of such a trend and to remove it if deleterious or to enhance it if beneficial.) Here, we elaborate on the possible use of capture–recapture methods for such a purpose, but we urge investigators to consider whether a simpler approach is more appropriate, especially for surveillance analysis (see, for example, Hook [1990]). Sometimes enhancing capture–recapture methods with data from an additional source, especially data obtained by sampling the population (if a frame can be specified), is preferable to the full capture–recapture methods (see Hook and Regal, 1999 for elaboration and an example).

ESTIMATING PREVALENCE FROM TWO SOURCES

Suppose data are available from two sources (two overlapping, incomplete lists of cases), labeled *1* and *2*. Suppose also that presence is indicated as subscript 1 and absence as subscript zero. If n_{11} cases are reported by, or located in, both *1* and *2*, n_{10} are in source *1* only, n_{01} are in source *2* only, and n_{00} are unobserved (listed in neither source), then n_{00}, the number missing from both sources, may be estimated by:

$$\tilde{n} = n_{10}n_{01} / n_{11} \qquad (13\text{–}1)$$

This number is the maximum likelihood estimator (MLE).

A small-sample adjustment, which under some circumstances may improve an estimate of n_{00}, can be made by adding 1 to the denominator; that is, by dividing $n_{10}n_{01}$ in Eq. 13–1 by $1 + n_{11}$, rather than by n_{11} (see Wittes, 1973, 1974 for a discussion of both the MLE and this adjustment). Another adjustment, implied by the analysis of Evans and Bonnett (1994), is to add 0.5 to each of the 3 terms n_{10}, n_{01}, and n_{11}. It is usually impossible to determine whether either of these adjustments improves the estimate in any particular case. In most surveillance applications either adjustment would have a marked effect only if n_{11} is zero or very small. We have reservations about attempting any capture–recapture estimate in such cases; that is, cases wherein a small sample adjustment seriously alters an estimate. In deriving two-source estimates in our examples below, we do not use a small-sample adjustment.

The MLE of the population total N, is:

$$\tilde{N} = n_{10} + n_{01} + n_{11} + (n_{10}\, n_{01} / n_{11}) \qquad (13\text{–}2)$$

or, equivalently,

$$\tilde{N} = (n_{10} + n_{11})(n_{01} + n_{11}) / n_{11} \qquad (13\text{–}3)$$

Such an estimate presumes—and this is a key assumption—that the sources are independent; that is, that observing a case in one source, X, is as likely for cases in the other source, Y, as for those not in the other source, Y.

Data from Hook et al. (1980) on spina bifida in upstate New York for the years 1969 to 1974 provide an example of a two-source estimate. In this example, we consider cases from the files of a medical rehabilitation (MR) bureau that provides statewide services and cases reported on birth certifications (BC). In these years, 389 cases were noted on the BC forms but not in MR files, 64 were reported in MR but not in BC forms, and 124 cases were reported in both. If we denote BC as source *1* and MR as source *2*, then $n_{11} = 124$, $n_{10} = 389$, and $n_{01} = 64$. The estimate of unobserved cases from Eq. 13–1 is 201, and the estimate of the total from Eq. 13–2 or 13–3 is 778 affected persons. (If we use the small-sample adjustment of Wittes or of Evans and Bonnett, the estimate would be 776 or 779, respectively.) The estimate assumes that MR and BC are independent. Our knowledge about these sources gives us no reason to reject this assumption, but it might be incorrect. With additional sources, one can often test for and adjust for the possible dependencies of sources.

ESTIMATING PREVALENCE FROM THREE OR MORE SOURCES

For data from multiple sources, we limit consideration to log linear methods whose application to capture–recapture estimates was first suggested by Fienberg (1972). We regard these methods, or some modification of them, as optimal. Several other methods have been developed for capture–recapture estimation, some of which are discussed by the International Working Group for Disease Monitoring and Forecasting (1995). Some complex methods for adjusting log-linear estimates by combining them with logistic regression (when considerable information is available on covariates) are discussed by Ahlo (1990, 1994), Ahlo et al. (1993), and by Tilling and Sterne (1999).

With three or more data sources, the structure and notation of the observed data may be presented as in Table 13–1. With data on three sources, three different two-source estimates may be generated by ignoring the data on the other list. The example in Estimating Prevalence from Two Sources, above was such a case because data from a third source, death certificates, was ignored in reaching our two-source BC-MR estimates. As explained below, there may be advantages to ignoring the information in the unused source.

When data from three sources are used, eight different models of the affected population are generated, each making different assumptions about the dependencies among the sources, and each associated with a possibly different estimate (see Table 13–1). A question immediately arises as to which estimate is optimal or whether the estimates can be combined. Numerous methods have been developed for deriving an estimate from these eight models, or, more generally, from models using k sources, where $k \geq 3$ (see Hook and Regal, 2000 for an extended discussion). This discussion is limited to two such methods.

One method is to select the estimate generated by the model with the minimum Akaike Information Criterion (AIC) statistic (but see the exception below). If m represents a particular model, its associated AIC statistic is:

$$\text{AIC}_m = (G^2)_m - 2\ df_m \tag{13–4}$$

Table 13–1 Notation and models for estimating prevalence from three independent data sources

	Notation		

	Case included in		
Source 1*	Source 2*	Source 3*	Frequency
yes	yes	yes	n_{111}
yes	yes	no	n_{110}
yes	no	yes	n_{101}
yes	no	no	n_{100}
no	yes	yes	n_{011}
no	yes	no	n_{010}
no	no	yes	n_{001}
no	no	no	$n_{000} = x$

*The total in Source 1 is denoted as n_{1++}, in Source 2 as n_{+1+}, and in Source 3 as n_{++1}. $N_{Obs} = n_{001} + n_{010} + n_{100} + n_{011} + n_{101} + n_{110} + n_{111}$.

Model*	Degrees of freedom	Estimator ($\tilde{N}$ or $\tilde{n}$ where $\tilde{N} = N_{Obs} + \tilde{n}$)
Independent	3	$\tilde{n} = \tilde{N} - N_{Obs}$ where $\tilde{N}$ is the solution of $(\tilde{N} - n_{++1})(\tilde{N} - n_{+1+})(\tilde{N} - n_{11+}) = \tilde{N}^2(\tilde{N} - N_{Obs})$
1-2 Interaction	2	$\tilde{n} = (n_{110} + n_{100} + n_{010})n_{001}/(n_{111} + n_{101} + n_{011})$
1-3 Interaction	2	$\tilde{n} = (n_{101} + n_{100} + n_{001})n_{010}/(n_{111} + n_{110} + n_{011})$
2-3 Interaction	2	$\tilde{n} = (n_{001} + n_{010} + n_{011})n_{100}/(n_{111} + n_{101} + n_{110})$
1-2, 1-3 Interactions	1	$\tilde{n} = n_{010}\, n_{001}/n_{011}$
1-2, 2-3 Interactions	1	$\tilde{n} = n_{100}\, n_{001}/n_{101}$
1-3, 2-3 Interactions	1	$\tilde{n} = n_{100}\, n_{010}/n_{110}$
1-2, 1-3, 2-3 Interactions (The "saturated" model)	0	$\tilde{n} = n_{111}\, n_{100}\, n_{001}\, n_{010}/n_{110}\, n_{101}\, n_{011}$

*The estimate associated with the independent model is derived by assuming that all sources are independent of each other in this population. The estimate associated with the *1-2* interaction model is based on the assumption that the only dependency in the population involves source *1* and source *2*; that is, that sources *1* and *3* are independent and that sources *2* and *3* are independent. (Analogous assumptions apply to estimates associated with the *1-3* and the *2-3* interaction models.) The estimate associated with the *1-2, 1-3* interaction model is based on the assumption that, in this population, dependencies exist between source *1* and source *2*, and between source *1* and source *3*, but not between source *2* and source *3*. (Analogous assumptions apply to estimates associated with the *1-2, 2-3* and *1-3, 2-3* interaction models.) The estimate associated with the *1-2, 1-3, 2-3* interaction model is derived on the assumption that each of the sources has a dependency with the others in this population.

Here, df_m is the degrees of freedom of model m. If there are three sources, the model that assumes independence of all three sources has 3 degrees of freedom; the model that assumes one two-source interaction has 2; the model that assumes two two-source interactions has 1; and the model that assumes all two-source interactions (the saturated model in this log-linear application) has zero degrees of freedom (see Table 13–1).

G_m^2 is the likelihood ratio statistic associated with model m, (sometimes called the *deviance*); that is, for model m:

$$G_m^2 = 2 \sum O_i \ (\ln(O_i / E_i)) \qquad (13\text{–}5)$$

where O_i is the observed number in the ith cell, and E_i is the expected number in the ith cell predicted by model m. For the saturated model, the observed and predicted values are always the same, so G^2 is zero. As df is also zero for this model, the minimum value of AIC_m will always be zero or less. For reasons explained in detail in Hook and Regal (1997, 2000), if this criterion selects the saturated model, it is recommend that *no* capture–recapture estimate be attempted using the saturated model or any other method.

Assuming that the saturated model is not selected, it is suggested that a semi-Bayesian method, which is denoted as "weighted AC," also be considered. This method, which is a modification of an approach suggested by Draper (1995), derives a weighted estimate from the estimates of all models. The lower the value of AIC of a model, the higher the weight given to its associated estimate.

If $\tilde{n}_m$ is the estimate for the unobserved number in the population associated with model m, then the weighted *AIC* estimate for $\tilde{n}$, the number in the unobserved cell x, is:

$$\tilde{n} = \sum ((\exp(-AIC_m / 2) \ x_m) / \sum (\exp(-AIC_m / 2)) \qquad (\text{Eq. } 13\text{–}6)$$

As a practical matter, to avoid a possibly unbounded estimate with this method if a null cell is present, using the correction suggested by Evans and Bonnett (1994), which involves adding $(1/(1/2^{k-1}))$ to each cell where k is the number of sources is recommended. (See also Hook and Regal, 1997, 2000 for further comment on small-sample corrections with three or more sources.)

Note that, with four or more sources, the saturated model estimate is also unstable in the presence of null or small cells. The all-two-way-interactions model with four or more sources is not saturated, however, and the associated estimate is less unstable than in the three-source case. Despite its instability with null or small values in any cell, the saturated model has some optimal properties. For a full discussion of the nuances of its properties as applied to capture–recapture estimation, see Hook and Regal (1997, 2000).

The number of possible estimates using log-linear methods quickly rises as the number of sources increases beyond three. With four sources, there are 113 different models, and thus the same number of estimates. With five sources, there are 6893 models and associated estimates, and with six sources, tens of thousands. For four or more sources, the same criteria may be used for model selection as discussed above (or other criteria, as in Hook and Regal, 1997, 2000). Alternatively, numerous sources may be collapsed into no more than three sources before analysis. This notion of pooling sources to overcome potential dependencies in epidemiologic applications, appears to have originated with Wittes (1974).

As discussed extensively elsewhere, the concept of a source is somewhat arbitrary (Hook and Regal, 1995). Pooling the names in some sources to construct a single list may make good sense. For instance, if three large hospitals in a jurisdiction all report a certain type of case, the cases may be pooled to construct a single natural source, the list of all hospitalized cases. Often, however, cases may be reported in numerous small sources with no natural shared characteristics. A *gemisch* is designated as a source constructed from two or more sources with qualitatively different community dynamics. A gemisch may be the only reasonable manner in which to treat source with very small numbers.

There are $_kC_{(k-3)}$ different methods of generating 3 different sources from data distributed among k sources, each associated with a possibly different optimal estimate. Thus, 4 sources generate 4 different three-source structures, 5 sources generate 10, 6 sources generate 20, and so forth. If there are many sources, this approach reduces markedly the calculational complexity, without making much practical difference in the final estimates. (We have found that the 3-source estimates constructed from different types of pooling of 4 or more sources are fairly similar. We also suspect one could construct examples that provide exceptions.)

We prefer to work with no more than three sources, because we find that conceptualizing interactions and dependencies among four or more sources is very difficult. Even with three sources, difficulties may arise. Pooling many sources in some manner to produce three or fewer lists often provokes further difficulties in conceptualizing interactions if one of the lists is artificially constructed (i.e., if it is a gemisch source, which must be formed, to reduce the total number to three). Even with three well-defined, distinct nongemisch sources, we have still experienced difficulties in thinking about possible dependencies (see Regal and Hook, 1998 for elaboration).

SOURCES OF UNCERTAINTY IN MAKING ESTIMATES AND IN EVALUATING TRENDS

Statistical fluctuation over time in the underlying rates of events in the population is a major concern in surveillance. Capture–recapture analysis introduces an additional source of uncertainty into the procedure. For surveillance purposes, it is suggested that the investigator simply choose what appears subjectively to be the optimal capture–recapture approach to the data, assuming that one can be established (see example below and Hook and Regal, 1999 on this point), and analyze the trends in the estimates over time as if the capture–recapture process had no uncertainty.

If the derived statistic on the trend in such point estimates crosses a decision boundary for follow-up, at this point, the investigator can examine the issue of whether the uncertainty in capture–recapture undermines the rationale for further investigation. In such an endeavor, we prefer not to entangle ourselves with the usual issue of establishing precise statistical criteria for conducting a follow up field investigation, using either exact data or capture–recapture estimates.

Even statistical procedures that use exact or other distribution-free methods to derive uncertainly about a capture–recapture estimate almost always underestimate the true extent of that uncertainty. In our experience, the accuracy of matching the names of individuals listed in various sources provides the largest potential problem, which is rarely addressed by investigators in estimation. In many cases, unique or close-to-unique identifiers, such as names, are not available because of confidentiality considerations. One can undertake a form of probabilistic matching or related procedure, as in Roos and Wajda (1991) or Frischer et al. (1993), but ultimately one can only guess at the magnitude and direction of the bias. As long as this bias is consistent over time, it does not present a serious problem for surveillance.

Matching was likely close to 100% in the upstate New York spina bifida example in Estimating Prevalence from Two Sources, above but such close matching is atypical and arose only because the information was derived from health department records with full identifying information. Use of birth certificates and other heavily monitored data sources enable name changes and other changes to be detected.

The nature of uncertainly of matching is particularly noteworthy for elusive populations, such as adolescents and adults addicted to drugs of abuse, for whom a constant name is of little concern and often a detriment to a chosen lifestyle (Lambert, 1990; Korf et al., 1994). Yet it is precisely for estimating the size of these elusive populations that many investigators seem to find capture–recapture methods particularly attractive. Direct ascertainment is often simply not possible. On this point, see Korf et al. (1994) and Frischer et al. (1993). Even for nonelusive populations, matching may be a hidden problem (see Hook and Regal, 1999) for a likely example. Matching problems do not arise in traditional ecology, as long as the identifying marks, such as tags, stay on the animal and are not defaced, but even here problems may arise (Schwarz and Stobo, 1999).

Formal confidence intervals for capture–recapture estimates may be calculated using several methods (see Hook and Regal, 1995 and Regal and Hook, 1999). If a model selection criterion, such as AIC is used, the derived interval about the estimate is an underestimate, because this method does not adjust for model uncertainty (see Regal and Hook, 1991 on this point).

For the semi-Bayesian method, such as the weighted AIC, in the absence of any sanctioned procedure, we have used, as a rough guide to measuring the uncertainty of the estimate, an interval whose bounds are calculated by weighting the confidence limits associated with the estimate of each model. In this derivation, we weight the limits associated with each model as we did those applied to the associated estimate. However, as intuitively attractive as this approach appears, we know of no formal justification for using it.

As in the example below, many different estimates may be made from the same data. For this reason, we use subjective judgments in interpreting estimates derived from capture–recapture data, searching for consistencies and inconsistencies, and taking into consideration our expectations about the nature of the sources used. Full Bayesian methods using Markov chain-Monte Carlo methods (MCMC) may eventually enable such subjective considerations to be incorporated into formal calculations of uncertainty.

MULTI-SOURCE EXAMPLE

Few examples have been found in the literature of authors providing raw data by source intersection over time, which enables some type of surveillance analysis. Indeed, the only example that presented sequential data from more than two sources was published by one of the authors of this chapter (Hook et al., 1980).

Spina Bifida in Upstate New York, 1969–1974

Here, data are reconsidered from the example of a two-source estimate, above. These data report the frequency of clinically important spina bifida, a congenital defect notable at birth, in live births in upstate New York from 1969 to 1974. (This frequency may be termed the incidence in each year, although in another sense it is best regarded as livebirth prevalence [Hook, 1982]). The focus is on surveillance of the year-to-year trends. Table 13–2 provides data from these three sources of the type likely to be readily available to the epidemiologist who is studying birth defects: birth certificates (BC), the records of a state medical rehabilitation program providing services to those affected (MR), and an additional source, reports on death certificates (DC) (see Hook et al. [1980]).

Table 13–2 Number of live infants born with spina bifida, upstate New York, 1969–1974, by year of birth and permutation of sources of ascertainment

Source type			Year of birth						
BC	DC	MR	1969	1970	1971	1972	1973	1974	All years
yes	yes	yes	0	0	5	4	1	2	12
yes	yes	no	37	30	22	20	14	19	142
yes	no	yes	14	25	22	18	19	14	112
yes	no	no	64	60	33	23	29	38	247
no	yes	yes	1	0	1	1	0	1	4
no	yes	no	12	11	9	6	6	5	49
no	no	yes	8	4	11	14	18	5	60
					Totals				
All BC			115	115	82	65	63	73	513
All DC			50	41	37	31	21	27	207
All MR			23	29	39	37	38	22	188
BC and/or MR			124	119	94	80	81	79	577
BC and/or DC			128	126	92	72	69	79	566
DC and/or MR			72	70	70	63	58	46	379
All			136	130	103	86	87	84	626
All livebirths			161,088	165,192	149,640	134,196	126,241	126,786	863,143

BC, birth certificates; DC, death certificates; MR, Bureau of Medical Rehabilitation files.

The data in Table 13–2 indicate primarily a fall in rates of spina bifida between 1969 and 1974, not a public health concern, although of some interest (and a national trend in that time interval, still unexplained). If the example is deemed not pertinent to the usual interest in surveillance—detecting an increase in rate—we suggest that, as an exercise, the trends be considered as if the time sequence were reversed.

Simpler Alternatives to Capture–Recapture Analysis

Before considering capture–recapture methods for surveillance, the investigator should examine what trends are suggested by the data using simpler methods, that is on readily available data without such analysis. For example, suppose data from only one of the three sources are available. Each source might be useful for surveillance in the sense of providing data that signal a change in the birth prevalence of the condition. As a practical matter, among the three sources, the use of birth certificate data alone, is optimal from the perspective of timeliness. Waiting for death to occur, or for referrals to state agencies for support, could delay matters indefinitely. The collection of data in the spina bifida example used a cut off of an achieved age of 3 years in ascertaining cases in DC and MR reports.

Nevertheless, the number of cases reported to a single source may change for reasons other than an increase in the actual rate of occurrence. An increase or decrease in rate based on death certificate reports alone might merely reflect a change in the seriousness of the cases reported; for example, a greater proportion of less serious cases of spina bifida might be included. Changes in the number of cases reported to a health department program, such as one that supports medical rehabilitation, may reflect varying efforts by outreach programs, or changes in eligibility. Changes in reports on birth certificates, which in principle should ascertain all cases of congenital defects evident at birth, may simply reflect changes in reporting compliance by hospitals.

Pooling all sources in this example might begin to form a registry of cases. Simply tracking the number of cases in such a registry (the sum of distinct cases reported in all available sources) may well be sufficient as long as one source does not provide a high proportion of unique cases that are not ascertained by other sources. In our example, pooling all three sources is limited by including only records available in a department of health and collected (rather passively) for other purposes. A more active effort might seek other sources to expand such a registry.

With these caveats, consider the live-birth prevalence data and rates by year of birth and source in Tables 13–3 and 13–4. These data indicate the changes in rates of infants born with spina bifida each year, using only the data available from each source, and from various combinations of sources, without attempting any capture–recapture methods. For the largest single source, all BC, the rate appears to drop by about 20% after 1970. After this drop, changes in data are compatible with statistical fluctuation. If we consider the cases only in BC and MR, the trend is similar to that in the rates of cases in all three sources. If we consider the number of cases in all sources, the drop from 1970 to 1971 is less, but overall there is drop of about 20%

Table 13–3 Rates of spina bifida per 1000 livebirths in upstate New York by year of birth and source intersection

Source type			Year of birth						
BC	DC	MR	1969	1970	1971	1972	1973	1974	All years
yes	yes	yes	0.00	0.00	0.03	0.03	0.01	0.02	0.01
yes	yes	no	0.23	0.18	0.15	0.15	0.11	0.15	0.16
yes	no	yes	0.09	0.15	0.15	0.13	0.15	0.11	0.13
yes	no	no	0.40	0.36	0.22	0.17	0.23	0.30	0.29
no	yes	yes	0.01	0.00	0.01	0.01	0.00	0.01	0.00
no	yes	no	0.07	0.07	0.06	0.04	0.05	0.04	0.06
no	no	yes	0.05	0.02	0.07	0.10	0.14	0.04	0.07

BC, birth certificates; DC, death certificates; MR, Bureau of Medical Rehabilitation files.

Table 13–4 Rates of spina bifida per 1000 livebirths in upstate New York by source and year of birth

Source	Year of Birth						
	1969	1970	1971	1972	1973	1974	All years
All BC	0.71	0.70	0.55	0.48	0.50	0.58	0.59
All DC	0.31	0.25	0.25	0.23	0.17	0.21	0.24
All MR	0.14	0.18	0.26	0.28	0.30	0.17	0.22
BC and/or MR	0.77	0.72	0.63	0.60	0.64	0.62	0.67
BC and/or DC	0.79	0.76	0.61	0.54	0.55	0.62	0.66
DC and/or MR	0.45	0.42	0.47	0.47	0.46	0.36	0.44
All Sources	0.84	0.79	0.69	0.64	0.69	0.66	0.73

BC, birth certificates; DC, death certificates; MR, Bureau of Medical Rehabilitation files.

from 1969 to 1971. In the following section, these inferences are compared with those from a capture–recapture analysis of the same data.

Capture–Recapture Estimates

Two-source approaches

First three different two-source surveillance analyses are examined because each illustrates separate problems with, and advantages of, two-source analysis. Our main interest is biases in a known or predicted direction.

Analysis of birth certificates versus death certificates should in principle be unbiased. Experience with vital record reports has suggested, however, that institutional factors affect reporting of birth defects. Although there is no hard evidence, it is suspected that a hospital that reports defects inaccurately on birth certificates is likely to do the same on death certificates. Children with spina bifida tend to die in the same hospital in which they are born. These factors would predict an expected positive association of the two sources used, and thus to a net underestimate with two-source capture–recapture. (This prediction occurred only *after* further experience with vital record reports, not before the original analysis in Hook et al. [1980]. For illustrative purposes here, it is assumed that this positive dependence is suspected *before* the analysis.)

There are strong grounds for believing that analysis of death certificates versus medical rehabilitation files is biased to a negative association. Many infants with spina bifida die shortly after birth, before enrollment in the rehabilitation program can be arranged. Therefore, two-source capture–recapture analysis should overestimate the numbers affected.

We know of no reason to expect reports on birth certificates and diagnoses in a medical rehabilitation program to depend on one another. We expect the two-source estimate to be unbiased and to be intermediate between the other two-source capture–recapture estimates.

With one exception, the estimates in Table 13–5 confirm the latter prediction. As expected, for each year, the BC versus MR estimate is below (in some cases, markedly below) the DC-MR estimate. For each year except 1970, the BC versus MR estimate is above the BC-DC estimate. Over all years, the BC-MR estimate is about 11% higher than the BC-DC estimate and only about one-third of the DC-MR estimate. In view of these results, and their consistency with our expectations, we ignore the two-source DC-MR estimate for surveillance. The other analyses suggest a clear drop in rate between 1969 and 1971. For BC versus DC, the drop occurs almost entirely between 1970 and 1971; for BC versus MR it occurs almost entirely between 1969 and 1970. Also of interest is that, with BC-MR, the rate for 1973 is a clear outlier from the relatively steady trend after 1970.

Table 13–6 indicates the amount of increase of the capture–recapture estimate over the total number of cases ascertained in the two sources. Variations in this ratio over the years explain, in another sense, how the two-source capture–recapture estimates differ from those derived by simply adding the numbers in the sources.

The two-source capture–recapture analysis has not changed markedly any of the suggestive trends between 1969 and 1971 derived by considering the number of cases in BC alone, in BC and MR together, or in all sources. However, the BC-MR capture–recapture analysis has drawn attention to a suggestive increase in 1973 that would have been overlooked otherwise. The estimated rate in 1973 is now 15% to 20% higher than that in any other year between 1971 and 1974. This two-source capture–recapture analysis has heightened suspicion about a possible outlier in that year.

Table 13–5 Two-source capture–recapture estimates of numbers and rates of spina bifida per 1000 livebirths in upstate New York, 1969–1974, by year of birth and generating sources

Source combination		Year of birth						All years
		1969	1970	1971	1972	1973	1974	
BC versus DC	Number	155	157	112	84	88	94	690
	Rate	0.96	0.95	0.75	0.63	0.70	0.74	0.80
BC versus MR	Number	189	133	118	109	120	100	778
	Rate	1.17	0.81	0.79	0.81	0.95	0.79	0.90
DC versus MR	Number	1150	—*	241	229	798	198	2432
	Rate	7.14	—*	1.61	1.71	6.32	1.56	2.82

*Unbounded high estimate.

BC, birth certificates; DC, death certificates; MR, Bureau of Medical Rehabilitation files.

Table 13–6 Ratio of estimated rates derived from two-source combinations to observed rates by year of birth.*†

Source combination	Year of birth						All years
	1969	1970	1971	1972	1973	1974	
BC versus DC	1.21	1.25	1.22	1.17	1.28	1.19	1.22
BC versus MR	1.52	1.12	1.26	1.37	1.48	1.27	1.35
DC versus MR	15.97	—	3.44	3.64	13.76	4.30	6.42

*The "observed" rate for any two source combination in any year is the sum of all live infants born with spina bifida in such a year reported in either source divided by the number of livebirths in that year.

†The closer the ratio to 1, the better the agreement.

BC, birth certificates; DC, death certificates; MR, Bureau of Medical Rehabilitation files.

Three-source approaches

Tables 13–7 and 13–8 present the live-birth prevalences and prevalence rates, respectively, derived using several different models. Here, choosing an estimate using the minimum AIC criterion becomes complicated, because the optimal model varies from year to year. The BC-MR model is optimal in 1969, 1970, 1971, and 1974; and the BC-MR, BC-DC model is optimal in 1972 and 1973 and over all years combined. This inconsistency indicates why, at least for surveillance purposes, the semi-Bayesian method, which weighs results over all models is preferred. Fortunately, in this example, such trends are consistent with minimum AIC estimates in trend by year, whatever the method, and confirm the conclusion derived by confining capture–recapture analysis to data from two sources only: a suggestive fall in 1969 to 1971, and a suggestive outlying high in 1973.

Comment

Among the few reports of temporal trends in capture–recapture epidemiologic data over time, only one illustrates a point similar to that made in our example. In surveillance of tetanus mortality in the United States from 1979 to 1984, Sutter et al. (1990) used data from two large sources but did not pool the sources. Results from one source suggested a modest decrease over time, while the other suggested no change. However, a graph of the derived estimates from two-source capture–recapture analysis implies an outlier, an increase in one year (1981), and a more pronounced drop in mortality in all of the years analyzed (Sutter et al., 1990). Without examining the raw data by year, we cannot comment further. But the thrust and even the direction of the trends in this example are similar to that illustrated by the New York spina bifida data and reemphasize the potential use of capture–recapture analysis for surveillance.

Table 13–7 Three-source capture–recapture estimates of the frequency of livebirths with spina bifida in upstate New York, 1969–1974

Method of estimation	Year of birth						All years	Sum of estimates over all years
	1969	1970	1971	1972	1973	1974		
Minimum AIC	163*	147*	117.5*	104.2†	114.7†	96.6*	758.7†	743
Model selected	(BC-MR)	(BC-MR)	(BC-MR)	(BC-DC, BC-MR)	(BC-DC, BC-MR)	(BC-MR)	(BC-DC, BC-MR)	
Model (BC-MR)	163	147	117.5	97.8	107.8	96.6	731.4	729.7
Model (BC-DC, BC-MR)	173.2	140.1	119.8	104.2	114.7	98.1	758.7	750.1
Saturated Model (BC-DC, BC-MR, DC-MR)	138.4	133.8	132.4	105.1	147.8	90.9	758.4	750.2
Weighted AIC	158.9	144.9	121.8	102.4	119.1	95.6	740.3	742.7

*Minimum AIC is associated with Model BC-MR.

†Minimum AIC is associated with Model BC-DC, BC-MR.

AIC, Akaike Information Criterion; BC, birth certificate; BC, death certificate; MR, Bureau of Medical Rehabilitation files.

Table 13-8 Three-source capture–recapture estimates of the frequency of infants born with spina bifida per 1000 livebirths in upstate New York, 1969–1974

Method of estimation	Year of birth						All years	Sum of estimates over all year
	1969	1970	1971	1972	1973	1974		
Minimum AIC	1.01	0.89	0.79	0.78	0.91	0.76	0.88	0.86
Model (BC-MR)	1.01	0.89	0.79	0.73	0.85	0.76	0.85	0.85
Model (BC-DC, BC-MR)	1.08	0.85	0.80	0.78	0.91	0.77	0.88	0.87
Saturated Model (BC-DC, BC-MR, DC-MR)	0.87	0.81	0.88	0.78	1.17	0.72	0.88	0.87
Weighted AIC	0.99	0.88	0.81	0.76	0.94	0.75	0.86	0.86

AIC, Akaike Information Criterion; BC, birth certificates; DC, death certificates; MR, Bureau of Medical Rehabilitation files.

CONCLUSION

To detect a newly introduced hazard, surveillance should be a regular, on-going process. In this example and discussion, there has been no attempted to construct the analogue to this process in which, after collecting the 1969 data, one would analyze the data by successive years as they were reported. Rather, in a certain sense a type of retroactive surveillance exercise, using data collected over many years was undertaken. Nevertheless, an attempt was made to present clearly the general implications for a cautious and pluralistic approach to deriving estimates. Further, it is emphasized that capture–recapture analysis may lead to the conclusion that *no* useful estimate is derivable. It may instead stimulate an ad hoc attempt to collect a representative sample of the population, hence enabling a ratio-estimator estimate, which is an analogue of a capture–recapture method (see, for example, the case discussed in Hook and Regal [1999]). Another question concerns the effort expended in gathering data from an additional source. To our knowledge, only LaPorte et al. (1995) have analyzed this issue systematically. Last, the Deming approach bears repeating. Consider the ultimate goals of the exercise before you start, and ask the question, "What difference can any altered rate derived from capture–recapture analysis make, anyway?"

We are aware of very few examples of capture–recapture analyses in which the derived estimates have had any significance whatsoever for the health of the public. Capture–recapture methods have typically been used to refine prevalence or incidence rates. Other than in studies of elusive populations, where such refinement may be important, capture–recapture analysis strikes us as having had little, if any practical significance in any reported jurisdiction. Moreover, it has not substantially altered any inference about the frequency of disease reached by more traditional methods. Nevertheless, the use of capture–recapture analysis in timely surveillance analysis may be one of the few epidemiologic applications in which this approach may contribute to the ultimate goal of public health.

REFERENCES

Ahlo, J.M. (1990). Logistic regression in capture–recapture models. *Biometrics* **46,** 623–635.

Ahlo, J.M. (1994). Analyses of sample based capture–recapture experiments. *Journal of Official Statistics* **10,** 245–256.

Ahlo, J.M., Mulry, M.H., Wurdeman, K., and Kim, J. (1993). Estimating heterogeneity in the probabilities of enumeration of dual system estimation. *Journal of American Statistical Association* **88,** 1130–1136.

Brenner, H. (1994). Application of capture–recapture methods for disease monitoring: potential effects of imperfect record linkage. *Methods of Information in Medicine* **3,** 502–506.

Deming W.E. (1938). *Statistical Adjustment of Data*. Mineola, New York: Dover. Cited in Orsini, J.N. (1997). Deming, William Edwards. In Johnson, N.P. and Kotz, S., eds., *Leading Personalities in Statistical Sciences from the Seventeenth Century to the Present*. New York: Wiley, p. 360.

Deming, W.E. (1986). *Out of the Crisis*. Cambridge, MA: MIT Center for Advanced Engineering Study.

Draper, D. (1995). Assessment and propagation of model uncertainty (with discussion). *Journal of the Royal Statistical Society Series B* **57,** 45–98.

Evans, M.A. and Bonnett, D.G. (1994). Bias reduction for capture–recapture estimators of closed population size. *Biometrics* **50,** 388–395.

Fienberg, S.E. (1972). The multiple-recapture census for closed populations and incomplete 2^k contingency tables. *Biometrika* **59,** 591–603.

Frischer, M., Leyland, A., Cormack, R., Goldberg, D. J., Bloor, M., Green, S.T., Taylor, A., Covell, R., McKeganey, N., and Platt, S. (1993). Estimating the population prevalence of injection drug use and infection, with human immunodeficiency virus among injection drug users in Glasgow, Scotland. *American Journal of Epidemiology* **138,** 170–181.

Hook, E.B. (1982). Incidence and prevalence as measures of the frequency of birth defects. *American Journal of Epidemiology* **116,** 743–747.

Hook, E.B. (1990). Timely monthly surveillance of birth prevalence rates of congenital malformations and genetic disorders ascertained by registries or other systematic data bases. *Teratology* **41,** 177–184.

Hook, E.B., Albright, S.G., and Cross, P.K. (1980). Use of Bernoulli census and log-linear methods for estimating the prevalence of spina bifida in livebirths and the completeness of vital record reports in New York State. *American Journal of Epidemiology* **112**, 750–758.

Hook, E.B. and Cross, P.K. (1982). Surveillance of human populations for germinal cytogenetic mutations. In Sugimura, T., Kondo, S., and Takebe, H., eds. *Environmental Mutagens and Carcinogens*. Toyko: University of Tokyo Press, and Tokyo and New York: Alan R. Liss, pp. 613–621.

Hook, E.B. and Regal, R.R. (1995). Capture–recapture methods in epidemiology: methods and limitations. *Epidemiologic Reviews* **17**, 243–264. (Corrigenda in *American Journal of Epidemiology* **148**, 1219, 1998.)

Hook, E.B. and Regal, R.R. (1997). Validity of methods for model selection, weighting for model uncertainty, and small sample adjustment in capture–recapture estimation. *American Journal of Epidemiology* **145**, 1138–1144.

Hook, E.B. and Regal, R.R. (1999). Recommendations for presentation and evaluation of capture–recapture estimates in epidemiology. *Journal of Clinical Epidemiology* **52**, 917–926.

Hook, E.B. and Regal, R.R. (2000). Accuracy of alternative approaches to capture–recapture estimates of disease frequency: internal validity analysis of data from five sources. *American Journal of Epidemiology* **152**, 771–779.

International Working Group for Disease Monitoring and Forecasting. (1995). Capture–recapture and multiple record system estimation I. history and theoretical development. *American Journal of Epidemiology* **142**, 1047–1058.

Korf, D.J., Reijneveld, S.A., and Toet, J. (1994). Estimating the number of heroin users: a review of methods and empirical findings from the Netherlands. *International Journal of the Addictions* **29**, 1393–1417.

Lambert, E.Y., ed. (1990). *The collection and interpretation of data from hidden populations*. NIDA Research Monograph 98, 158. Rockville, Maryland: National Institute of Drug Research, U.S. Department of Health, Education and Welfare.

Laporte, R.E., Dearwater, S.R., Chang, Y.F., Songer, T.J., Aaron, D.J., Kriska, A.M., Anderson, R., and Olsen, T. (1995). Efficiency and accuracy of disease monitoring systems: application of capture–recapture methods to injury monitoring. *American Journal of Epidemiology* **142**, 1069–1077.

Orsini, J.N. (1997). Deming, William Edwards. In Johnson, N.P. and Kotz, S., eds. *Leading Personalities in Statistical Sciences from the Seventeenth Century to the Present*. New York: Wiley, pp. 355–360.

Regal, R.R. and Hook, E.B. (1991). The effects of model selection on confidence intervals for the size of a closed population. *Statistics and Medicine* **10**, 717–721.

Regal R.R. and Hook, E.B. (1998). Marginal versus conditional versus "structural source" models: a rationale for an alternative to log-linear methods for capture–recapture estimates. *Statistics and Medicine* **17**, 69–74.

Regal R.R. and Hook, E.B. (1999). An exact test for all-way interaction in a 2^M contingency table: application to interval capture–recapture estimation of population size. *Biometrics* **55**, 1241–1246.

Roos, L.L. and Wajda, A. (1991). Record linkage strategies. I. Estimating information and evaluating approaches. *Methods of Information in Medicine* **30**, 117–123.

Schwarz, C.J. and Stobo, W.T. (1999). Estimation and effects of tag-misread rates in capture–recapture studies. *Canadian Journal of Fisheries and Aquatic Sciences* **56**, 551–559.

Sutter, R.W., Cochi, S.L., Edward, W., Brink, E.W., and Sirotkin, B. (1990). Assessment of vital statistics and surveillance data for monitoring tetanus mortality, United States, 1979–1984. *American Journal of Epidemiology* **131**, 132–142.

Tilling, K. and Sterne, J.A. (1999). Capture–recapture models including covariate effects. *American Journal of Epidemiology* **149**, 392–400

Wittes, J.T. (1972). On the bias and estimated variance of Chapman's two-sample capture–recapture population estimate. *Biometrics* **28**, 592–597.

Wittes, J.T. (1974). Applications of a multinomial capture–recapture model to epidemiological data. *Journal of the American Statistical Association* **69**, 93–97.

Index